UNDERSTANDING LUNG CANCER

Also by Naheed Ali

Understanding Alzheimer's: An Introduction for Patients and Caregivers

The Obesity Reality: A Comprehensive Approach to a Growing Problem

Diabetes and You: A Comprehensive, Holistic Approach

Arthritis and You: A Comprehensive Digest for Patients and Caregivers

Understanding Celiac Disease: An Introduction for Patients and Caregivers

Understanding Chronic Fatigue Syndrome: An Introduction for Patients and Caregivers

Understanding Fibromyalgia: An Introduction for Patients and Caregivers

UNDERSTANDING LUNG CANCER

An Introduction for Patients and Caregivers

Naheed Ali

ROWMAN & LITTLEFIELD
Lanham • Boulder • New York • Toronto • Plymouth, UK

Published by Rowman & Littlefield
4501 Forbes Boulevard, Suite 200, Lanham, Maryland 20706
www.rowman.com

10 Thornbury Road, Plymouth PL6 7PP, United Kingdom

British Library Cataloguing in Publication Information Available

Library of Congress Cataloging-in-Publication Data

Ali, Naheed
Understanding lung cancer : an introduction for patients and caregivers / Naheed Ali.
pages cm
Includes bibliographical references and index.
ISBN 978-1-4422-2323-3 (cloth : alk. paper) — ISBN 978-1-4422-2324-0 (electronic)
1. Lung—Cancer—Popular works. 2. Caregivers—Popular works. I. Title.
RC280.L8.A44 2014
616.99'424—dc23
2013036194

∞™ The paper used in this publication meets the minimum requirements of American National Standard for Information Sciences Permanence of Paper for Printed Library Materials, ANSI/NISO Z39.48-1992.

Printed in the United States of America

CONTENTS

IV: RESOLUTIONS

V: HOMESTRETCH

DISCLAIMER

This book represents reference material only. It is not intended as a medical manual, and the data presented here are meant to assist the reader in making informed choices regarding wellness. This book is not a replacement for treatment(s) that the reader's personal physician may have suggested. If the reader believes he or she is experiencing a medical issue, professional medical help is recommended. Mention of particular products, companies, or authorities in this book does not entail endorsement by the publisher or author.

PREFACE

Lung cancer is a disorder characterized by the rapid advance of malignant cells in the lungs. Like every cell, except mature red blood cells, a lung cell houses genetic material called *deoxyribonucleic acid* (DNA), which is duplicated every time a cell matures. When a mutation occurs during the process, an abnormal cell is born.[1] As these cells multiply aggressively, they eventually form a cancerous tumor that can spread from the lungs to other tissues in the body.[2] An understanding of lung cancer in this capacity is useful, whether or not someone knows another who suffers from it. Lung cancer is one of the leading forms of cancer mortality, and it can happen to anyone.[3] Signs and symptoms are not clearly recognized, and in many cases, patients are completely unaware that they have lung cancer until it has advanced to the later stages, making it more difficult to successfully treat. Lung cancer caused almost 30 percent of all cancer-related deaths in the United States in 2012.[4]

WHAT READERS WILL GAIN FROM READING THIS BOOK

Reading about lung cancer will provide an in-depth understanding of it, how it can be treated, and what specific roles a caregiver can provide. This will also help people ascertain what signs and symptoms to watch for, especially for those who are exposed to the following risk factors:

- Smoking or secondhand smoke.[5]

- Personal history of respiratory-related diseases, such as bronchitis, emphysema, asthma, or any respiratory disease that weakens the lungs.[6]
- History of lung cancer in the family. This was the subject of a case study conducted in 2006 wherein researchers concluded that lung cancer can be hereditary.[7]
- Exposure to air pollutants, such as radon and asbestos.[8]
- Living in particularly concentrated areas, such as major cities.
- Residing in areas near large industrial buildings known to emit thick polluted gases.
- Excessive alcoholism.[9]

For people who are exposed to these risk factors, knowing which signs and symptoms to watch for will enable them to be proactive and get tested or diagnosed earlier. Becoming equipped with knowledge about lung cancer can make a huge difference in avoiding lung cancer or preventing the escalation of its malignant stages. Furthermore, a unique book on lung cancer, such as this one, offers a variety of information not only for the patient but also for caregivers. This will enable both the patient and the caregiver to better understand the treatment process. Reading the lung cancer literature will also help patients and caregivers cope with the disease process.

LUNG CANCER LITERATURE: PATIENT BENEFITS

When patients understand or are at least familiar with the terminology that health care professionals use, they will be able to converse better with their doctors. This is especially beneficial when doctors explain treatment progress. In this way, a patient will be able to ask more effective questions. Being able to interpret basic information from laboratory findings will also help the patient know what particular questions to ask his or her doctor. It is always advisable to ask medical personnel about lung cancer as a disorder in general, but with personal knowledge about such a cancer, patients will assume full involvement in the management process. In this way, patients will learn more about their options in terms of medication and treatment process and thus reduce complications.

Lung cancer patients will also learn more information about clinical trials. A clinical trial, which is one stage in research about certain diseases, enables doctors and specialists to explore medical strategies involving new medications, treatment, and medical devices.[10] Reading more about this will help patients analyze viable decisions with regard to a particular treatment that has undergone such trials. Information presented in a book on lung cancer will also enable patients to ask the right questions regarding this process, including the following:[11]

- How is the new treatment going to possibly help?
- What intervention will they receive, if really needed?
- What are the rights of patients undergoing clinical trials?
- What are the risks, if any, with the new treatment?

Gaining knowledge about lung cancer will also enable the patient to discover appropriate support groups that will help one cope with the disease process.[12] Communicating with other individuals who have lung cancer will give the patient more information about certain medications and the treatment process. This is especially helpful when trying new medications. Patients will have an idea of which reactions, signs, or symptoms to look for so that they can converse with their health care professionals. The *symptomology* (study of symptoms) of cancers, such as those of the lung, are subjective and numerous. For this and other reasons explained in chapter 3, I refer to lung cancer throughout this book as a *disease process* rather than just a disease.

LUNG CANCER LITERATURE: CAREGIVER BENEFITS

A lung cancer caregiver helps a sufferer in more ways than one—from helping with daily housecleaning, laundry, cooking, and driving around for appointments to assisting him or her with medications and other medical needs. Well-informed caregivers can make a big difference in a patient's recovery. They understand the importance of monitoring all medications taken by the patient. They also know the importance of noting reactions such as vomiting, nausea, or pain—information that is vital for doctors in monitoring the progress of the patient's treatment process and in introducing new medications to their patients.

Providing lung cancer patients with an improved diet based on re-search on the subject will also aid in their recovery.[13] A healthier diet can help patients counteract or lessen the strains of the medications.[14] Unfortunately, the different treatment processes available for treating lung cancer also affect the patient's appetite. Not only do lung cancer patients partially lose their sense of taste, but they can also have sore throats, dental and gum issues, and nausea, making it more challenging for them to consume foods properly.[15] Caregivers will be able to help patients more if they are aware of these issues by reading more on the topic.

Caregivers also provide emotional assistance to lung cancer patients. There are times when patients feel guilty of what caused the disease process, such as excessive smoking or working in an environment that is known to expose one to radon or asbestos.[16] Guilt can cause stress in the patient and eventually will affect how he or she responds to treat-ment and medications. Studies show that feelings of shame and guilt about the cause of lung cancer, particularly smoking, affect how the patient proceeds with diagnosis and treatment.[17] Such times have to be handled with attentiveness to maintain cooperation between caregiver and patient. When the caregiver reads on the topic and comes to under-stand lung cancer, the patient will be more likely to follow medications and trust the caretaker in helping him or her recover much more effec-tively. Another way a caregiver provides emotional support is by orga-nizing family gatherings for the individual with lung cancer. This nor-mally helps both the patients and other family members who do not understand what the lung cancer patient is facing.[18] As a caregiver, reading more about lung cancer in the form of a book will provide tips on how to appropriately handle the disease process.

Lung cancer treatment is a lengthy phase, and it can be expensive for both the patient and the family. Thus, it helps to know more about the health management protocols of the patient and other family mem-bers that may be applicable. Moreover, caregivers will be able to com-pletely participate in the treatment process by reading more on the topic. They will be able to talk to patients about different options for addressing their lung cancer issues and participate in discussions with doctors about the progress of treatment. They will also be able to ask doctors questions that the lung cancer patient may have overlooked during a doctor's visit. Simply put, the lung cancer patient and the caregiver form a strong team that can enhance the progress of the treatment.

Further reading about lung cancer permits caregivers to have a better understanding of how to maintain financial support to carry on with the expenses of treatment. This includes reviewing the patient's insurance policies and those of family members that may be applicable to covering treatment expenses. Reviewing public and nonprofit organizations that advocate certain lung cancer approaches is also an option. Caregivers will additionally learn that they need to take care of themselves in order to take care of their patients more efficiently.[19] Time, effort, and love given when taking care of a loved one with lung cancer is immeasurable; sometimes they care so much that it can be mentally draining while subconsciously creating a feeling of bitterness over time. A book about lung cancer such as this one also helps when it comes to taking care of the caregivers themselves.

A COMPREHENSIVE APPROACH TO LUNG CANCER

When a patient is diagnosed with any type of chronic disorder, such as lung cancer, information is the first installment to the best clinical defense. Comprehensive knowledge of lung cancer will give patients a better understanding of the different stages and what types of treatments are available.[20] A study conducted in England showed that a lung cancer patient's recovery was inversely related to the use of surgical resection.[21] However, a peer-reviewed journal article stated that different procedures in surgical resection offer a different probability of survival.[22] A patient who is well versed in lung cancer research and its potential contradictions will be able to talk to doctors more effectively about the choices they have and be better informed making decisions with regard to medication and surgery, if needed.[23] With all the above in mind, I hope this comprehensive writing will help patients and physicians make educated decisions about the disease process known as lung cancer.

I

Groundwork

I

INTRODUCTION TO THE LUNG CELL

The extensive study of any malady—whether lung cancer or another disorder—involves utilizing the system and methods of biology, biochemistry, and genetics of the cell. These tools will assist in the accurate study of lung cancer, a disease process that results from the rapid, uncontrollable expansion of anomalous cells in the lungs. In an article published in the *British Medical Bulletin,* the authors established that researching the biology of lung cancer—including the investigation of cells—would help immensely in early diagnosis and treatment, thus increasing the survival rate of lung cancer.[1] Because DNA mutations in the lung can lead to lung cancer, patients and caregivers should understand that genes (which are a major component of lung cells) are another risk factor, whether a person is a smoker or not.[2]

Studies on lung cancer cells continue in the hopes of discovering possible improvements that can be made in current treatments, particularly at the cellular level.[3] Thus, to understand all of this research—past, present, and future—one must have good understanding of the basic information regarding cell structures and how they behave and perform overall in the lung cancer sufferer's body.

BASICS OF THE CELL

The cell is a common component of all living organisms; it accomplishes a multitude of tasks, including absorbing nutrients and converting them to energy. A living organism can have just a single cell to about 1 trillion cells differentiated into the following two classes:[4]

- Unicellular organisms are single-celled organisms that are some-times called monads. Some fungi and bacteria are classified as unicellular.[5]
- Multicellular organisms are those that consist of more than one cell, such as humans.[6] For multicellular organisms, the different cells in the body perform different functions but are intercon-nected within a complex communication structure.

The cell is the functional and structural unit of life. It comprises the body's hereditary material of genes (DNA) and the cell's machinery (RNA) essential for generating enzymes and various proteins. It has three parts: the cell membrane, the cytoplasm, and the nucleus.[7]

Three Major Types of Cells in the Human Body

Although the human body contains more than 300 types of cells, three major types are based on their main functions:

- Epithelial cells facilitate the transfer of nutrients and act to pro-tect the core tissues. These cells are classified on the basis of their shape.[8] Squamous epithelial cells, found profusely in the lungs, are thin and flattened, aiding in the transfer of nutrients through the cells. The lung's air sacs are composed of this type of cell. Cuboidal epithelial cells have a cube-like shape and are found in glands dispersed throughout the body.
- A muscle cell's role is to facilitate muscle contraction for bodily processes, such as movement, digestion, and heart functions. Skeletal muscle cells connect the skeleton and facilitate body movements. Cardiac muscles cells are found in the heart, accom-modating the functions of that organ. Smooth muscle cells make up the string of cells in the organs and tissues of the body and are located in the digestive tract.
- Nerve cells facilitate communication in the central nervous sys-tem through the synapses or tiny intercellular spaces.[9]

Nucleic Acids: The Hidden Role Players

DNA is a polymer molecule that supplies a blueprint for the cell's development, function, reproduction, and death. It contains biological information, making each cell function distinctively. Normal cells undergo *replicative senescence*, a process by which cells will grow, reproduce to a certain number, and then fade away.

The chemical compounds (in this case, amino acids) adenine (A), guanine (G), cytosine (C), and thymine (T) make up DNA. These bases pair accordingly and bind with sugar molecules and phosphate molecules, forming a *nucleotide*. The nucleotide is arranged into two long strands, creating a spiral called a double-helix strand.[10] DNA is found in the nucleus of the lung cell and other cells, but it is also found in the mitochondria. The term used to refer to this type of DNA is *mitochondrial DNA* (mtDNA).[11] Each DNA molecule is composed of genes (the body's genetic information). It is the pattern that controls the development of a certain species, and every time a cell splits in two, DNA is replicated in an exact manner.[12] The information stored in DNA consists of roughly 3 billion bases and is connected in a double helix by the four chemical bases adenine, guanine, cytosine, and thymine.[13] Approximately 99 percent of the total bases making up DNA are the same for all humans.[14] The differences seen in all organisms are brought about by the sequence in which the bases are interconnected. This pattern is analogous to a parallel code where letters are assorted to create different words.

Ribonucleic acid (RNA) is the principal ingredient in replicating DNA or lung cells as a whole. In many ways similar to DNA, RNA is composed of at least one molecule called a *nucleotide*, which is the basic constituent of both RNA and DNA. The four chemical bases that make up RNA's nucleotide are adenine (A), cytosine (C), guanine (G), and uracil (U).[15] In the duplication process, RNA plays a major role in sifting out related genes and noncoding components of DNA. RNA ensures that the noncoded DNA parts are removed before it is transported from the nucleus for replication.[16] The term for this procedure is *transcription*. This is also the part of the process where mRNA is produced so that it can be converted by ribosome to protein.[17] This converted protein cannot be converted back to a nucleic acid, and this is all part of what is known as the central dogma of biology, to which lung cells are no exception.[18]

Organelles

Organelles are specialized subunits in the cytoplasm that are usually covered with lipid bilayers. The most significant organelles are the mitochondria, endoplasmic reticulum, Golgi apparatus, lysosomes, and nucleus. These organelles have explicit, vital roles in the lung cell.

Nucleus

The nucleus is a membrane-enclosed *organelle* that houses the genetic materials responsible for reproduction, growth, metabolism, and functions of lung cells. It is where DNA transcription, replication, and RNA synthesis occur. The nucleus regulates nutrient metabolism, controls the secretion of ribosomes, maintains the integrity of the cell's DNA against possible foreign bodies, intervenes in the copying of DNA during the cell cycle, and determines gene expression. It is the control center of the lung cell. The nucleus holds most of the DNA in the cell, and its main function is to control the processes taking place in the cells, such as cell division, growth and maturity, and death. It is enclosed in a nuclear envelope, or membrane, that shields and separates the nucleus from the other parts of the lung cell.[19]

Cytoskeleton

The cytoskeleton is the lung cell's "scaffolding" as well as "highway." It is a network of intricate patterns of protein fibers that give the lung cell its shape. It also serves as a pathway for the motor proteins to transport "cargo" inside the cell. The cytoskeleton allows movement of organelles from place to place and aids in cellular motility. Its organized arrangement plays an important role in cell division. The cytoskeleton is found within the cytoplasm and is similar to a system of fibers, and although its primary function is to maintain the cell's structural framework, it also helps cells move autonomously and spontaneously.[20]

Cytoplasm

The cytoplasm or cytosol is where most of the processes of the lung cells take place. This is a fluid similar to jelly that holds most of the internal parts of a cell. Cytoplasm, or the space inside the cell, houses cytosol and organelles. Cytosol is an intracellular (within the cell) fluid, a gel-like substance composed of water, dissolved nutrients, ions, salts, organic molecules, and *macromolecules* (large molecules). Cytosol contains protein, proteasome, ribosome, and *cytoplasmic ribonucleoprotein*.[21]

Endoplasmic Reticulum

The endoplasmic reticulum is an organelle that acts as a molecule transporter for the lung cells through a protein's individual signal sequence.[22] It is the site of active protein synthesis, lipid metabolism, carbohydrate metabolism, and detoxification. The two types of endoplasmic reticulum, which are classified according to their appearances, are the rough endoplasmic reticulum and the smooth endoplasmic reticulum. The smooth endoplasmic reticulum has a smooth surface; the rough endoplasmic reticulum's rough surface is due to tiny structures called *ribosomes* surrounding it. The ribosomes that contain RNA templates are attached to the endoplasmic reticulum, translated accordingly, and converted into new proteins for the lung cell to use. These proteins are brought to the Golgi apparatus for further processing and packaging. The smooth endoplasmic reticulum, on the other hand, synthesizes and metabolizes steroids, lipids, and phospholipids. It facilitates the attachment of receptors on cell membrane proteins as well as detoxification.

Golgi Apparatus

The *Golgi apparatus* is also called the Golgi body or Golgi complex. It is an organelle that sorts, modifies, and packages the proteins processed in the lung cells before they are transported either inside the cells or to other parts of the body.[23]

Lysosomes

Lysosomes are organelles that process bacteria in the lung cells. They remove harmful components that permeate cells and are responsible

for revitalizing worn-out cell parts.[24] Lysosomes have been described as
the "digestive system" of the cell. They contain enzymes that facilitate
the breakdown of waste materials and cellular debris, digest bacteria
that infect the cell, and help repair damaged plasma membrane.

Mitochondria

Mitochondria are organelles that convert nutrients to energy from food
and other forms that the lung cell can utilize. They possess an independent genetic component (DNA) and can duplicate themselves.[25]

Plasma Membrane

The plasma membrane is a semipermeable casing that protects the
cell.[26] Also known as the cell membrane, one of the functions of the
plasma membrane is binding cells to other cells; it thus plays an integral
role in sustaining multicellular configuration. Plasma membranes also
serve as ion conductors or solid electrolytes, which are useful during the
oxidation process in the lung cells. Another function of the plasma
membrane is to facilitate communication between lung cells through
cell signaling.

Ribosomes

Ribosomes are cell structures that process proteins based on genetic
information in the lung cell. Ribosomes are either attached to the endoplasmic reticulum or floating in the cytoplasm.

Cell Membrane

The cell membrane is a thin cellular structure that encloses the cytoplasm. It functions as a protective "wall" that supports and retains the
contents of lung cells. The transport of energy, nutrients, and waste
products occurs across the cell wall. The membrane aids in cellular
communication by binding with the signals or ligand. It also has receptors that allow the transmission and reception of signals from the environment or from nearby cells that are triggering a cellular response. A
lung cell's membrane has attributes of self-recognition—the ability to
identify "self" and "nonself." The cell membrane consists of embedded
proteins and lipids, which are organic molecules made up of hydrocar-

bons. The primary lipid of the cell membrane is *phospholipid*, a derivative of fatty acids. It has two ends: the *hydrophobic* ("water-fearing")
tails projecting inward and the *hydrophilic* ("water-loving") heads
pointing to the exterior surface. This arrangement results in the formation of two layers of phospholipids, commonly called the phospholipid
bilayer. The phospholipid bilayer contributes to the lung cell membrane's selective permeability to ions and molecules.

A FURTHER LOOK INTO HUMAN LUNG CELL ORGANIZATION

The lungs are the organs responsible for supplying oxygen to the body.
Humans have two lungs: the left lung is slightly smaller and is made up
of two lobes, and the right lung has three lobes. The major parts of the
lungs are the pleura, lobes, trachea, bronchioles and alveoli, and diaphragm. Pleura are thin sacs that contain the lungs. They are attached
to the trachea, which is the main passageway of air connected to the
nose, mouth, and the lungs. The trachea branches off to a smaller passageway: the bronchus (plural *bronchi*).[27] Bronchi split to tiny passageways named *bronchioles*, the ends of which are the openings of the
alveolus (plural *alveoli*). The alveoli are tiny sacs in the lungs that facilitate the exchange of air whenever humans breathe. The diaphragm
contributes by facilitating the inflation and expansion of the lungs.

Trachea

The *trachea*, also called the windpipe, is the tube that connects the
lungs to the mouth and nose.[28] It is wide and elastic and is composed of
15 to 20 cartilages, also called *hyaline cartilages*. These C-shaped rings
contract while coughing, changing the diameter of the trachea to provide air when needed.[29] There are several types of cells found in the
trachea, one of which is the *chondrocyte*. Chondrocytes are found in
the tracheal cartilage but are also found in the joints, such as those of
the knee, and do not have blood vessels or lymphatic vessels. The trachea regulates the air that passes through the respiratory system by
producing mucus that traps unwanted particles, such as dust or bacteria. Mucus comes from the cells lined up in the interior of the trachea.

Both *goblet cells* and *ciliated epithelial cells* are found in the linings of the trachea and are responsible for the production of mucus in the trachea.[30]

Other cells found in the trachea include *cartilage lacunae*. This cell group, found in the cavities in between the tracheal cartilages, aids in the trachea's flexibility and strength. *Ciliated cells* are also found in the trachea.[31] Called *ciliated columnar epithelial cells*,[32] these rectangular cells have about 200 to 300 hair-like surfaces referred to as *cilia*. They often look "stretched out"; the mitochondria are found in the apex part of the cell, and the nuclei are found at the base. Cells in the trachea are bonded together by desmosome, also called *macula adherens*, which are found in between the epithelial lung cells.[33] This system of cells in the trachea is what causes the choking and coughing reflexes that also serve to protect the body of the lung cancer patient from unwanted substances.

Bronchi and Bronchioles

The bronchi and bronchioles make up part of the conducting zone of the respiratory system. They allow a continuous passage of air from the nose to the pharynx, larynx, trachea, and then bronchi and bronchioles.[34] The trachea branches off into the lungs through the bronchi in both lungs. The cell structure of bronchi is a combination of different cuboidal or columnar epithelial cells that may or may not have hair-like attachments. Such cells that possess hair-like attachments are called ciliated epithelium.[35] The cell structures combine to protect the lungs in the event of infection.[36] The epithelial cell structures function as a physical barrier for uninfected cells from the host cells. They also play a role in sustaining the proper circulation of air in the lungs. A paper published in the *American Journal of Respiratory Cell and Molecular Biology* stated that recent experiments have revealed that epithelial cells also react as immune effectors to infections and may actively cause inflammation responses.[37] Aside from these similarities to the trachea, bronchi are also enclosed in C-shaped hyaline cartilages.

Bronchioles are the tiny branches of the bronchi. They are lined with smoother muscle walls compared to bronchi. Similar to the trachea, these muscle walls help regulate the flow of air in the bronchioles by changing their diameter.[38] This also helps prevent unwanted substances from passing into the lungs. Bronchiole branches go deeper and further in that they become even smaller, leading to terminal bronchioles, where the alveoli are connected. The bronchioles continue to branch further in stages. When a person inhales, the oxygen passes through the lobular bronchiole and later goes through the terminal bronchioles, where the alveoli are connected. Bronchioles are made up mostly of epithelial cells that are more cuboidal in shape. Dome-shaped *clara cells* are also found in the ciliated epithelial cells in the bronchioles. Clara cells have been shown to actively participate in protecting the air passageways from unwanted elements in the bronchioles.[39] Goblet cells are situated in the larger parts of the bronchioles as an extension from the trachea and bronchus. These are cells that secrete mucus and are called such because they are shaped somewhat like goblets.

Alveoli

The human lung is the organ of respiration; it has alveoli containing collagen and elastic fibers that are responsible for the lung's flexibility—necessary for inhalation and exhalation actions. The alveolus is the part of the respiratory system where the swapping of oxygen and carbon dioxide happens. The alveoli are the hollow cavity endings of the bronchioles and are attached to the terminal bronchioles. They are connected by alveolar ducts, which are lined up with squamous epithelial cells. The exchange of oxygen and carbon dioxide happens in the alveoli and is common among mammals.[40] Typically, there are about 270 million to 790 million alveoli in adult human lungs.[41]

The two different types of cells in the alveoli are categorized as type I and type II cells. Type I cells consist of *pneumocytes (lung cells)* and squamous alveolar cells, which make up roughly 95 percent of the alveolar surfaces.[42] In 2001, a study indicated that the type I cells in the alveoli play an essential role in maintaining the balanced system of the lungs.[43] Type II cells consist of cuboidal epithelial cells and cover up the remaining 5 percent of the alveoli's cell composition. The main functions of type II cells include (1) the secretion of a surfactant that reduces the tendency of the surface to contract when the cells encounter a liquid surface and (2) the maintenance of fluid levels. They are also responsible for regenerating cells following an injury.

Each alveolus in the lung cancer patient's lungs consists of an epithelial layer and an extracellular matrix wrapped in a fine network of capillaries. The alveolar wall has three cell types. Type I, or the squamous alveolar cells, compose the alveolar wall. Type II, known as great alveolar cells, secrete a pulmonary surfactant composed of a phospholipid and protein mixture that decreases the surface tension of the thin fluid that coats the inside of each alveoli. This fluid facilitates the movement of gases between blood and alveolar air. An inadequate pulmonary surfactant contributes to lung collapse, or *atelectasis*. The type II cells also repair damaged endothelium. The macrophages, a third type of alveolar cells, are responsible for eliminating foreign material, such as bacteria.[44]

CELL DEVELOPMENT: SIMILARITIES AND DIFFERENCES

All cells, including those of the lung, have DNA imprinted in them and contain the chromosomes that can determine the gender of specific species. This chromosomal profile also allows one to determine gender simply by probing a single cell.[45] Male and female individuals have different chromosomes that are imprinted with their DNA. The DNA in the cells induces the glands to produce specific hormones that in effect create the differences and similarities between males and females. Testosterone is one such hormone.

Testosterone is an organic compound that falls under the classification of steroid hormones and that stimulates the development of the male reproductive system. All steroid hormones are converted from cholesterol.[46] It was commonly thought that testosterone is present only in males, being produced primarily in the *Leydig cells* in the testes.[47] For both males and females, however, testosterone is also produced in the outer portion of the adrenal gland, which is called the adrenal cortex. The adrenal cortex controls the balance of salt and water in the lungs by producing hormones derived from carbohydrates and fats.[48] In females, testosterone and its precursors are found in the ovary, but the concentration is far less in comparison to the testosterone produced in males.[49]

Testosterone plays a major role not only in the development of reproductive organs and deepening of voice in males but also in stimulating the development of male-dominant characteristics, such as increased rate of muscle production, bone mass, and growth of body hair, such as beards and axillary hairs. Some studies indicate that testosterone is essential in developing fetuses and plays a major role in fetal health.[50] It has also been found that testosterone causes the brains of male fetuses to develop larger compared to female fetuses.[51]

Another steroid hormone that affects the development of lung cells is estrogen. Estrogen is also an organic compound that is dominant in females. It can also be found in males, but the concentration is far less than that produced in females.[52] This hormone is produced by the *granulosa cells* found in the ovarian follicles of the ovaries. A granulosa cell is a type of somatic cell. Somatic cells make up the body parts of living organisms, such as internal organs, connective tissues, and bones.[53] The increased rate of estrogen in the female body affects the composition of body parts by reducing body and bone mass.[54]

Both testosterone and estrogen are found in male and females, and it is the level of production that affects the developmental differences in them. The differences in chromosomal composition in DNA also affect the rate at which the cells are reproduced.[55] The rates of evolution are deemed to be the fastest among male chromosomes.[56]

Studies have shown that the presence of these two organic compounds help maintain the body's defense in terms of fighting disease processes, such as cancer. One study stated that estrogen may be used effectively to prevent and treat breast cancer.[57] Another experiment maintained that undergoing testosterone treatment could produce positive results among prostate cancer patients.[58] In an article written for the *New York Times Magazine*, the writer stated that an apparently low testosterone count among HIV patients is common and that the usual treatment is to undergo regular intravenous doses of artificial testosterone.[59] Osteoporosis can also be prevented with appropriate amounts of testosterone in the body of the lung cancer patient.[60]

Cell Biology in Relation to Lung Cancer

Cells multiply through the process of division, where the exact DNA composition is being copied in each of the cells reproduced. During the process, however, mutations occur in the fundamental structure of DNA, and in some circumstances this leads to the production of cancer cells.[61] One process that causes these mutations in lung cancer cells is cell oxidation. Uncontrolled oxidation in the cells generates "free radicals" that can disturb the stability of molecules in the body.[62] This type of cancer usually causes the mutation in mtDNA, which is defenseless to these disturbances and has a restricted capacity to heal.[63]

Cell mutations are common during the process of cell division. A mutated cell in the lung may be restricted and will not cause any damage to its neighboring cells regardless of how unpleasant its properties may be. However, if a mutated cell starts to exponentially grow and damage other cells in the process, a neoplasm occurs, and a tumor is produced in the process. Uncontrolled tumors can damage and invade other cells around it, and this is where the lung cell starts becoming malignant and cancerous. Typically, a cancerous cell can be traced down to a primary tumor on a certain organ.[64]

Lung cancer frequencies often do not become apparent until 10 to 20 years after the incidence of heavy smoking. Even now, most cases are not detected until they have advanced to the later stages.[65] Speaking from a cellular standpoint, lung cancer is usually detected after it has formed new blood vessels that nourish the lump of abnormal cells, which also serve as a conduit for infecting other cells in the body. As the reader will deduce from the upcoming chapters, lung cancer starts with just one mutation in the lung cell, and this goes on to exponentially damage and overtake the healthy cells. To have a better grasp of the literature pertaining to cancer and lung cancer, one must have a basic understanding of what a lung cell is and what components are found in the lung cells.

2

LUNG CELL HEALTH VERSUS LUNG CELL DISORDER

Healthy cells play a vital role in stabilizing fitness levels of individuals at risk of developing lung cancer. These cells undergo a series of cellular communications and processes to maintain the normal operations of the body and achieve optimum wellness. They use energy to perform these metabolic activities and replenish themselves with nutrients to regain the utilized elements. Deficiency of elements essential in metabolism results in disrupted functioning and maturity of the cells, and constant disruption leads to damaged cell components, such as DNA, and may contribute to the development of cancer.[1] Therefore, understanding how lung cells work in healthy ways and comprehending what malignant cells require can help prevent severe medical disorder or death.

Going further, it is essential to know that the lung cancer sufferer's body is really a network of systems functioning interdependently. These body systems are a group of organs performing certain tasks. The organs are made of tissues grouped together, and these tissues contain a vast number of cells. In essence, cells are the building blocks of life with various characteristics and functions. Healthy cells contain DNA that "program" the cell's development. Alterations in DNA may lead to the development of abnormal cells, and these resultant, uncharacteristic cells will continue to replicate, producing more cells with damaged DNA and result in lung cancer formation.

CHARACTERISTICS OF A HEALTHY HUMAN LUNG CELL

The normal, healthy cell engages in various processes throughout its life span. These include the following:

- Cell proliferation
- "Cell deletion"
- Cellular recognition
- Active and passive transport
- Gene programming
- Signal transmission within and among cells
- Basic energy generation and consumption
- Oxygen delivery and combustion
- Defense mechanisms

These complex events require several methods of intracellular and extracellular communication to maintain equilibrium. Understanding the normal behavior of cells, tissues, and body organs such as the lungs provides knowledge about how the body functions to maintain balance of the internal environment as well as how the body responds to any disturbance in its stability. Furthermore, understanding how cells work helps one understand how lung cancer arises and how it can be managed.

The human body is multicellular, and all the different cells have various purposes. Cells such as those found in healthy lungs can act as vehicles of information, as protection from infection, or as a component that helps the individual convert food into energy to survive. Every organism starts out with a single cell and goes through a process called the cell cycle to multiply to either make a colony of single-celled organism or create a multicellular organism, such as a human being. A sequence of biological checkpoints ensures that the cell is established for the next process. When a cell is deemed healthy, it is permitted to multiply in moderation; otherwise, it is typically repaired or destroyed.[2]

Cell Cycle

The cell cycle, sometimes termed *cell life*, is a series of changes that involves cell growth and replication of DNA, providing daughter cells from cell division. There are two phases in this cycle: interphase and nuclear division, called *mitosis*.[3] Interphase, described as the "living" phase of a healthy cell cycle, is a stage where growth and DNA duplication occur. A cell's life is dependent on the free energy it acquires from its surroundings.[4] Lung cells by themselves cannot produce energy to perform every action, but the food that humans eat and also the energy derived from sunlight are the primary sources of the energy needed to complete each of the cells' tasks.[5]

A healthy lung cell does not immediately use all the energy that is stashed in the nutrients. Cells, including those localized in the lung, go through a process called oxidation.[6] This is the process when cells are aided by oxygen and enzymes to convert nutrients to compounds needed by cells. Such nutrients are then stored and transported as energy molecules known as *adenosine triphosphate* (ATP).[7] When a healthy lung cell reproduces, an exact replica of its genetic coding is delivered onto the new cell. This is called *template polymerization*, a process that lets the lung cell follow a certain pattern for a species' characteristic and development.

Healthy individual lung cells act as "minifactories" and can make nucleotides and proteins composed of common subcomponents. Cells not only have the blueprint of the body but also control the processes that are required in sustaining life.[8] Management of simple sugars, amino acids, and nucleotides as well as other chemical components is a part of these cellular processes. Lung cells are protected by a cell lining called *plasma membrane*. This part of the lung cell is partially permeable and allows only those ions, nutrients, and other organic molecules that are useful to cells to pass through.[9] All cells require proteins to aid other cells. Healthy lung cells go through the oxidation mentioned earlier, but to complete that process, they also make use of proteins delivered in the form of enzymes. Mitosis, or nuclear division, is a process where the healthy nucleus splits in two. At this stage, there is a complete distribution of replicated DNA to the daughter cells.

A Look Inside

In reality, the cycle of the healthy cell, whether lung or other cell, consists of the birth of a new cell, carefully regulated periods of cell division to create more new cells, and eventual cell death (*apoptosis*) to get rid of aged cells. Each cell (not mature red blood cells) possesses its own "brain," called the nucleus. The nucleus is composed of chromatin, which works with DNA strands to preserve the genetic makeup of the cell via the chromosomes, prevents DNA strands from encountering damage, and oversees how the genetic information is copied and carried over when the cell begins to reproduce through the process of cell division.[10] Healthy lung cells divide in one of two ways: *mitosis* or *meiosis*. Mitosis is the most common cell division process. A single cell splits, and two identical "daughter" cells are produced, containing the same genetic data as their predecessor. Mitosis accounts for the symmetrical growth of the body, as it is responsible for the replication of cells in the internal organs and external body parts, such as limbs and facial features. It is also responsible for the proper development of the fetus. Meiosis, on the other hand, is a process open only to the reproductive system. The daughter cells that are generated in meiosis are formed from two sets of genetic information (coming from the sperm and egg cells, respectively), and thus the resulting lung cell combines these sets of data, resulting in a genetic string that is distinct from the original cells. This allows children to be differentiated in terms of gender and makes them different from their parents.[11]

A healthy lung cell undergoes mitosis only about 50 times in its lifetime. The chromosomes possess "body clocks" to keep track of a cell's aging process—two at each end of a chromosome for a total of 96 body clocks. These internal clocks work thusly: Every time a cell divides, part of the chromosome that is being copied to the new cell gets cut off—literally—resulting in a shorter chromosome. Chromosomes have a minimum length standard to adhere to, and once this length is reached, the cell is alerted as to the end of its ability to reproduce and enters a period of "retirement," where it stops undertaking the work of constantly splitting. Lung cell aging reaches its zenith when the cell begins to decrease in size and detach from its neighboring cells. The process of apoptosis begins when the lung cell's surface starts "bubbling" and parts of it begin to break off. The act of "dying" commences when the nucleus itself crumbles, followed by the rest of the cell.[12]

Proper Cell Communication

Healthy lung cells "communicate" with each other to facilitate cellular activities and to organize cell actions. This capability ensures development, tissue repair, and immunity and sustains homeostasis. This complex system of communication is called cell signaling. Failure in the transmission or processing of information leads to certain disorders, such as uncontrolled autoimmunity, diabetes, and cancer. Cells transmit and receive signals. The source of the signals can be from the cell's environment or from other cells. These signals must pass through the cell membrane in order to trigger a cellular response. They may readily cross the membrane or may need to interact with receptor proteins acting as messengers embedded along the cell membrane. Only cells with correct corresponding receptors on their surfaces will react to that certain signal.[13]

When Cell Communication Fails

Cells communicate continuously and constantly. Because of this, various mechanisms are maintained for appropriate cell growth: (1) cell division takes place as a reaction to external signals; (2) cells connect, communicate, and interact with their neighboring cells (neighboring cells send out an alert when changes in connection exist); (3) cells group together and remain within their tissue boundaries; (4) enzymes reconstruct damaged DNA; and (5) if a cell is irreparable, it commences self-destruction.[14]

Disease

Disease begins when there is an interruption of at least one transmission in the lung cell signaling course. Absence of signals, excessive signals, disregarding of a signal by the target, signals failing to arrive at their target, and multiple breakdowns can all disrupt cellular communication.[15]

Absence of Chemical Signals

The pancreas discharges insulin, thereby instructing the liver, fat cells, and muscle cells to store sugar for later consumption. In type 1 diabetes, there is an absence of pancreatic cells that produce insulin; in this manner, the insulin signal is also absent. There is a sugar buildup, reaching toxic levels in the blood, and the resulting condition can further lead to kidney failure, blindness, and heart disease. Healthy lung cells can also be disrupted in this manner.

Excess of Chemical Signals

Stroke occurs when there is obstruction in blood vessels resulting in the death of brain cells. *Excitotoxicity* exists when dying cells in the brain discharge huge amounts of *glutamate*, a neurotransmitter facilitating neural communication, memory, cognition, learning, and regulation. It also regulates muscle tone in humans. High concentrations of glutamate kill cells, including brain and lung cells unaffected by the blockage.[16]

Indifference to Signals

On occasion, signals in the lungs fail to arrive at their target or are completely disregarded by the latter. *Multiple sclerosis* is a nervous system disease affecting the brain and spinal cord. This condition is characterized by a damaged myelin sheath, a protective material surrounding nerve cells. The damage slows down the transmission of messages between the brain and the body. Multiple sclerosis contributes to muscle weakness, visual disturbances, difficulty with coordination and balance, uncontrolled movements, and depression. By extension, lung cancer can aggravate this condition.[17]

Multiple Breakdowns

Cancer arises from multiple breakdowns in cellular communication. When there is disruption in cell signaling, cells may be able to grow and divide continuously even in the absence of signals that instruct healthy lung cell growth. Uncontrolled growth typically stimulates a signal for self-destruction. However, in multiple breakdowns, cells are unable to respond with certain signals, including those for cell death, resulting in uninterrupted cell division and creating a tumor. As the breakdown progresses, blood vessels sprout from the tumor and promote further enlargement. More signals evolve, and eventually unhealthy (i.e., cancerous) lung cells gain the capacity to invade and spread to other areas of the body.[18]

CELL MALIGNANCE AND CANCER CELLS

Normal cells have distinct traits: they regulate reproduction, mature or become specialized, and later undergo apoptosis or self-death, especially when damaged. These traits and cellular processes are programmed in the DNA, but a change (mutation) in the DNA disturbs the cell cycle. This mutation can lead to the formation of cancer cells. These cells have unregulated, increased rates of growth and division. Lung cancer cells result in altered function and cellular characteristics. The characteristics are hyperplasia, dedifferentiation, metastasis, invasiveness, and angiogenesis.[19]

Characteristics

Hyperplasia

Normal lung cells have a regulated rate of growth wherein they cannot divide indefinitely. On the other hand, cancer cells produce their own enzymes (such as *telomerase*) that add another set of DNA sequence that continually rebuilds chromosomes. The cells do not stop dividing, and this uncontrolled cell division results in hyperplasia, or the uncontrolled growth of tissues, which are—after all—comprised of cells.

Dedifferentiation

Differentiation is a mechanism by which a generic cell matures into a more specific cell type. The transition changes the simple cell's membrane potential, size, shape, metabolic activity, and responsiveness to signals. Dedifferentiated lung cells regress and remain unspecialized in function and structure.[20]

Metastasis

Normal cells remain in the right place at the right time, whereas cancer cells do not. When cancer cells replicate, they produce excessive amounts of collagen-dissolving enzymes. These enzymes separate the collagen and thus stimulate the lung cancer cells to invade and travel. As they travel, they form new cells in the body—cells that should not be there.

Invasiveness and Angiogenesis

Cancer cells develop the ability to pass through the basement membranes of some organs. They obtain the capacity to penetrate and destroy other cells and tissues. In the context of lung cancer, angiogenesis is when lung cancer cells create new blood vessels, enabling them to access nutrients from nearby tissues or organs needed for their growth.[21]

Benign versus Malignant Growth

Cell growths are classified as either benign or malignant. Benign "tumor" growth is a mild, nonprogressive lump of cells with no invasive properties of cancer and lacks the ability to metastasize. Malignant growth is a condition where there is a progressive growth of cells forming large masses that metastasize to distant parts of the body, preventing the affected organs from functioning efficiently. Cancer cells may spread locally through blood circulation, through the lymphatic system, or through the body cavity.[22] For what is considered "localized" spread, lung cancer cells grow randomly where they originated and progress to new environments more conducive for their survival and further proliferation. As they mature, they utilize the space and the nutrients of the surrounding tissues. They also produce larger amounts of enzymes that can cause death to the cells around them.[23] Lung cancer cells have the ability to detach themselves from their origin and spread through the bloodstream, and as they enter into the blood vessels, they flow along with the blood and then attach to other organs.[24] There, the atypical cells multiply to grow into another tumor in other regions of the body.

Cancerous cells arising from severely malignant lung cancer can also penetrate the lymphatic system.[25] The lymphatic system controls the movement of lymphatic fluid in the body. This fluid contains oxygen, proteins, sugar, and lymphocytes. The lymphatic vessels contain portals for immune cells, which can be accessible to the cancer cells as well. Once the cancer cells have reached the small channels of the lymph nodes, they travel along with the fluid and form additional new growth in a particular area. Cancer cells can also spread through the body cavity via the pericardial, pleural, peritoneal, and subarachnoid spaces.

This type of spread is described in cases of ovarian tumors that move to the liver via the peritoneal cavity.[26]

SIGNIFICANCE OF KNOWING ABOUT LUNG CELL HEALTH

Healthy cell life within the lungs creates a healthy energy level, which is resistant to stress. Lung cells partially supply the body's energy, and the inability to produce this energy leads to declines in health, and degenerative conditions emerge. *Disease* can be perceived as a product of alterations in cells that may involve a deficiency in the energy needed by mitochondria, or a malfunction of the nucleus. For instance, an inadequate supply of "fuel," be it in the form of vitamins or other cell factors, leads to coronary heart disease. Knowing how and why nutrients are needed in converting food to cellular energy to be used in different cellular metabolic reactions in the lungs can help prevent disease. In heart failure, for instance, insufficient fuel and nutrients in the cells impair the pumping function of the heart muscle, causing shortness of breath and accumulated fluids in the body. Another cause of disease is the alteration of metabolic "software" in the nucleus of the cell. This alteration causes cell multiplication and disruption of collagen structure. Such an altered state promotes the development of infectious diseases and cancer.[27]

With that in mind, it is important for patients and caregivers to know that food intake has a profound influence on overall health of cells, including those of the lungs. The lungs are responsible for providing oxygen to the bloodstream, transporting essential nutrients throughout the body, and removing the waste product carbon dioxide. A healthy lung also manipulates the concentration of prescription drugs and other substances in the bloodstream. It filters out small blood clots and gas microbubbles in the veins produced from decompression (as in underwater diving). It serves as shock-absorbing protection for the heart and acts as a blood reservoir containing almost 10 percent of the total blood volume of the entire circulatory system.[28] It produces mucus and secretes *immunoglobulin* (a cell protein molecule) necessary in fighting infection. Therefore, any disruptions in the normal functioning of the lungs affect other organs and the entire body as well.

During respiration, the lungs take in air that contains a mixture of oxygen and other pollutants or toxins. Exposure to these toxins causes the production of free radicals in the lungs, so knowing how to avoid certain environmental factors certainly helps. Free radicals are unsafe molecules that destroy healthy lung cells. To protect the lungs from damage, the body needs enough of a supply of the antioxidant vitamins C and E. Vitamin D keeps lung tissue healthy and promotes cell growth in the lung linings. Selenium and magnesium reduce inflammation and relax the lung muscles, facilitating healing and effective breathing. However, even some people who lead healthy lives and who take vitamins and eat healthfully may still fall victim to lung cancer.

HEALTHY LUNG CELL DEVELOPMENT AND AGING

Lung development involves different stages.[29] During gestation, human lungs appear as a protrusion of the primitive gut. They form into two buds on the left side of the body and three buds on the right. This formation commences the embryonic stage of lung development and ends with the formation of the pulmonary vasculature. In the *pseudoglandular* stage, the diaphragm forms, and columnar cells with glycogen lining the airways emerge. This stage relates to the advancement and complete separation of the airways into smaller branches and lasts from weeks 6 to 16. During weeks 16 to 26, the *pulmonary* (respiratory system) *acini* (conjunctions) grow as capillaries proliferate while the pulmonary epithelium decreases. Premature babies have a chance of survival at the end of this stage. In the *saccular stage*, at weeks 28 to 38, the alveolar ducts and sacs are generated from the saccules. The epithelial cells differentiate, transforming into flat type I cells and larger type II cells. During the final weeks of gestation, these type II cells release *surfactant*, a mixture of proteins and lipids necessary for the reduction of fluid surface tension. The alveolar stage begins at the last two weeks of gestation, and alveoli emerge and develop continuously. At birth, the lung transforms from a fluid-secreting structure to an organ that absorbs fluid.

The function of healthy lung cells deteriorates with age as structural changes take place, and suffering from lung cancer fails to improve the situation. The thoracic cage becomes rounder, the intercostal cartilages calcify, and arthritis in the costovertebral joints often occurs. The large bronchial tubes enlarge even further, while the opening of the bronchioles decreases after age 40. The alveolar sacs turn shallow, and the alveolar wall remains intact, but their surface area decreases by 15 percent by the age of 70.[30] In addition, diffusion of oxygen across the alveolar wall is limited. Major age-related changes in the otherwise healthy lung are associated with a progressive transformation of lung elasticity. The lung loses the recoil pressure that is exerted by an unusually expanded lung, and distensibility increases. Conversely, chest wall expansion decreases with age, resulting in increased functional residual capacity. The respiratory muscles have decreased force generation and tenacity, and such changes limit the maximal expiration.[31]

Finally, a healthy respiratory system secures gas exchange as the oxygen necessary for cellular metabolism reaches the various organs with the help of the pulmonary capillaries. Carbon dioxide, a product of mitochondrial tissue metabolism, travels toward the lung capillaries and is expelled outside the body. The ability of the rib cage to inflate (lungs expand due to the breathing in of air) and deflate (contraction from breathing out air) facilitates gas transport between mouth and alveoli. The process of inspiration (breathing in air) in an otherwise healthy lung cancer patient utilizes the diaphragm and the *parasternal* (next to the sternum bone) and *scalene* (triangle) muscles. Distension of the rib cage increases depression in the pleural space and distension of the lung, thus transporting gas molecules from the mouth or nose along the bronchial tree to the alveoli described in chapter 1. Expiration occurs when inspiratory muscles relax and the chest wall restores, resulting in a decreased volume of the respiratory system, and when a person suffers from lung cancer, these dynamics are definitely disturbed.[32]

3

REAL MEANING AND ANATOMY OF LUNG CANCER

Lung cancer has been cited as the most common cancer causing death.[1] The most well-known cause for it is cigarette smoke, but there can be other chemical and genetic factors.[2] This chapter seeks to clarify (1) what lung cancer is *really* all about as well as (2) how and why it surfaces as a process rather than a single straightforward disease. The chapter also discusses the types of lung cancer tumors that have been identified and how lung cancer affects one's body from an anatomical perspective.

Cancerous growths can be—but are not necessarily—classified into the following categories: carcinomas, sarcomas, leukemias, lymphomas, and germ cell tumors. Some tumors, however, do not clearly fall into these distinctions but rather are a mixture of characteristics from different scientific classes. An example of this is a *carcinosarcoma*, found in parts of the body that contains both epithelial cells and connective tissue while satisfying the requirements for both carcinomas and sarcomas.[3] Since part III of this book describes specific types of lung cancer in detail, it is imperative for patients and caregivers to now comprehend the broader categories into which some lung cancer variations fall.

CANCER CATEGORIES

Carcinomas

Carcinomas are malignant tumors that originate from epithelial cells. Epithelial cells make up most of the body, lining internal organs and forming the skin, thus accounting for 80 to 90 percent of all carcinomas.[4] Carcinomas are further subdivided into two types: *adenocarcinomas* and *squamous cell carcinomas*. Adenocarcinomas originate from the glands (*adeno* = gland) and epithelial tissue and are responsible for lung cancer and other common cancers, such as those of the breast and prostate. Adenocarcinomas commonly develop in parts of the respiratory system that produce mucus and other secretions, such as milk. and manifest with pale, thick mucus.[5] Adenocarcinoma of the lungs is the type of lung cancer often experienced by nonsmokers, with women being affected more than men.[6] Asians are also more susceptible to this type of cancer.[7]

Sarcomas

Sarcomas are tumors originating in connective tissue, including bones, cartilage, and soft tissue, such as tendons, ligaments, blood vessels, muscles, and fat. Sarcomas are more common in young adults and are responsible for cancers of the bone, brain, and stomach.[8] *Angiosarcomas* are tumors found in the blood and the bone marrow, *chondrosarcomas* are responsible for cancers of the cartilage, *fibrosarcomas* affect tendons and ligaments, *liposarcomas* develop from fat tissue, and *gastrointestinal stromal tumors* target the connective tissue of the intestinal tract.[9] While soft-tissue sarcomas typically develop in the extremities of the body as noted by clinical reports, they most often spread to the lungs.[10]

Leukemia

Leukemias are not solid tumors but are more like "liquid" cancers.[11] They originate in the bone marrow, with mutant cells inducing the production of ineffective white blood cells. They also cause anemia by affecting the ability of red blood cells to propagate properly and hence decrease the oxygen content of the bloodstream. Subsequently, when oxygen is diminished in the bloodstream, the lungs are affected. Leukemia is categorized into two types: acute and chronic. *Acute leukemia* involves underdeveloped white blood cells that cannot perform their assigned tasks in the body, while *chronic leukemia* involves more evolved cells that can still perform. Chronic leukemia degenerates over time and affects the sufferer gradually. Those who have suffered leukemia in the past or are suffering from it currently have a higher chance of eventually developing lung cancer.[12]

Lymphomas

Lymphoma tumors (or simply *lymphomas*) are formed in the lymph system and affect anatomical regions, such as the lymph nodes, spleen, tonsils, and the bone marrow.[13] Lymphomas are identifiable by the lumps they raise on the lymph nodes near the neck, the underarms, and the breast, to name a few. Lymphomas affect the cells in the immune system, particularly the white blood cells called lymphocytes, and are categorized into two types: Hodgkin's lymphoma (also known as Hodgkin's disease) and non-Hodgkin's lymphoma. Hodgkin's lymphoma patients are rarer than non-Hodgkin's patients and are prone to the subsequent development of lung cancer.[14]

Germ Cell Tumors

Germ cell tumors are commonly found in youth and adults, targeting reproductive organs, such as ovaries and testes.[15] They commonly metastasize to vital organs, such as the brain, the liver, the lymph nodes, the bone marrow, and the lungs. However, in rare cases, germ cell tumors can be found in these areas as well. These tumors, called *extragonadal germ cell tumors*, occur as a result of germ cells being left at different sites while traveling through the body to the reproductive areas. Extragonadal germ cell tumors are similar to normal germ cell tumors, but they are formed mainly outside the reproductive system rather than being only a result of metastasis.[16]

A "DISEASE PROCESS"

Cancer itself is not a disease that is caught or entirely genetically inherited as it is. It is a process of cell mutation that begins when cells do not undergo the natural process of apoptosis (programmed cell death). In the case of lung cancer, these mutated cells eventually form into lumps of tissue, and these lumps amass into a neoplasm, more commonly known as a tumor. The tumor is considered benign if it does not invade other parts of the body and remains in the area where it was birthed. It is considered malignant if the tumor begins to spread cancer cells via the circulatory and lymphatic systems and starts disrupting body functions outside the original tumor site in a process called invasion.[17]

Cell mutations occur in two ways: the activation of *oncogenes* and the inactivation of *tumor-suppressor genes*.[18] Oncogenes are genes that have a predisposition to cause cell mutation. When active, they encode proteins, called *oncoproteins*, into a cell that cause cell activity and disrupt the normal programmed cell cycle. Since it is unable to die as planned, the abnormal cell then undergoes rapid and unbridled cell division (mitosis), resulting in the formation of cancerous tissue.[19] Tumor-suppressor genes also encode proteins; however, the proteins they produce are geared to fighting cancerous cells. When it comes to the real meaning of lung cancer, the function of tumor-suppressor genes is nullified or weakened. Without opposition, lung cancer cells can spread freely.[20]

Left as they are, mutated lung cells continue to increase and "invade" other healthy cells nearby, creating masses of damaged tissue. These masses form into cancerous tumors that continue to grow in size as more lungs cells become abnormal. Cancerous tumors become self-sustained by forming their own blood vessels during angiogenesis. The malignant tumor, on reaching a critical level of growth, begins to migrate some of the "daughter" cancer cells (new cells created as a result of mitosis) to different parts of the body in a process called metastasis.[21] Metastatic cancer cells release their grip on the original tumor and follow other cells through the bloodstream and the lymph system until another site conducive to tumor growth is found. When a desirable site is reached, the cells stick themselves onto the new tissue and cause another tumor to grow. Rather than the original tumor, these new tumors, called metastatic tumors, are often the culprits behind cancer-related deaths.[22]

UPPER ANATOMY AND LUNG CANCER

Lung cancer is particularly deadly because of its ability to stay undetected for a long time and thus affect areas of the upper body anatomy. The lungs are not sensitive to pain and are capable of functioning normally via their reserve capacity for a long time in spite of tumor growth. By the time a sufferer starts displaying symptoms of lung cancer, it is often too late.[23] The lungs can function effectively even in disease because they work together closely with the upper parts of the body that help sustain them.[24] Unfortunately, this also means that when the lungs are afflicted with sickness, other anatomical structures are affected as well.

Brain

This is one of the most common sites for cancer cells to metastasize to, occurring in about half of lung cancer sufferers. It happens more often with *small cell lung cancer* sufferers than *non–small cell lung cancer* sufferers and within one year of lung cancer onset. Both are described further in chapter 11.[25]

Lung tumors that somehow find their way into the brain are debilitating—the pressure on the cranium due to swelling and direct brain cell damage can cause problems with memory, coordination, vision, speech, and comprehension.[26] Symptoms of brain tumors include severe headache, nausea, fatigue, and fever. In worse cases, the problem can include seizures and paralysis.[27] Psychological illness can also occur when tumors lean on the parts of the brain that control personality, bringing about personality disorders and severe mood swings.[28]

Tumors in the brain traceable to lung cancer can also lead to a disorder called *syndrome of inappropriate antidiuretic hormone secretion*. Common in those with small cell lung cancer, this syndrome occurs when the pituitary gland overproduces antidiuretic hormones, causing the sodium levels in the blood to go down and too much water to be retained in the body. The syndrome results in an increased tendency to urinate and grow thirsty quickly. It also causes weight loss due to lack of appetite loss, nausea, lethargy, and arrhythmia and in acute cases can render one comatose. Encephalopathy, or inflammation of the brain, can also be brought about by the attack of abnormal white blood cells against healthy cells.[29]

Vocal Cords

Tumors in the lungs can cause a lung cancer sufferer to develop a perpetually hoarse voice. This is because the nerves connected to the vocal cords are being choked, resulting in their weakening or complete paralysis.[30] This symptom is called unilateral vocal fold paralysis, and lung cancer sufferers are forced to speak in soft, harsh, and breathy tones because the vocal fold needs so much more air than normal to produce sound. Sufferers experience sore throats whenever they speak because other muscles in the neck must now support the work of the vocal fold, and speaking normally leaves them breathless. The act of swallowing also results in coughs and voice changes.[31] Vocal cord trouble is one of the signs of advanced lung cancer.[32]

Airways

Anatomically, the airway structures, such as the bronchi and the trachea described in chapter 1, are often affected by lung cancer early on due to their proximity to the lungs. The damage usually manifests in a chronic cough or bronchitis, which may grow more serious as tumors lean harder on the airways and produce bloody phlegm called haemoptysis.[33] Blockage in the airways can also result in dypsnea or chest pain as a result of the increased effort to get the necessary amount of air circulation.[34] The difficulty in breathing can also result in wheezing as air attempts to move past the blockage.[35]

Esophagus

When lung tumors enlarge and begin to lock the esophagus, the patient suffers from swallowing dysfunction, known as dysphagia.[36] This points to the cancer's advanced state and can lead to a loss in appetite and liquid intake due to the pain of swallowing. Secondary physical effects of dysphagia include kidney failure, malnutrition, and a weakened immune system as a result of the loss of proper eating habits. Dysphagia can also lead to depression and antisocial tendencies in sufferers as they find it difficult to consume food and mingle in public.[37]

Heart

The right side of the heart is anatomically affected by lung cancer, as it is the side of the heart that supplies blood to the lungs to be oxygenated. However, lung cancer also causes the rest of the circulatory system damage by not being able to properly cleanse the blood of carbon dioxide before it is to be distributed throughout the body. The left side of the heart may also fall victim to lung cancer due to high blood pressure in the lungs as a result of the blood not being able to flow smoothly.[38] Metastases of lung cancer tumors to the heart can also occur through growth on major blood vessels, causing swelling of the face and trachea as well as heavily visible veins in the neck and chest area.[39] When the right atrium of the heart is affected, this symptom is called *superior vena cava obstruction* or *superior vena cava syndrome* because of the way the vena cava blood vessel is "choked," preventing it from delivering blood back to the heart and vice versa.[40] Aside from the superior vena cava, tumors can also invade the heart via the pulmonary veins, which are connected to the blood vessels on the left atrium of the heart.[41] The blood pumped by the heart can also carry the effects of lung cancer. *Anemia* can occur as a result of the lack of normal red blood cells, and high platelet counts result in blood clots. The clotting can clog the arteries (*arterial thrombosis*) and lead to inflammation from clotting of the veins (*thrombophlebitis*).[42]

Externally, the chest area can be affected by hormonal imbalances triggered as a result of lung cancer. Gynecomastia occurs in males and manifests as the enlargement of the breast area. It develops due to the increase of estrogen levels and the decrease of testosterone.[43] Females may experience galactorrhea, which is characterized by the sudden production of milk from the breasts.[44]

Shoulders and Arms

Some lung cancer patients may experience constant ache in their shoulders, with occasional numbness in the arm, and the hand may also follow.[45] These are indicators of Pancoast's syndrome, which is a result of tumors that have developed near the apex, or topmost part, of the lung.[46] Known also as *Pancoast tumors*, *pulmonary sulcus tumors*, or *superior sulcus tumors*, these tumors are typically non–small cell carcinomas and can often cause the suppression of nearby nerves and arteries. Left untreated, the Pancoast tumor can end up affecting the brachial plexus, which is the network of nerves located in between the shoulder and the collarbone.[47] It connects the central nervous system to the arm and, when damaged, can compromise the function of the arms and hands, causing loss of feeling and tingling. This band of symptoms is called *thoracic outlet syndrome*.[48] Additional effects to the hands include the metastasis of cancer cells to the bones in the hand, leading to a painful swelling of the fingers referred to as *digital (finger) clubbing*.[49]

Diaphragm

The diaphragm, which assists in expanding the lungs while inhaling, can be paralyzed as a result of lung cancer. Diaphragmatic paralysis occurs when tumors press on or grow on the phrenic nerve, located between the lungs and the heart, which controls the diaphragm's function.[50] When lung cancer cells invade the diaphragm and penetrate the muscle, it is a sign of advanced-stage cell malignancy since it is considered irreversible.[51]

Liver

The liver is another popular anatomical site for the metastasis of lung cancer cells because all the blood from the body passes through it for filtering. Cancerous growths in the liver are detected because they cause the liver to become enlarged. This is as a result of its limited size and capacity.[52] The liver is tender when prodded, and, a result, the lung cancer sufferer experiences pain below the rib cage area.[53] Tumors in the liver can result in unexpected weight loss due to the body's inability to regulate waste as well as *jaundice* (yellowing skin) due to accumulation of *bile*, a yellowish digestive fluid found in the liver.[54] Once the lung cancer has reached the liver, the prognosis is poor, as it is a sign of how far the disease process has already progressed. Most patients suffer liver failure as the cancer reaches its last stages.[55]

Adrenal Glands

Lung tumors spreading to the adrenal glands can cause pain and tenderness in the anatomical region near the ribs.[56] Hormonal abnormalities as a result of cancer cells in the adrenal gland also lead to Cushing's syndrome, which causes cortisol levels to rise. The result is high blood pressure, edemas, myopathy or muscle disease, obesity of the thorax and face ("moon face"), mood swings, and weight loss.[57]

Kidneys

When the lungs fail to clear carbon dioxide from the blood, the kidneys try to help compensate for regulatory failure by increasing acid levels in the body so that the excess carbon dioxide can be removed via urination. The kidneys also try to increase oxygenation in the blood by increasing *erythropoietin*, a protein hormone involved in red blood cell production, which leads to the proliferation of red blood cells in order to provide more vessels for oxygen to run through.[58] While metastasis to the kidney is rare, it has occurred on occasion. In a well-documented case in China, a renal tumor originating from a squamous cell lung carcinoma was detected in a patient who was in remission.[59]

LOWER ANATOMY AND LUNG CANCER

Pelvis

The pelvic bone near the waist is one of the bones commonly invaded by cancer cells originally rooted in the respiratory system.[60] The invasion comes as a result of the pelvis's connection to the vertebral venous system, which links the parts of the thorax and allows lung cancer cells to spread easily to the lower body.[61] The pelvic bone usually feels painful, though it is often written off as a strained muscle.[62] It can fracture easily, which signifies that the pain may be the result of the presence of *osteolytic (bone-destroying) lesions*. These lesions (severe grazes that destroy bone) are one of the hazardous symptoms of metastasis to the bone, as they cause holes to be formed in the bone, making it brittle. Pain in the bone can also be the result of osteoblastic or osteoclerotic lesions, which are abnormal growths of bone. These growths are also brittle and break easily.[63] Tumors of the bone usually develop in stage 3 or stage 4 cancer, and thus by the time pelvis invasion is detected, chances of survival are quite low.[64]

Aside from bone invasion, the pelvis is also affected by *Lambert-Eaton myasthenic syndrome*, which is an autoimmune syndrome targeting the muscles near the middle of the body (proximal muscles). The syndrome causes the proximal muscles on the lower half of the body to weaken, making actions such as sitting, climbing stairs, and walking normally difficult. Joint reflexes are slowed, and in later stages the respiratory muscles can be weakened as well. This is one way in which the lower anatomy of the body plays an indirect role in a disease process such as lung cancer.[65]

Stomach

Pancoast's syndrome, aside from affecting the hands and the shoulders, also affects the abdomen by causing stomach pain and tenderness.[66] Abdominal fluid buildup, or *ascites*, is another result of Pancoast's syndrome and is an indication of terminal-stage cancer. Ascites is caused by a number of tumor-related factors, including pressure on the nerves, infections, and blockages. It can impede the diaphragm and cause breathing to become labored.[67] Signs of ascites include tightened skin over the stomach, immediate feeling of fullness despite minimal food intake, and the veins of the abdomen becoming visible.[68]

Digestive System

Some of the aftereffects of cancer are caused not by lung tumors but by their by-products on the lower anatomy of the patient. The digestive system, for instance, is directly affected not by tumor growth from the lungs but by intestinal secretions.[69] These symptoms may occur early on the onset of lung cancer but are often diagnosed as other illnesses. Vasoactive intestinal peptides released within the gastrointestinal tract activate *adenylate cyclase*, an enzymatic secretion that has muscle-relaxant capabilities and causes diarrhea.[70] Constipation can also occur due to increased blood calcium levels, or hypercalcemia.[71] Hypercalcemia incites increased gastrin production, which is a peptide that inhibits the digestive function of the stomach and delays bowel movement.[72] This leads to increased acidity, which in turn results in the constant need to urinate.[73] In some unusual cases, the intestinal walls are ripped open due to blockage within the intestine, causing bowel perforation.[74] This can affect either the small or the large intestine and cause body waste to enter the abdomen. This leads to severe stomach pain and fever as the waste infects the blood.[75]

Pancreas

Lung cancer invading the pancreas is uncommon.[76] On the occasion that it does, it often occurs in those with advanced small cell lung carcinoma or stage 4 non–small cell carcinoma.[77] Metastatic pancreatic tumors can cause the pancreas to become inflamed, a condition known as pancreatitis. This manifests as strong stomach pain and requires medical attention as soon as possible.[78] Pancreatitis is connected to the failure of the lung to oxygenate the blood, a sickness known as *hypoxemia*,[79] and also causes blood sugar levels to fluctuate.[80]

Feet

One of the more serious anatomical and physiological features of lung cancer is *edema*, or accumulated fluid in the feet and ankles that causes swelling.[81] Known obsoletely as dropsy, edema is another sign of advanced-stage cancer of the lungs or other cancer, as they are signs that the heart and the lungs are having difficulty functioning normally. The inability to keep the circulatory system running smoothly results in fluids being retained, and the kidneys have to work more diligently to properly get rid of the excess fluids. In the meantime, the fluid is concentrated at the extremities of the lower body. Edemas are aggravated by salt intake, as salt regulation places even more strain on the kidneys, and thus fluid retention can be even greater.[82] When at its worst, an edema can cause mental problems such as confusion and render the person suffering from lung cancer comatose.[83]

4

HISTORY OF LUNG CANCER

Oncology is the branch of science that studies and deals with tumors and cancer.[1] In relation to lung cancer, oncology is concerned with cancer diagnosis, screening efforts including relatives of patients and the population, treating the disorder, following up with cancer patients after successful therapy, giving palliative care for terminal malignancy cases, and dealing with ethical issues of cancer care. Medical history taking goes hand in hand with physical assessment and the identification of signs and symptoms.

HISTORICAL DEVELOPMENTS AND ORIGINS OF CELL MALIGNANCY

Cancer in general has been present throughout history. Its existence is seen among the remnants of human mummies in ancient Egypt, where people discovered fossils of bone tumors and damaged skulls, as seen in head and neck cancers. At about 3000 BC, scholars described cancer partially in an early Egyptian "textbook" on trauma surgery. It mentions eight cases of breast tumors and prescribes a primitive form of *cauterization* (burning) as the palliative treatment to this disease process.[2]

The word *cancer* is really accredited to Hippocrates (460–370 BC), a Greek physician who is known as the Father of Medicine. He used *carcinos*, a Greek word that translates to *crab*, in describing tumors, probably because of their crab-like appearance as seen in spreading tumors that have projections. Some theories suggest that it was because of the hardness of a tumor, which may have brought to mind the feel of a crab's shell. Others think that the difficulty of removing a tumor reminded Hippocrates of the strength of a crab's grip.[3] In AD 47, Celsus, a Roman doctor, agreed with Hippocrates' comparison and subsequently translated *karkinos* into the Latin word now universally known as *cancer*.[4] It was Galen (AD 130–200), a Roman physician of Greek ethnicity, who introduced the term *oncos*, the Greek word for *swelling*. He used it to describe benign tumors and used *carcinos* for *malignant tumors*.[5]

Sixteenth to Seventeenth Centuries

During the Renaissance of the fifteenth century, scientists contributed to enhancement in understanding the human body, and this is when Galileo and Isaac Newton started using the scientific method for anatomy. William Harvey published the book *Exercitatio Anatomica de Motu Cordis et Sanguinis in Animalibus* (*An Anatomical Exercise on the Motion of the Heart and Blood in Living Beings*), which gives a better understanding about the circulatory system as well as foundational knowledge about how cancers, such as those of the lung, might use the system as a means to spread.

Eighteenth Century

In 1761, Giovanni Morgagni of Padua performed autopsies to determine the cause of death by relating the patient's illness with the *pathologic* (disease-related) findings. His discoveries led researchers in understanding the development of tumor cells found in lung and other cancer types. It became the foundation for scientific oncology. John Hunter, a Scottish surgeon, pioneered in the surgical removal of tumors. Different theories regarding the causes of cancer had risen. Wilhelm Fabray believed that the milk clots in the mammary duct caused breast cancer. The Dutch professor Francois de Boe Sylvius stated that acidic lymph fluid caused cancer and that diseases were a result of chemical processes occurring in the body. In the late 1770s, British surgeon Percivall Pott discovered that cancers of the scrotum became a common disorder among the chimney sweepers. This discovery served as the first cause of cancer identified.[6]

Nineteenth Century

During the nineteenth century, tremendous advances in cancer research led to the field of oncology. Well-developed microscopes enabled researcher Rudolf Virchow to study the growth of the tumors—including those with similar features seen in the lung—on a cellular level. Improved *aseptic* (hygienic, sanitary) practices during surgery on tumors increased the survival rate of cancer patients. In the same period, different theories on chemical imbalances in the body were being formulated, and cellular pathology was born. English surgeon Campbell De Morgan made observations of the disease between 1871 and 1874. He believed that this so-called cancer poison eventually detaches from the primary tumor and travels through the lymph nodes, reaching other sites in the body. William Stewart Halsted developed the *radical mastectomy* (removal of breasts, usually for anticancer purposes) during the last decade of the nineteenth century.

In 1878, Thomas Beatson discovered the relevance of ovaries to the formation of milk in the breasts of rabbits. He performed a test removal of the ovaries, also called an *oophorectomy*, in patients with advanced breast cancer. This resulted in an improvement for breast cancer patients. He suggested that the ovaries might trigger the formation of *carcinomata*—the pluralized form of a cancer discussed extensively in chapter 9—in the breast. He also found that female ovarian hormone, known today as estrogen, stimulates breast cancer. This breakthrough became the foundation of hormone therapy practiced today, such as using tamoxifen and the aromatase inhibitors in treating or preventing breast cancer.[7]

Twentieth Century

In the 1900s, the genetic basis of many forms of cancer, including lung cancer, was recognized. German zoologist Theodor Boveri revealed that cells regenerate, containing multiple copies of a cellular structure he named *centrosome*. He hypothesized that chromosomes, though unique in nature, pass on different inheritance factors. According to his ideas, modifications in the chromosomes can breed a cell that has un-regulated growth potential and that transmits this trait to its daughter cells. He stated that cell cycle checkpoints, tumor suppressors, and oncogenes really do exist. He also claimed that exposure to radiation and contact with any physical or chemical insults or *pathogenic* (dis-ease-causing) microorganisms can lead to and promote cancer.

Marie and Pierre Curie introduced radiation, leading to a new, non-surgical therapy for lung cancer. Now, surgeons collaborate with hospi-tal radiologists when treating cancer instead of doing surgical opera-tions independently. Patients need treatment and admission to the hos-pital facility. Because of this, patient data are compiled in hospital files, a method spearheading the creation of statistical patient studies.

Historically, several researchers and organizations surfaced in rela-tion to treatment and management to cancers such as lung cancer. Fifteen physicians and businessmen founded the American Cancer So-ciety under the name American Society for the Control of Cancer. In 1926, Janet Lane-Claypon issued a study for the British Ministry of Health in which she compared 500 breast cancer cases and 500 control patients having similar backgrounds and lifestyles. Her works on cancer epidemiology were the inspiration behind the publication of *Lung Can-cer and Other Causes of Death in Relation to Smoking*. For over 50 years, tremendous efforts were made to gather data among medical practices, hospitals, provinces, states, and even countries to analyze and learn the correlation between environment and culture on the inci-dence of cancer. During this period, the Japanese medical community noticed that the bone marrow was destroyed among the victims of the Hiroshima and Nagasaki atomic bombings. They concluded that radia-tion could eliminate diseased bone marrow if protocols were carried out correctly. This contributed to the advancement of bone marrow trans-plants for leukemia.

It was also during the World War II that studies arose about the therapeutic effect of nitrogen mustard, an otherwise toxic chemical, in lymphomas. This served as the model for creating alkylating agents that destroy rapidly growing cells characteristic of cell malignancies such as lung cancer. Sidney Farber of Boston showed that *aminopterin* (an anticancer drug) terminates the progression of acute leukemia in chil-dren.[8] In the late 1950s, *methotrexate* (a chemotherapy drug explained in chapter 15) was used to try to cure metastatic cancer. The era of chemotherapy had begun. In the late 1960s, Anthony Epstein, Bert Achong, and Yvonne Barr identified the first human cancer virus, named Epstein-Barr virus.[9] Starting in the 1970s, ultrasound, computed tomography (CT), magnetic resonance imaging, and *positron emission tomography* (PET) replaced exploratory surgical operations in diagnosing lung cancer. Experts then began to extensively use CT scans and ultrasound to guide biopsy needles into tumors. Today, the field of oncology continues to (1) investigate lung cancer and its corresponding management, (2) carry out the latest anticancer drugs for chemotherapy, (3) identify correct radiological dosages, and (4) determine many environmental, chemical, and physical factors that cause lung cancer.

CAUSES OF CANCER THROUGHOUT HISTORY[10]

Early Egyptians attributed or "blamed" what is known today as cancer on gods. It puzzled people and professional caregivers, inspiring them to formulate different theories on the causes of cell malignancies such as lung cancer.[11]

Humoral Theory

According to Hippocrates, the body contains four "humors," or bodily fluids: blood, phlegm, yellow bile, and black bile. Balanced humors make a person healthy, and deviations in any of the humors cause disease, such as an excess of black bile in the body causing cancer. The Roman named Galen adapted this idea, and this theory was applied for over 1,300 years throughout the Middle Ages, during which medical knowledge improved little because the study of the body through autopsies was restricted by the Church.

Lymph Theory

It was considered that life exists because of the constant and precise flow of the body's fluid, the blood and lymph, through the solid parts. Stahl and Hoffman hypothesized that fermented and degenerated lymph, varying in density, acidity, and alkalinity, constitutes cancers such as lung cancer. Scottish surgeon John Hunter acknowledged that tumors develop from lymph and spread by the blood. [12]

Chronic Irritation Theory

Rudolph Virchow, the famous German pathologist, concluded that all cells, including cancer cells, come from other cells. He mentioned that cancer is brought on by chronic irritation and spreads, much the way a liquid behaves. In the 1860s, German surgeon Karl Thiersch illustrated how malignant cells spread without acting like a fluid.

Trauma Theory

Regardless of the advances made in the understanding of cancer, from the late 1800s until the 1920s trauma was considered a factor that caused cancer. This belief remained despite other, obvious factors causing cancer formation in experimental animals.

Infectious Disease Theory

Zacutus Lusitani (1575–1642) and Nicholas Tulp (1593–1674), two physicians in Holland, argued that cancer was communicable, as evidenced by the occurrence of breast cancer in members sharing the same household. Lusitani declared the contagion theory in 1649 and Tulp in 1652. To them, preventing the spread of cancer warrants isolation of patients, preferably outside cities and towns. Throughout the seventeenth and eighteenth centuries, people considered cancer as contagious. In the late 1770s, the first cancer hospital in France was forced to move away from the city because of fear within the general population. [13]

NOTABLE LUNG CANCER PATIENTS THROUGHOUT HISTORY

Fame is no protection against lung cancer, as this deadly disease process can strike anyone at any age. Lung cancer targets actors, artists, and musicians whose lifestyle choices have included smoking cigarettes.

The following list includes many famous figures who were struck down by lung cancer at the height of their careers:[14]

- Peter Jennings, age 67: Longtime anchor of the ABC newscast *World News Tonight*, Jennings was a lifelong smoker who announced in 2005 that he had been diagnosed with lung cancer. Jennings handled his diagnosis with dignity and grace. He died four months later on August 7, 2005.
- Steve McQueen, age 50: Despite being an internationally known "bad boy" actor, McQueen did not develop lung cancer as a result of smoking cigarettes alone. In 1979, McQueen was diagnosed with *pleural mesothelioma*, a type of cancer associated with asbestos exposure. Even today, there is no known cure for this type of lung cancer.
- Dana Reeve, age 44: Actress and wife of *Superman* star Christopher Reeve, Dana tragically was diagnosed with lung cancer in 2004. According to her, she had never smoked cigarettes.
- Walt Disney, age 65: Creator of Mickey Mouse and the massive Disney entertainment empire, Disney was a beloved figure who was diagnosed with a tumor on his left lung during an examination for an unrelated ailment. The tumor was malignant, and Disney's lung was consequently removed. He lived for another five weeks.
- Lou Rawls, age 72: A renowned singer, Rawls was diagnosed with cancers of the lung and brain. Although he had been a smoker earlier in life, Rawls quit smoking 35 years before his death in 2006.
- John Wayne, age 72: Arguably the most famous actor of his generation, Wayne smoked six packs a day before developing lung cancer in 1964.
- Paul Newman, age 83: A great actor in his day, Newman was diagnosed with lung cancer in June 2008 and died in September of that year. Newman was a heavy smoker, though he had quit 30 years before his death.
- Claude Monet, age 86: One of history's greatest painters, Monet died in 1926. Monet had been a smoker for many years.
- Warren Zevon, age 56: An internationally known musician, Zevon was diagnosed with inoperable *peritoneal mesothelioma*, a type of lung cancer usually associated with asbestos exposure.

- Vincent Price, age 82. Master of horror and well-known actor, Price was a lifelong smoker who died from lung cancer in 1993. He had suffered from *emphysema* for many years.
- George Harrison, age 58. One of the four legendary members of the Beatles, Harrison, a longtime heavy smoker, was first treated for throat cancer in 1997. He underwent surgery for lung cancer in May 2001, but the cancer later metastasized to his brain. He died in 2001.

ANOTHER LOOK AT THE PAST AND PRESENT

For the period 2006–2010, the median age for cancer of the lungs and bronchus was 70 years.[15] This determination refers to the median age at diagnosis, meaning that it includes only the moment of diagnosis regardless of the stage in which the lung cancer was at that time. The following provides some understanding of the magnitude of lung cell malignancy in the said time period:[16]

- People under 20 years of age who were diagnosed with cancer of the lungs and bronchi: about 0 percent
- Between ages 20 and 34: about 0.3 percent; between ages 35 and 44: about 1 percent; between ages 45 and 54: 9 percent; between ages 55 and 64: 21 percent; between ages 65 and 74 (which includes the median age): about 31 percent; between ages 75 and 84: 28 percent; over age 85: almost 9 percent

Currently, it is estimated that about 230,000 men and women will be diagnosed with cancer of the lung and bronchus during 2013 alone. Of this number, almost 200,080 will be men, and roughly 110,100 will be women. From the total number of diagnoses, one can assert that a vast number of people of both sexes will unfortunately expire from lung and bronchial cancer.[17]

II

Clinical Picture

5

CAUSES AND RISK FACTORS OF LUNG CANCER

Lung cancer has always been incurable, and even today it is treated with inordinate difficulty. The mortality rate is considerably high, especially if the cancer is diagnosed late and patients do not have proper treatment. When people are found to have lung cancer in its minor stages, their life quality will be influenced greatly by the illness even if the tumorous growths are removed in totality. This is due to (1) the psychological impact of the illness, (2) medication used for management of the disease process, and (3) other factors. This chapter therefore presents the causes of lung cancer and suggests ways to prevent them.[1]

The chances of a normal cell turning cancerous can increase because of two main factors: faulty genetic data inherited from a family member and carcinogen exposure. Damaged genetic data can be passed on to the younger generation by blood, which increases the predisposition for cancer onset even though it does not become the direct cause. Carcinogens, on the other hand, are substances that facilitate the creation of free radicals in the body and that can directly disrupt a cell's chemical makeup. Examples of carcinogens are tobacco, radiation, ultraviolet radiation, and exhaust fumes.[2] The carcinogenic contents of tobacco have (1) made cigarette smoking the leading cause of lung cancer, accounting for 85 percent of such cases, and (2) contributed to making lung cancer the most prevalent cancer in recent years.[3]

MAIN CAUSES OF LUNG CANCER

Tobacco Smoke Exposure

Reports show that smoking is the cause of 80 to 90 percent of cancer cases.[4] The more a person smokes, the higher the chances of falling ill. Also of importance is how *long* the person has been smoking—not only the *number* of cigarettes smoked in a given day. Cigarettes contain many dangerous components, both natural and artificial. Moreover, the content of tar in cigarettes is high. Tar residues can accumulate in lung tissue, causing different kinds of lung illnesses, including lung cancer. The longer a person smokes, the more harmful elements are contained in the lungs. Thus, the risk of lung cancer is increased in those individuals who have been smoking for a longer time, and quitting reduces one's chances.

It was commonly believed that only cigarette smoking leads to lung cancer while pipe and cigar smoking is not as perilous, but recent research shows that pipe and cigar smoking also can lead to lung cancer, though the risk is not as high as it is from cigarette smoking.[5] The reason for that is that in cigarettes, the number of artificial chemical elements that endanger health is much higher than in pipe tobacco or cigars. It does not matter whether one smokes inexpensive or expensive cigarettes, as all of them contain dangerous substances. Those who start smoking at a younger age can be sure that they have a higher chance of contracting lung cancer, as the immune systems of young people are not as resistant to illnesses as those of adults. The period of smoking experience should also be considered.[6]

Passive, or secondhand, smoking increases the risk of lung cancer, although the damage is still much less than by active smoking. Some people believe that the impact of passive smoking is not so high because, for obvious reasons, the exposure is less frequent. The immune systems of nonsmokers are not as accustomed to the dangerous elements of smoke as are those of smokers. Besides, people can be heavily exposed to passive smoking at home or in the workplace, and young children can be especially affected by passive smoking. Simply put, if a person does not want to be among the 80 to 90 percent mentioned earlier, he or she would need to cease smoking.[7] It is also useful to participate in physical exercise to reduce the risk of lung cancer.

Exposure to Toxins

The lung is among the most important organs exposed to environmental agents and has the ability to protect itself by both immunological and nonimmunological mechanisms. It has efficient immunological ways to defend itself and the body. When exposed to irritants, the highly efficient *mucociliary* (mucus and tiny "hairs") clearance system activates and returns the irritants to the posterior *pharynx* (throat). When the irritant is enormous, the traditional immune cells or pulmonary *parenchymal* (functional) cells increase the production of mucus secretions and release mediators employing inflammatory cells, incorporating more *phagocytes*, or cells that engulf foreign materials. These foreign irritants include nitrates, sulfur dioxide, formaldehyde, smoke, particulate matter, volatile organic compounds, and indoor allergens, such as dust mites, domestic pets, and fungi.[8]

Radon is the main cause of lung cancer in people who work in uranium mines, being one of the decay products of uranium.[9] Radon is radioactive and can be found just about everywhere in rocks and soil. The primary concern is that it is somehow able to build up in homes and other buildings. It can enter homes through cracks in foundations, openings in drains, and gaps around pipes. It also can be present in the water supply in homes where well water is used. People can be exposed to radon gas every day in their homes without suspecting any danger. Many homes in the United States have elevated levels of radon gas, and individuals living in older buildings should be especially careful about potential exposure to the gas. Residents of such older buildings could have their radon levels checked by a specialist who is able do this. One can also purchase a test kit.[10]

One of the most common dangers of lung cancer is exposure to asbestos. Asbestos particles can stay in lung tissue for an entire lifetime and thus increase the risk of lung cancer significantly over time. Although asbestos is limited in use and even banned in most developed countries, factory workers in poorer countries are still being exposed to asbestos in their workplaces. That is why it is important to read and follow carefully all safety rules at the workplace, especially if one works in a dangerous environment and deals with asbestos regularly.[11]

Diesel exhaust affects people in particular professions, such as professional drivers. Although measures are now taken to prevent damage to one's health caused by diesel exhaust, this dangerous substance is still among the factors that increase the overall risk of lung cancer. All safety requirements should be followed while performing such work. Today, some engines foil dangerous diesel exhaust and decrease or eliminate exposure to this harmful substance.[12]

Contact with materials such as silica, arsenic, and chromium can increase the risk of lung cancer. Most affected by these are people working at factories located in developing nations, where health care systems may not be advanced enough to protect workers. Exposure to arsenic is also common in regions where groundwater is saturated with these substances, and many people the world over drink well water every day.

Lung cancer risk is strongly associated with exposure to the following:[13]

- Arsenic and its compounds
- Hexavalent chromium and its compounds
- Talc containing asbestos fibers
- Iron and steel founding
- Cadmium and its compounds
- Coal gasification
- Beryllium
- Ionizing radiation
- Crystalline silica
- Chlormethyl ether, both technical and nontechnical grade
- Aluminum production
- Cola production
- Underground hematite mining (radon)
- Nickel refining (nickel oxides and sulfides)

While exposure to these chemical elements is much lower than it was in the past, it is still among the major causes of lung cancer by people who work in particular industries, especially in factories. Miners and professional drivers are exposed to diesel exhaust, while factory workers are exposed to asbestos and silica. If possible, people who are at risk of developing lung cancer should try to protect themselves from these harmful chemical factors. The use of protective gloves, proper ventilation, masks, and other preventive methods can lower the risk of lung

cancer significantly. If a person works in an industry know
exposure to these chemicals, he or she should make sure t
dietary habits and exercise regularly. Routine visits to the
certainly help ensure that "things are in check" for the worke.

Air Pollution

Air pollution from factories, vehicles, power plants, and other venues is
the cause of up to 5 percent of all cases of lung cancer.[14] Scientists
believe that living in polluted areas permanently is comparable to being
exposed constantly to cigarette smoke. In many cases, people who live
in areas with high levels of nitrogen oxides eventually suffer from lung
cancer. The use of coal in homes for heating and cooking increases the
level of smokiness in the house, and therefore the risk of lung cancer
increases. These factors are common in industrial areas of developing
regions.

The risk of becoming ill with lung cancer is higher for people residing in industrial areas close to plants and factories regardless of what
products are manufactured. Although the air pollution outdoors is beyond anyone's control, people can try to reduce smoke pollution in their
homes. If the opportunity arises, a person might be wise to relocate to
an area with cleaner air. Furthermore, specific measures can be taken
at the government level to prevent or reduce air pollution.

Genetic Factors

Clinical lung cancer researchers believe that at least one heritable gene
is responsible for lung cancer. That is why people who have a direct
relative who is ill with lung cancer are 5 percent more likely to suffer
from the malady.[15] This risk does not depend on whether one is a
smoker, though smoking increases the risk significantly. Scientists have
also discovered some genes that are responsible for susceptibility to the
development of other lung diseases, and these also can be regarded as
increasing the risk of lung cancer, as they damage lung tissue. In addition, the risk of lung cancer is increased for someone who has a sibling
who has that cancer. It is strongly recommended to avoid any harmful
habits, as the immune system is weakened due to gene mutations, and
hence genetic susceptibility to lung cancer could remain elevated.

Scientists have come to the conclusion that disorders in genetic structure make up one of the major obstacles to the smooth proliferation of cells. DNA code analyses and medical studies have confirmed that abnormal cell mutation causes apoptosis, which indicates the premature death of cells and tissues in the lungs.[16] Other experts claim that DNA is mainly damaged mainly by overexposure to carcinogenic components. These harmful elements are found in tobacco, narcotic substances, and asbestos.[17] Destructive carcinogenic materials enter into the body and affect the lungs through inhalation.

Previous Existence of Malignant Cells

People who once suffered from lung cancer are more likely to fall ill with the same disease process again. Lung cancer, even if treated properly in the form of surgical removal of tumor tissue, leaves scars in lung tissue that are highly susceptible to lung cancer all over again. The immune systems of such people are weaker as well since medications used for treatment have long-term effects on the body. It is worth also taking into consideration the mental and physical condition of people who experience lung cancer. All these factors increase the risk of lung cancer significantly. For people who had these "close calls" with lung cancer, it is advisable to avoid working in conditions known to increase the risk of lung cancer. Furthermore, the diets (chapter 14) of such people should include, to a certain extent, products rich in antioxidants, which are known to prevent lung cell damage.

Previous Treatments Related to Other Cancers

If a person has been previously treated for a different form of cancer, the medicines used seem to increase the risk of lung cancer within a number of years.[18] Especially predisposed to lung cancer are patients who have had radiation therapy to the chest, such as a woman with breast cancer or an individual who has suffered from Hodgkin's disease. Once lung cancer in such patients is diagnosed, it tends to have a more formidable clinical course. When considering previous treatments for other cancers as a potential cause for lung cancer, it is important to know that patients should not refuse any treatment suggested by the cancer physician. If one has been treated for cancer in the past, it is necessary to avoid any kind of smoking (active or passive) and visit the doctor regularly to prevent the illness or to get diagnosed at the earliest precancerous or cancerous stage possible.

Previous Infections and Viruses

Scientists claim that any infection or virus, such as the human papillomavirus, can increase the risk of lung cancer.[19] The evidence may not be 100 percent clear, but caregivers should understand that all infections do influence the immune system in some way or another and thus can lead to further disorders, including lung cancer. Viruses such as HIV and AIDS increase the risk of lung cancer, as they influence the human immune system irrevocably. People with AIDS and HIV should be especially vigilant about lung health at the cellular level (chapter 2). They can use management techniques to cope with constant mental and physical exertion since these forms of stress can diminish the capabilities of the immune system.

Drug Use

Clinical research validates that the use of prescription drugs such as aspirin is associated with the risk of lung cancer.[20] Especially dangerous are those drugs used after organ transplants, as they suppress the immune system to avoid the rejection of the transplanted organ. The immune system is accordingly suppressed, and the risk of lung cancer increases. Drugs used in combination with harmful habits, such as smoking, constant stress, and improper diet, add to the causative effect of lung cancer.

Diet as a Potential Risk Factor

It may sound ridiculous at first, but some dietary habits can also lead to an increased risk of lung cancer. Research proves that beta-carotene supplements used by smokers *increase* the risk of lung cancer, though it has been previously asserted that beta-carotene is beneficial to one's health overall.[21] People who drink water with arsenic in it have an increased risk of lung cancer, and some scientists believe that there is a correlation between cancer and the use of products rich in cholesterol and fat.

Cooking Fumes

Finding the true "cause" of lung cancer also concerns women in regions where wok cooking is common (e.g., Asia). Wok fumes seem to be one of causes of lung cancer in women. The simplest way to avoid this is to use other equipment, such as a type of stove that does not involve an open fire.

Sedentary Lifestyle

Recent studies have shown that lung cancer and other types of cancer are more likely to develop in people who tend to have sedentary lifestyles.[22] This fact cannot prove that a sedentary lifestyle can directly cause lung cancer, though one should consider that sedentary lifestyle influences the general health of a person, as lung ventilation and function is decreased. All these factors increase the risk of general lung disease as well as lung cancer.

Pesticides

The use of pesticides cannot be regarded as a direct cause of lung cancer. However, constant exposure to these chemicals, even in limited amounts, can lead to many health disorders, including breast and liver cancer. Considering that people who have been ill with any kind of cancer are at a higher risk of becoming ill with lung cancer, it is possible to say that pesticides can be regarded as a risk factor of lung cancer as well. Today, strong pesticides are used worldwide to increase the productivity of plants and to fight off insects. These chemicals are considered relatively harmless if not overused, but scientific research shows that they can lead to serious illnesses and significantly increase the risk of lung cancer.[23] This is why, if a person is unsure whether pesticides are present, fruits and vegetables should be washed prior to consumption.

Physical and Mental Stress

Some believe that physical and mental stress can lead to cancer. Although there is no direct connection between these factors and lung cancer cases, admittedly stress does influence the immune system and can lead to serious illnesses as well as lung cancer. The risk increases if a close relative is diagnosed.[24] People under stress tend to develop unhealthy types of behavior, such as smoking. Solid clinical research also proves that alcohol consumption, which is sometimes initiated by patients to relieve physical and mental stress, plays a pivotal role in respiratory cancer.[25]

It is worth mentioning, however, that in people already diagnosed, the recovery process is much more difficult if they are under stress. Those who suffer from stress produce some hormones that can promote metastasis. People who suffer excessively from physical stress can undergo proper stress management, training in relaxation, and social therapy if needed. *Mental* stress and its role in lung cancer is covered in more detail in chapter 16.

CLINICAL CAUSES OF LUNG CANCER

Tuberculosis

When it comes to causes and risk factors for lung cancer, individuals suffering from *tuberculosis* fall into a rather special category. This disorder, even if cured properly, leaves scars in the lung tissue that can seriously predispose someone to lung cancer. Individuals who have experienced tuberculosis are 11 times more likely to become ill with lung cancer than those who never had tuberculosis.[26] Lung cancer can often be mistaken for tuberculosis, and a wrong or missed diagnosis of the latter can be a straightforward cause for late lung cancer and, possibly, death of the patient.

It is worth remembering that tuberculosis is a more common illness in developing countries with unusually large and congested populations. Tuberculosis is also commonly observed in prisoners since during incarceration people become infected easily, and proper diagnosis procedures and treatment either arrive too late or are not available at all.

Thus, this illness is closely connected with social and living conditions and can, in that way, be an ancillary cause of lung cancer.

Pneumonia

One more illness that is not as dangerous and damaging to health as tuberculosis is pneumonia, but the latter disorder should be given more attention today because it damages lung tissue and can cause lung cancer if treated improperly or if lung tissue scars are neglected in the long run. In some cases, pneumonia can be (1) a cause or a symptom of lung cancer or (2) developed *with* cancer.[27] That is why if someone has pneumonia, special attention to his or her lung health might be offered. Concomitant lung cancer and pneumonia make the treatment more intense and could worsen the results of managed care of the patient.

Chronic Bronchitis

Despite being an illness that increases the risk of lung cancer, *chronic bronchitis* (long-term inflammation of the chest airways) is often ignored by most people suffering from it, as it is common during the winter months and usually does not cause as much trouble as other, more serious illnesses. Nonetheless, research shows that almost all patients suffering from lung cancer have suffered from chronic bronchitis as well.[28] This should not come as a surprise since chronic bronchitis is an illness caused by bronchial inflammation. This illness damages airways and increases the risk of lung cancer, which is why it should never be ignored and should always be treated properly and in time.

SOCIAL AND CULTURAL CAUSES OF LUNG CANCER

Sociocultural causes of lung cancer must be discussed separately in this chapter, as there is a wide spectrum of categories involved here.

Economic Situation

As one can imagine, people in certain countries lack enough resources to provide themselves and their families with a proper level of health care and effective diagnoses and treatment opportunities. Also, living in damp environments, such as those seen with flooded basements, can make a person more susceptible to lung cancer. When healthy but expensive food is unavailable, people tend to eat more fast food or other affordable items known to be high in cholesterol and fats and fewer fruit and vegetables. This can indeed heighten the risk of lung cancer.[29]

Limitations with Public Assistance Programs

In the United States, public assistance programs provide treatment to both citizens and noncitizens. However, the main problem is that such programs are limited to emergencies. The major disadvantage here is that the treatment is available only after the soon-to-be lung cancer patient submits particular documents, and this also takes time and worsens the situation. Moreover, there are still groups of people who are not eligible to receive free treatments, depending on the type of program. Even if the person can be treated, sometimes the disease process is already at the stage when the best treatment protocols are ineffective.[30]

Problems with Insurance Coverage

There are regions in the world that do not provide insurance coverage on a regular basis, and most people living there cannot afford themselves a proper cancer treatment and diagnosis. Although it may not be a direct cause of lung cancer, the absence of insurance often leads to cases when people get diagnosed with lung cancer in emergency rooms but the illness has developed to a stage when the treatment is ineffective. In poorer countries, the cost of cancer diagnoses and treatment is so high that people cannot afford the much-needed insurance. Things may turn to the point where sufferers prefer to work and earn sustainable incomes rather than receive appropriate treatment.[31]

Transportation Issues

In some instances, people still lack a proper transport system that would otherwise make the delivery of a patient to the hospital a difficult and expensive task. This is also one of the excuses for people not to visit a health care professional to check their health and take preventive measures when necessary. In addition, transporting a person afflicted with lung cancer to the hospital and providing him or her with proper treatment may be beyond the financial capabilities of some families.[32]

Exposure to Dangerous Chemicals

In relation to the topic of how chemicals can cause lung cancer, individuals of lower socioeconomic status are known to work in dangerous industries and are exposed to the influence of carcinogenic elements. In some manufacturing plants, no sufficient measures are taken to protect people from dangerous materials, or it is possible that employers really do not take the health of their workers into consideration. Overall, those of lower economic and social status live in more polluted areas, as accommodation is usually much cheaper in industrial areas where air, soil, and water pollution levels are higher than ideal. In addition, such people do not have access to healthy food since the costs of these foods are relatively higher.[33]

Lack of Preventive Information

Both education and life satisfaction can play a crucial role when it comes to a person's susceptibility to lung cancer. The main problem is that due to educational restraints, people may not have proper knowledge of how to prevent the advance of lung cancer and how to recognize it at early stages. Lack of information about the ecological condition of a given area where people live or of a particular building where destructive chemicals aggregate can also be a risk factor for lung cancer by extension.[34]

As one can see, almost all causes and risk factors of lung cancer can be traced back to sociocultural elements. In reality, everything starts from the time a woman gets pregnant. The health of her future child, including lung cancer susceptibility, will depend on whether (1) she smokes, (2) uses alcohol, or (3) has a proper diet and obtains enough vitamins and minerals to provide a good immune response to her child. It also depends on the number of lung cancer cases in the family. Living in a clean atmosphere early in life, providing a proper diet, and developing healthy lifestyle habits will (1) provide a good basis for a healthy lifestyle and (2) support the immune system so that he or she will be able to resist the circumstances of cell malignancy, such as that seen in cancers of the lung.[35]

6

PATHOLOGY OF LUNG CANCER

Pathology is the scientific study of disease that warrants diagnostic procedures that subsequently help doctors in the detection of medical disorders for treatment. In some ways, pathology lays emphasis on the cause, diagnosis, structural, or morphological changes in the sizes of cells and the method of pathogenesis. Pathology can also be seen as the symptoms of a disorder itself, and while signs and symptoms have different medical bases, a "sign" is considered the same as a symptom for the purpose of this chapter. Pathological study is important for understanding the causes and nature (in this case, the symptomology) of a deadly disease process such as lung cancer. If professional caregivers are unable to find the major symptoms in the lungs, they will most certainly have problems managing the patient.

PATHOLOGY OF LUNG CANCER AT THE GENERAL LEVEL

Patients can be too afraid to express their troubles and sorrows to their doctors, and they might hesitate to reveal to the physician what they truly feel as result of *white-coat syndrome* or *white-coat hypertension.*[1] However, it is important to disclose all symptoms when seeing a doctor for any ailment. Any information a patient can provide will help with diagnosis and treatment. While symptoms of various *types* of lung cancers are discussed in part III, the lung cancer patient and caregiver should understand that the appearance of lung cancer symptoms develops over time.

At a primary level, a patient with lung cancer at an initial stage eventually experiences *dyspnea* (difficulty breathing), wheezing, and coughing, with sticky phlegm containing blood. A sudden loss of weight is also a prominent symptom of lung cancer. Patients feel uneasy while breathing forcefully, and the patient suffers from fatigue and anxiety. Following diagnosis, depression and mental exhaustion can greatly weaken patients as well.

Malignant cancer at various phases bears similar symptoms and signs. A patient who feels ill simply breathing should see a doctor immediately. If there is a constant coughing tendency, chest pain, overflow of sputum with blood from the lungs, and unusual discomfort, patients should pay the doctor a visit for close observation. Generally, lung cancer in its benign state is embedded without obvious symptoms. Due to colds, people can experience coughing with spasm. In the event that symptoms persist for more than a month, it might be wise for the patient to talk to a health care consultant stating his or her preexisting maladies. Authorities unanimously agree that smoking is a bad habit that hastens the occurrence of lung cancer in certain individuals. Carcinogens that contribute to lung cancer are present in tobacco, aluminum, and asbestos, to name a few.

An individual with lung cancer might suffer from regular coughing and for a number of reasons. The early symptoms of bronchitis, asthma, *chronic obstructive pulmonary disease*, and *gastrooesophageal* (stomach and esophagus) reflux are characterized by uninterrupted coughing, so lung cancer might not be the first thing a doctor or a patient considers. However, if symptoms persist, even after treatment for the suspected cause, further tests should be conducted. It is important for patients to keep track of their symptoms to better guide their doctors in making a diagnosis.

Furthermore, pain is a general symptom that makes a patient feel uneasy and lose concentration. Due to the spread of cancer in the lungs, nerves become injured to some extent, and this causes mild to moderate pain in the backside and shoulder. The nature of pain at different stages of lung cancer can be similar in magnitude. Reporting this kind of pain is also important.

PATHOLOGY OF LUNG CANCER AT THE DETAILED LEVEL

After extensive pathological research, a group of experts has prepared a medical survey report in which they have stated that the symptoms of lung cancer at the more detailed level, such as depression, are inconspicuous.[2] When lung cancer starts to progress, the symptoms include too much calcium, *syndrome of inappropriate antidiuretic hormone* (SIADH), chest pain, excessive appetite, and obstruction in the respiratory system.[3] Muscle stiffness and weakness is another symptom that may worsen over time. Chest X-rays and other forms of screening and analysis will help doctors decide what may be happening and will help in any diagnosis.

Symptomatically, lung cancer spreads steadily to "deactivate" patients from performing tasks comfortably. While it is a slow death for a patient who is in the middle stages of lung cancer, the quality and quantity of life may be extended by the management of symptoms. Symptoms at the advanced level are much more palpable. At this final stage, patients are weak. They may have difficulty communicating with family and friends. Solid clinical evidence suggests that this type of social isolation can also result in hallucinations.[4] Proper medications and therapies reduce mental setback and physical uneasiness to some extent. Shortness of breath is a general symptom that alerts patients about the negative impact of malignant lung cancer. The patient's weight abruptly decreases to the point where he or she feels feeble and weak.

Clinical reports and studies have confirmed that when lung cancer spreads all over the body, important organs start functioning improperly. Due to the rapid progression of the disease, various organs of the body "get a jolt" over time but not when general symptoms first begin to appear. The brain, liver, adrenal glands, and kidneys will soon face a sudden decrease in function. Chest pain becomes serious and frequent, weakening the cancer patient's body.

Structural and Morphological Changes in Cancerous Cells of the Lungs

After lung cancer attacks, the shape of cellular structures in the lungs abruptly changes, then proceeds slowly. Doctors try to monitor this progression through analyses and lab tests. When cancer does harm to different layers of the lungs, the epithelium swells and becomes large via a process known as hyperplasia (chapter 2). Prior to initiating any therapeutic procedure or treatment to reduce the pain of lung cancer patients, doctors try to track this irregularity in tissue form and structure as much as possible.

In addition, there is higher possibility of proliferation in the development of basal tissues and cells that are deeply embedded in the lungs. Doctors define this morphological change as dysplasia. They try to check and resist the speedy outgrowth of nuclei and *basal cells* (cells located deep within the epithelium) in the lungs. As time passes, cells in the lungs lose the ability to multiply at the appropriate rate. Until the malignant cells penetrate deeply to rip through the basement membrane, however, the lung will not be considered fully metastatic or malignant. If patients are under special care prior to the onset of the symptoms of lung cancer, such as basal proliferation, there will be greater hope for recovery.

COMMON SYMPTOMS OF LUNG CANCER

Weight Loss, Fever, Fatigue, and Dehydration

While some research studies maintain that lung cancer causes weight loss, others argue that the patient can *gain* a substantial amount of weight from chemotherapy.[5] Either way, it is important to know that lung cancer patients often ignore the cause of rapid weight loss within a few weeks. If a patient loses 10 pounds abruptly, weight loss is obviously a grave concern for him or her, and therefore no one should neglect it. To summarize, weight loss is a common primary symptom of lung cancer.

Individuals with lung cancer experience fevers that make them physically very weak.[6] They are unable to concentrate and might not be able to complete their work. As a result, they have low energy levels, and mental exhaustion or fatigue can soon set in. In case the fevers and extreme fatigue spiral out of control, it is necessary to reach out to professional caregivers, such as a physician or nurse, immediately. A person suffering from lung cancer who has a couple of months to live feels extreme fatigue, and days can become dull and meaningless.[7]

Dehydration is another common sign of lung cancer. Patients who have severe lung cancer that seems to be unbeatable slowly lose interest in eating food and drinking water. Although their bodies need nutrients, vitamins, and proteins in adequate amounts on regular basis, patients can't eat nutritious food and consume water as they would were they healthy.[8]

Coughing, Vomiting, and Clotting of Blood

Hemoptysis (coughing with blood) is a major symptom of lung cancer.[9] Some patients cough constantly throughout the day, and there is also the possibility of a voice break situated in the *larynx* (voice box). At the time of hemoptysis, patients feel chronic pain in the abdominal regions and backside of the body. It is up to the doctors to establish whether lung cancer exists once the patient presents with symptoms of hemoptysis. In some cases, however, the symptoms disappear after a few days. If symptoms of hemoptysis linger for a long time, repeated observations may be necessary to assert whether it is the cause of the cancer since hemoptysis does not *always* confirm the existence of malignant cells in the respiratory system. Clinical cases have proven that patients who have entered into the last stage of lung cancer go through *hematemesis* (vomiting blood).[10] The individual with advanced lung cancer who tries his or her best to eat meals—however nutritious they may be—tends to vomit blood. At advanced phases, emboli and free radicals increase and mingle with other constituents of the bloodstream. This blood clotting is a severe symptom, as it obstructs the smooth flow of blood in the circulatory system.

Cachexia and Bone and Joint Pain

Cachexia is when muscles begin losing strength. When lung cancer occurs and damages muscle tissues as well as the airways of the lungs, patients have to bear pain, mental anguish, weakness, fever, and other difficulties simply to breathe fresh air so that oxygen can activate the body. However, cachexia is a symptom that warns patients about the destructive impact of lung cancer. Muscles becomes lean, and therefore lung cancer patients will have to take medication to enhance normal muscle growth. Muscle cramps and pain in different joints of the body can surface concomitantly in lung cancer.[11]

Lung cancer spreads to the bones, and when metastatic bone cancer is discovered without an obvious source, it can be linked to an underlying lung cancer. Bones that lung cancer often spreads to include the upper bones of the arm and leg (the *humerus* and *femur*), the spine (especially the vertebrae in the chest and lower abdominal areas), and the pelvis. Lung cancer is also unique in that it can spread to bones in the hands and feet. The pain may feel similar to that of a stinging strain or muscle pull at the start but steadily exacerbates and can become serious. When bone metastases reach the arms and legs, pain is often worse with rapid muscle movement. Pain due to the spread of lung cancer to the spine and surrounding areas is often worse after sundown and following prolonged bed rest.[12]

Headaches and Other Neurological Symptoms

Researchers have devised new methods of ridding the world of lung cancer. Modern science and technology have enabled scientists to upgrade diagnostic procedures and treatments for alleviating the severity of respiratory cancer symptoms, such as headaches. Headaches, which lung cancer patients might experience often, and neurological symptoms create a diverse range of problems along both the caregiving and the patient spectrum. Lung cancer can make a patient nervous and his or her facial expressions pale. Memory dulls as the cancer metastasizes to the brain. A severe pain in the head region ensues—a symptom that can be alleviated by antimigraine and standard headache-relieving medications.[13]

Neck and Facial Inflammation

Research has proven that lung cancer can cause neck pain. The neckline area, including the face, swells and correspondingly disfigures the upper anatomy (chapter 3) of the patient. Patients with lung cancer need guidance and advice for detecting the sole cause of such inflammation. At first sight, doctors may not get immediate answers when attempting to learn these specific symptoms of lung cancer, and inflammation of the face as a direct result of lung cancer remains questionable in current research circles.[14]

Pain and Insomnia

A patient whose lung cancer is painful needs special care. Pain varies, depending on the severity of the cancer. A patient who has malignant lung cancer loses interest in doing just about anything, mainly because of the physical and mental pain at hand. When the pain becomes unbearable, experts advise patients to use helpful gestures to express their displeasure. Doctors often calculate the intensity of pain in the last stages of lung cancer by applying a measurement parameter. For instance, a score of 1 to 3 might indicate average or mild pain, and a score of 7 to 10 might indicate severe, relentless pain that could very well constitute a medical emergency. The remaining few months can be challenging for patients fighting for their lives in spite of all the pain.[15]

Chronic pain can prevent a lung cancer patient from sleeping properly, a condition called *insomnia*. Patients whose lung cancer is worst face a number of health hazards as a result of improper sleep patterns. At night, they do not possess enough stamina to fall asleep. Patients might wake up at very short intervals. Insomnia causes them to become restless and noisy.[16]

Swallowing, Breathing, and Voice Symptoms

Dysphagia (difficulty swallowing) is one of the important symptoms of advanced lung cancer and can cause discomfort in a patient while eating. Eating complications become severe after the onset of malignant cancer in lungs, and when a bedridden lung cancer patient tries to swallow food the right way, pain in the thoracic region can appear. Moreover, he or she might be reluctant to consume any hard foods.[17]

At the most advanced stage of lung cancer, the sufferer starts breathing rapidly, putting much pressure on the entire respiratory system. He or she doesn't feel at ease to inhale and exhale air properly and might

groan while trying to breathe strongly or talk loudly. Dyspnea under-
standably puts patients in an uncomfortable situation when with
friends. Rapid breathing can also be painful. Finally, case studies confirm that voice disorder is one symptom of lung cancer. [18]

7

LUNG CANCER SCREENING AND DIAGNOSTICS

Lung cancer is a disease process characterized by uncontrolled cell growth that if left untreated can extend to regions of the body beyond the boundaries of the lung—all through a harmful process called *metastasis*. This is why *diagnosing* it early, before it has spread, is important, as it boosts the patient's chance for successful resolutions (part IV).

As of January 1, 2010, approximately 340,000 men and women in the United States had a history of cancer of the lung and bronchus. Of this total number, about 180,000 were men and just over 215,000 were women—numbers that include all the people who were diagnosed with lung or bronchial cancer before January 1, 2010, regardless of (1) their current condition, (2) whether they were "cured" of these disorders, or (3) whether these disorders were still active in their organs.[1]

Of all the cancers worldwide, lung cancer is the most commonly diagnosed, and its incidence still grows. In 2007 alone, there were 1.5 million new lung cancer cases diagnosed worldwide, representing 12 percent of all cancer cases. Also, in 2007, there were approximately 1.35 million lung cancer deaths globally, giving this cancer the highest mortality rate. The greatest incidence of lung cancer diagnosis is found in the United Kingdom and Poland, where there are more than 100 cases per 100,000 people, and the lowest incidence is found in Senegal and Nigeria, where there are fewer than 1 death per 100,000 people. The numbers for lung cancer diagnosis are directly correlated to smoking, and in addition to developing countries where smoking has increased, the incidence of lung cancer cases will notably rise over the next few years in nations such as India and China.[2]

EARLY DETECTION AND INTRODUCTION TO METHODS

Clinical research continues to attempt to find better ways to detect lung cancer at the molecular level.[3] Because lung cancer is usually detected after it has compromised the functions of the lungs at both the detailed and the general level, it has become increasingly important to detect it early and to act before it has spread and affected other parts of the body. When found in time, in an early stage of its development, tumorous growths are much easier to stop.[4] However, lung cancer symptoms (chapter 6) may not always be perceived as those of lung cancer itself but as being the effect of some other manifestation (chapter 12) in the patient. The "other" disorder may lead to a failure of early detection and consequently the spreading of the cancerous growth until it destabilizes the functions of the lungs, at which point treatment might also need to be more invasive. This is why early detection is so vital and why recognizing the warning signs and taking prompt action can lead to early diagnosis and treatment of the disease with better outcomes.[5]

Unfortunately, solid symptoms that may aid in the detection of an early-stage lung cancer do not exist. Persistent coughing with small amounts of blood, chest pain, weight loss, and shortness of breath are some symptoms that, if investigated in time, may lead to the early diagnosis of lung cancer and its removal. The longer a cancer goes undetected, the more time it has to grow and spread, and the harder it is to treat.[6] Sadly, this is the case with many lung cancer patients; they report the symptoms too late or don't take action in time, and the cancer grows and develops until its presence is obvious. At that point, the cancer requires less effort to diagnose officially but is more difficult to effectively remove later. Bringing awareness of lung cancer to the public is one of the most important methods of early detection and can have a great impact on the disease.[7]

A LUNG CANCER PATIENT'S CLINICAL HISTORY

It is important to remember the role that a patient's clinical history plays in diagnosing lung cancer. Thus, relaying the details of a person's full medical background is imperative. A clinical history, also called *anamnesis*, is gathered by the physician, who asks specific questions to the lung cancer patient or other people close to the patient, such as family or friends, who can give suitable information. Such questions inquire about the patient's name, measurements, weight, and age but also about (1) the main symptoms they are presenting with, (2) a family history of the disease (if it has occurred before), and (3) risk factors (smoking, alcohol use, and work conditions). At this point and after an examination, the doctor may arrive at a *provisional diagnosis*, where he or she may suggest what might be going on; other possible causes for the symptoms will be explored as well.[8]

Providing such a clinical history is important to patients with lung cancer because the process may uncover some problems from the past that may have led to the formation of the disease process. Because there is a significant overlap between the symptoms of lung cancer and *chronic obstructive pulmonary disease* (COPD), a complete clinical history is required of any COPD that the patient may have suffered in the past or is more vulnerable to contracting.[9] This can help the attending physician determine if the symptoms are, indeed, coming from one such COPD or some other constituent that may pose as lung cancer. A study in the Netherlands has shown that many patients diagnosed with lung cancer also had a coexistent COPD but without any evidence that suggested lung cancer or that prompted physicians to test further.[10] This shows that the more complete the patient's clinical history, the greater the chances are for various COPDs to be excluded. This in turn narrows the range of possible diseases that may have caused the symptoms of those COPDs and reduces the amount of testing that has to be done to reach the source of the symptoms, be it lung cancer or not. A complete clinical history helps doctors determine if a potential lung cancer patient is more susceptible to other diseases that may have run in the family or if the patient has had a family member with lung cancer in the past. All this leads to swifter decision making and less valuable time wasted because when defying cancer, even if it has an "incubation period," a detailed history taking may allow some room for waiting. A quick response to the threat is what makes the difference between early removal of the cancerous growth or a long, arduous diagnostic course that has dangers of its own.

SCREENING PROCEDURES

The entire process of screening, at its most basic medical level, is all about (1) searching for the lung cancer before a person has shown any symptoms, (2) performing tests, and (3) eventually offering a positive or a negative conclusion.[11] Lung cancer continues to have one of the lowest survival rates simply because it is usually diagnosed when it has developed to the point where it shuts down the lungs and treatment becomes extremely difficult.[12]

There are some screening procedures that can be administered to those at higher risk of lung cancer. One such procedure is *sputum cytology*, the examination of sputum (mucus) under a microscope while searching for malignant or cancerous cells.[13] The patient is asked to cough forcefully into a cup—a required procedure because sputum is different from saliva. Sputum contains cells that line the respiratory passages, which in turn may carry some indication of lung cancer. Because it has been proven to be an unreliable method—since screening an *asymptomatic* (showing no symptoms) smoker does not necessarily mean that he or she is free of lung cancer—this is usually reserved for *symptomatic* (showing symptoms) patients.[14] There is a way to increase this method's accuracy, that is, collecting sputum samples over several days or in different parts of the day (morning, afternoon, or evening), but specimens from the early morning are most preferred. How adequate a specimen proves to be is dictated by how many pulmonary macrophages are found in the sputum.[15]

A macrophage is a white blood cell within tissues that is produced by the division of monocytes (a type of white blood cell).[16] The sensitivity of sputum cytology when used for diagnosing lung cancer increases with the number of samples taken from 42 percent with a single sample to 91 percent with five samples, and the positive predictive value is 100 percent, while the negative is only 15 percent.[17] Negative sputum results, however, don't guarantee the absence of lung cell malignancy, especially if the test is performed on patients suspected of being afflicted with lung cancer. The location of the lung cancer also plays a large role in determining the results of the test. If a malignant tumor is in the center of the lungs, the percentages vary between 46 and 77 percent but between 31 and 47 percent if it is in the periphery of the lungs.[18] In the end, this method is usually reserved for patients who have already shown some symptoms.

Blood Tests

A blood test is a laboratory analysis performed on a blood sample that is most often extracted from a vein in the arm using a needle, but a finger prick works equally as well. Because blood acts as "carrier" of waste products back to the excretory system for disposal, drawing a sample from a vein can provide much important information about its contents.[19] The bloodstream is affected by many medical conditions, so a blood test is the most common test to detect such conditions.

Proving its validity and high degree of success in detecting non–small cell lung cancer (the most common lung cancer) is a blood test that researchers at Kansas State University have developed. In less than an hour, the test can show results before the onset of symptoms (coughing and weight loss).[20] Symptoms usually manifest themselves in stage 2 of development, which is not necessarily too late for a relatively easy treatment. The researchers say that people who are currently listed as at risk for cancer, such as heavy smokers or people who have a family history of lung cancer, should have this test done to alleviate any doubt that lung cancer is developing.[21] They say that these at-risk people should visit their physicians and take this quick and simple test, which will be enough of an early indication of whether a cancer is developing. After a few such tests, and if cancer is confirmed, diagnostic imaging will begin. If the cancer is discovered at such an early stage, it will also be easier to treat.

A study was conducted that included 12 people with lung cancer between the ages of 27 and 63 and 12 cancer-free individuals who acted as a control group.[22] A blood sample was extracted from each of them and was then examined and tested three times before any conclusion was made. The test works by detecting enzyme activity in the body. Each type of cancer produces a specific enzyme pattern, also known as an enzyme signature, that can be identified by doctors. The enzymes are detected with the help of *iron nanoparticles* (tiny specks of iron) coated with amino acids and a dye. The nanoparticles are introduced to small amounts of blood or urine from the patient. The amino acids and dye have the properties of interacting with the enzymes in those blood or urine samples. The enzyme patterns help identify if there are other problems, such as lung inflammation from too much tobacco smoke or a lung infection, or if there is an even more serious underlying problem, such as end-stage cancer. Having a false-positive result for lung cancer is potentially dangerous from a financial standpoint and the amount of mental stress it can cause.

When all the testing was complete and conclusions were drawn from the study, there was a 95 percent success rate in diagnosing patients with first- and second-stage lung cancer, which proved to be the first step into a new arena of lung cancer diagnostics and early detection.[23]

Breath Analysis

Breath analysis focuses on detecting the presence of volatile organic compounds in the lungs of patients.[24] After the test has been completed, the data are compared to the results gathered from control subjects who are not afflicted with lung cancer. This is done by using *gas chromatography-mass spectrometry*, but the systems that allow for such tests to be performed are expensive, and medical personnel need to be specially trained to both use them and interpret the results in the end.[25] Other medical sensors can also be used for breath analysis that are much simpler, meaning that they are also much easier to use and more appropriate for the screening of a large patient population.

X-Ray

Some screening methods can be applied to *initially* identify the problem if cancer is suspected. *Chest radiography* or a chest X-ray is one of the first investigative steps taken after a patient has reported symptoms suggesting lung cancer.[26] The chest X-ray is a type of radiography that uses X-rays to screen for conditions that affect the chest area and nearby structures. X-rays are waves of electromagnetic radiation with short wavelengths and are comprised of photons. When passing through solid matter, the photons hit the atoms of the matter (in this case the human body and, more specifically, the lungs) and, depending on the matter's density, are absorbed or weakened.

The remaining rays that have passed through the matter freely are captured by a detector behind the object, after which a two-dimensional film is produced showing an image of the irradiated area.[27] Through this process, lung cancer can be seen as a solitary pulmonary nodule when it is in an early stage. However, this is not a sure sign that the node is cancerous because tuberculosis, fungal infections, organizing pneumonia, and many other diseases may have the same appearance on film when examined. Hence, further investigation is required to arrive at a definite conclusion.[28]

Computed Tomographic Scans

No matter what type of screening machine is used, the aim is always the same: to look for *pulmonary* (relating to the lungs) *nodules*, among others. The computed tomographic (CT) scan is a three-dimensional X-ray. The CT scanner is a machine that consists of a table for the patient to lie on along with a series of X-ray tubes that rotate around the patient to provide the three-dimensional image.[29] Each rotation of the tubes produces a cross-sectional image of the afflicted area (the lungs in this case), and after enough images have been collected, a three-dimensional image is constructed using digital geometry processing. After the scanning is complete and the image has been compiled, the pulmonary node, if there is one, glows as a white dot on the lungs.[30] This can help health care professionals identify the cause of the nodule and determine its malignance to see if it is cancer or some other formation.

Another screening procedure is a low-dose helical (spiral) CT scan. Helical CT scanning is a type of three-dimensional tomography in which the source of the X-rays and the detectors are mounted on a rotating gantry while the patient is moved back and forth at a uniform rate.[31] Until the 1990s, CT scanning was not considered a viable option for diagnosing lung cancer because the dose of radiation it delivered to the patient's body was too high (roughly 50 times more than the dose from an X-ray) to be used on an asymptomatic individual. This changed with the introduction of the low-dose helical CT, which was first mentioned in a study undertaken in 1990.[32] This method allowed for the images created by the CT scan to be at a resolution high enough for the physician to recognize lung nodules while irradiating the patient with a much smaller dose of radiation (approximately only five times that of a regular X-ray) than that of a regular CT, minimizing the patient's exposure to radiation and possible complications. [33]

A study launched by the National Cancer Institute reiterated the validity of low-dose helical CT. [34] Scientists compared the effects of the helical CT and standard chest X-ray and also conducted a nationwide trial of more than 53,000 heavy smokers between the ages of 55 and 74 who were randomly separated to receive either a normal X-ray or a low-dose helical CT. The experiment started in August 2002 and continued for several years. Participants were required to have a smoking history of at least 30 pack-years and to be either current or former smokers without any symptoms or history of lung cancer (a pack-year is the number of packs of cigarettes smoked per day multiplied by the number of years a person has smoked). The trial participants underwent screening tests with either the low-dose helical CT or the X-ray and were then assigned to two other annual screenings with the method they were administered the first time—once at the end of the first year and then again at the end of the second year of their participation in the trial. The study volunteers were then followed up for another five years, and each death was documented and examined, with special care and attention being given to the cause and whether it was lung cancer. After the trial was concluded, the results seemed to be more in favor of CT scans: there were a total of 354 deaths from lung cancer among the participants who were administered the CT scanning, while there were 442 deaths from lung cancer among the participants who had undergone the X-ray testing. [35] This showed a 20 percent difference between the two and showed that the low-dose helical CT is more reliable and beneficial to the general public and the battle against lung cancer. However, the trial investigators still insist that the single best way to prevent lung cancer death is to never smoke or to quit permanently if already smoking.

There are, however, some disadvantages of helical CT. [36] The cumulative effects of radiation from multiple CT scans can be harmful to the lung cancer sufferer's body. In addition, surgical or medical complications may occur with patients who have been proven not to have lung cancer but who demand additional testing through other diagnostic methods. The screening process itself can generate some findings that are not necessarily signs of cancer but that in turn cause unneeded anxiety, stress, and expense. In the end, one must look at the pros and cons of this screening procedure and decide if the advantages of significantly reducing mortality in lung cancer patients are worth dismissing because of minor flaws.

Magnetic Resonance Imaging

Magnetic resonance imaging (MRI) is another test that can be used to diagnose cancerous growths, using magnetism to reveal a picture of the inside of the body.[37] Although the MRI machine is noisy (it thumps and hums loudly), an MRI is painless and relatively safe. The patient is asked to fill in a checklist before undergoing a scan since some people cannot have an MRI, and the checklist ensures that no mistakes are made. Since the MRI uses magnetism, the checklist also ensures that patients do not have surgical clips, metal pins or plates, pacemakers, or any sort of piercing, as these can cause great discomfort or even severe damage if worn during an MRI.[38] Typically, a dye injection is given to the lung cancer sufferer beforehand so that the scanning will be more accurate. Some allergic reactions are possible because of the dye but are rare. Claustrophobia can also be an issue during an MRI because one is confined in a tight space inside the machine. The attending radiographers should be informed before the scanning day so that the patient may be given medication or a sedative to help with anxiety during testing.[39] Complete stillness is required during the MRI because any movements make the image less clear and may lead to problems in the final diagnosis.

The MRI machine is a long, large cylinder with a table that slides in and out of it. The scanning is done inside the machine. Since it uses a powerful magnet, the machine is completely radiation-free as well.[40] Once the patient is inside the scanner, the radiographer retreats to the observation room, and the scanning begins, taking anywhere from half an hour to an hour and a half. Because the machine is so noisy, some form of ear protection may be offered as well. This type of scanning is especially helpful in identifying lung cancer and is better than a CT scan since it produces clearer images. When the scanning is complete, the results are available after several weeks.[41]

Ultrasound

Medical sonography or *ultrasound* is a sound wave–based diagnostic medical imaging technique that is used to visualize various muscles, tendons, and internal organs of the body. It easily captures their size and structure and even identifies if any lesions exist.[42] This method's advantages, when compared to MRI or CT scanning, are that it is relatively inexpensive, it is portable, and it does not utilize any form of harmful mutagenic radiation; nor does it cause discomfort and anxiousness like the MRI machine does.

There are two potentially harmful physiological effects of ultrasound: it can enhance the inflammatory response in some lung cancer patients, and it can also heat soft tissue. Since ultrasound uses energy that can send mechanical pressure waves through soft tissue, it can cause molecular friction and heating of the cells, forming microscopic bubbles in the cell tissue and distorting the cell membrane.[43] Fortunately, this effect is usually minor because normal tissue *perfusion* (blood flow) dissipates most of the heat. With its high intensity, ultrasound can cause small pockets of gas to form in liquids or in tissues in the body that then contract or collapse. This is known as *cavitation*, but it is not known to be an issue at the diagnostic power levels used by ultrasound in the equipment that is used today.[44]

One use of ultrasound is determining the stage of lung cancer. This procedure, called *endobronchial ultrasound-guided transbronchial needle aspiration* (EBUS TBNA),[45] is similar to that of transbronchial biopsy described earlier: a tube, the bronchoscope, is inserted into the patient's large airways, but instead of extracting a piece of tissue right away, a probe is used to send sound waves through the surrounding areas, including the lungs and the *mediastinum* (the area of the chest between the lungs).[46] If any abnormal areas are located, a small grasping needle guided by the ultrasound takes a sample of the tissue, and the diagnostic process begins anew from there. Such a procedure is usually recommended to identify the stage of lung cancer or to either confirm or deny the malignancy of a pulmonary nodule in the lungs. It is also a less invasive method than, for example, an open lung biopsy, which is much more risky since it is a major operation.[47] EBUS TBNA can also spare the patient from undergoing the surgical removal of the cancerous growth since that may include removing surrounding lung

tissue when another method of cancer management, such as chemotherapy or radiation, is unavailable.

Thoracentesis

Thoracentesis is done to provide relief from symptoms, obtain specimens for analysis, and alleviate dyspnea and respiratory compromise
from pleural effusion (chapter 12) that could arise from lung cancer.
Often, a chest tube attached to a water-seal drain is inserted with or
without suction to remove fluid from the lung and allow its reexpansion.
However, if the underlying cause of the effusion is a malignancy, there
is a greater possibility of reoccurrence within days or weeks of effusion,
resulting in the need for repeated thoracentesis. This may cause pain
and imbalances in fluids and electrolytes and may increase the possibility of air entering the pleural space of the patient. To solve this dilem-
ma, *pleurodosis* can be performed to seal off the pleural space and
prevent reaccumulation of fluid. Talc or bleomycin, a chemically irritat-
ing agents, is instilled into the pleural space via chest tube or thora-
scope. Repositioning after instillation is done to promote uniform distribution of the agent. Surgical pleurectomy to remove the neoplasm or
implantation of a *pleuroperitoneal shunt* (a catheter that transfers fluid
from the chest to the abdominal area) may be done as well.[48]

Biopsy

Biopsy is an invasive diagnostic test that is performed by a surgeon. It is
a small operation that aims to remove a small bit of tissue from the area
of the body that is considered afflicted, in this case the lungs.[49] After a
tissue sample has been collected, it is examined by a *pathologist* (a
doctor who specializes in disease) to determine whether the extracted
sample has cancer cells present. If so, the pathologist can look at the
cancer's characteristics and file a detailed report of the findings. Biopsy
is a simple procedure and is very accurate.

The diagnostic accuracy of biopsy for respiratory cancers is supported by a study that was undertaken at the Western General Hospital
of Edinburgh in 1993.[50] The study involved several bronchial biopsy
specimens that showed positive results for lung cancer. These specimens were circulated among five experienced pathologists who wanted

to be more involved in lung cancer research. Each of them had to investigate all the specimens, note their conclusions, and conclude with a diagnosis. Then the specimens were compared to the biopsy extracts from which they originated, and the results were promising: for squamous cell carcinoma (cancer), the diagnostic accuracy was 75 percent, small cell carcinoma showed a 66 percent diagnostic accuracy, and adenocarcinoma showed a 50 percent diagnostic accuracy.[51] To further improve diagnostic accuracy, the *non–small cell, not-specified* classification category was introduced. Non–small cell carcinoma is a group of lung cancers that includes squamous cell carcinoma, large cell carcinoma, and adenocarcinoma, which are the most common types of lung cancer. Small cell carcinoma is an aggressive, fast-growing lung cancer that, when looked at under a microscope, has cells with an oval shape and the ability to spread to other parts of the body. The study mentioned above had less than a 10 percent chance of confusing small cell and non–small cell carcinoma, and the introduction of the non–small cell, not-specified category improved diagnostic accuracy by 10 to 15 percent.[52]

Several types of biopsy can be used to remove a piece from the afflicted lung tissue: transbronchial biopsy, needle biopsy, thoracoscopic biopsy, and open biopsy.[53]

Transbronchial Biopsy

Transbronchial biopsy is a type of biopsy that involves a long, thin tube with a close-focusing telescope at the end called a *fiber-optic bronchoscope*. A bronchoscope is a device that is used to see inside the lungs. It is inserted into the main airways through either the mouth or the nose and into the windpipe (trachea) and finally into the air passages of the lungs (bronchi). While the tissue sample is taken, the patient is asked to breathe out slowly.[54] After the tissue sample has been collected, it is given to a pathologist who examines it under a microscope, looking for any cancerous cells. Transbronchial biopsy can be considered a small procedure that is accurate to a certain limit.[55]

Needle Biopsy

Needle biopsy is one of the more commonly used biopsy methods for obtaining a tissue sample from the lungs in the case of lung cancer (and from the body in general). It includes a needle that is guided through the chest wall into the area that is suspected to contain the cancerous growth and is guided by CT. It also includes local anesthesia because the needle is large, and the procedure would otherwise be very painful.[56]

Thoracoscopic Biopsy

Thoracoscopic biopsy is similar to transbronchial biopsy in the sense that both utilize tools with flexible tubes. The main difference, however, is that unlike transbronchial biopsy, thoracoscopic biopsy is performed through the chest wall, giving more direct access to the lungs and bypassing the need for going through the trachea; this means that doctors can reach the afflicted place directly.[57] The device used for this is called an *endoscope,* and it is inserted through an incision in the chest wall, between the ribs, inside the chest cavity, and then into the lungs. This procedure is also called *video-assisted thoracoscopic surgery* since it is most commonly performed with the help of ultrasound and allows doctors to take a closer look at the suspected nodule. Like the other types of biopsy, it is also capable of obtaining a sample from the previously mentioned nodule itself.[58]

Open Lung Biopsy

This is the most invasive type of lung biopsy since it includes general anesthesia and involves a major surgical operation.[59] This method is performed less today because it poses the greatest amount of risk to the patient (e.g., blood loss and infection). However, open biopsy is still the standard by which all other biopsies are compared because the contact with the suspected pulmonary nodule is the most direct. Since this is a major surgical procedure, it requires a hospital stay and recovery time.[60] It is usually used only when other types of biopsy have failed to obtain a tissue sample or a larger sample is required. The open lung biopsy may require the surgeon to separate the ribs or even remove a portion of the rib to gain access to the lung itself. A tube is placed in the chest and lung to remove air and fluid postoperatively to avoid any complications that may subsequently occur. After the sample is obtained, the wound is closed with stitches, and after several days of recovery, the patient can be moved back to a hospital room.[61]

MORE ON SCREENING AND DIAGNOSTICS OF LUNG CANCER

The results of randomized trials that were published 20 years ago showed no significant reduction in deaths from lung cancer using screening that involved chest radiography in a combination of *cytologic* (cell) analysis of sputum. Methodological limitations in the studies, such as the frequent use of chest radiography in the control group as well as experimental groups' failure to comply with their prescriptions, may have been the reason for negative outcomes of these results.[62]

More recently, the early detection of lung cancer with high-resolution CT has revived interest in lung cancer screening.[63] Numerous CT screening studies have been conducted on individuals subject to higher lung cancer risk, including current and former smokers. Overall, baseline scans resulted in detecting 55 to 85 percent of cancers in stage 1. During annual follow-up scans, 60 to 100 percent of detected cancers are in stage 1. In contrast, routine clinical care in the United States resulted in diagnosing only 16 percent of cancers in stage 1.[64]

It is considered that stage 1 lung cancer has a 100 percent cure rate if the malignant cells are completely eradicated. The possible benefits of lung cancer screening must be weighed against the potential harm. Lung cancers can appear on spiral CT scans as *noncalcified (softer) nodules*, but screening leads to the detection of large amounts of noncalcified nodules, few of which are fully diagnosed lung cancers. Screening may expose people who do not have lung cancer to risks that include concern over probable abnormal findings, procedural complications, and substantial costs. CT screening may result in undertaking diagnostic procedures, including invasive surgery. The consequent morbidity and mortality might undermine the valuable effect of early-stage cancer diagnostics.[65]

Benefits and Risks of Lung Cancer Screening

A popular method of early lung cancer diagnosis, CT screening still raises questions over its positive effect on mortality rates and the patient's condition as a whole. International organizations involved in producing medical technology or manufacturing pharmaceuticals make continuous efforts in providing substantial evidence for or against the use of CT screening for secondary lung cancer prevention. Another strategy is to further evaluate suspicious formations using positron-emission tomography. Alternatively, for patients who screen positive for cancer with CT, *transthoracic needle biopsy* could be done as well. As a result of such a procedure, severely invasive surgery should be prescribed only in cases of confirmed lung cancer.[66] The benefits and risks of transthoracic needle biopsy as a screening method should be further compared to positron-emission tomography scanning; diagnostic costs and unavailability may add to limitations that could be alleviated by the support of corporations and government institutions (chapter 19).

Technical Advances in Lung Cancer Screening

The biotechnology industry, whether motivated by the population's health or by profit alone, are continuously investing in developing its lung cancer diagnostic products. Even the best evaluation of scanning methods may be complicated by the rapidly changing technology in this area.[67] A decade ago, a typical *single-detector CT* scanner provided 10-mm-thick "slices" of images in several minutes while the breathing motions of the chest compromised the image resolution. After years of refinement in multidetector CT scanners, the 64-row scanners of today can create an entire thoracic (chest) image with a 0.625-mm-thick slice in less than three seconds. These thinner slices enable better characterization of nodules and increase the ability to detect cases of central airway cancer.[68]

Nevertheless, data from clinical investigations fail to present solid, 100 percent evidence in support of using CT screening as the definitive screening process for lung cancer. According to the American Cancer Society, CT screening should not be performed in the event the person in question is not at risk in any way. Taking into account that many heavy smokers, past and present, are making their own decision to undergo screening, the American Cancer Society recommends that such people first discuss their decision with their physicians. Such screening manipulations should be done only in medical centers that employ multidisciplinary teams of specialists experienced in diagnosing and treating lung cancer. During such screening discussions with their patients, physicians are advised to explain to the patient the positive and negative outcomes, stressing the fact that no studies show that screening helps people live longer and pointing out that it is common to receive false-positive test results, which may cause unnecessary worry, medical procedures, and even surgery.

It is vital to note that lung cancer is one of the most elusive and difficult cancers to deal with, and because of that, diagnosing and detecting it early is of the utmost importance. This can be done in various ways, some involving more invasive methods than others. This is why patients should ask their attending physicians which one is best suited for them. The most certain way to diagnose lung cancer before it has had the time to develop and complicate treatment is for the patient to be aware of his or her physical condition and report any suspicious symptoms to a qualified caregiver.

8

OUTPATIENT AND INPATIENT EXPERIENCES

When attempting to gain an introductory understanding of a disease process such as lung cancer, it is important to differentiate between outpatient and inpatient management. Outpatients are those patients who are not hospitalized overnight but do visit hospitals, clinics, or other facilities to get treatment. Inpatients are those lung cancer patients who receive lodging and food in a health facility along with their treatment. Both types of treatment have some advantages and disadvantages. Being with one's family at home can be comforting for some patients, while for some, being in safe surroundings with doctors and other medical staff always close by can be a better option. In both instances, the stage of cancer may determine the level of care required.

INTERNISTS, FAMILY PHYSICIANS, AND ONCOLOGISTS

A plethora of caregivers, both formal and informal, are involved in treating a patient who is suffering from lung cancer. Family members, various doctors, nurses, social workers, friends, religious leaders, and others may all participate. The main task of professional caregivers is to help patients feel better, offer them support or guidance, and help them to maintain their health and comfort at various stages. Cancer patients are seen by a variety of physicians involved in different processes and stages and during different treatment phases. They include (1) oncologists, who diagnose and monitor the patient's physical health; (2) internists, who perform many tests for the patient; (3) anesthesiologists, who administrate anesthesia before surgery; and (4) other specialists who try to help the patient get better in different ways.

Internists

Physicians of internal medicine are experts who diagnose, treat, and take care of adults; the care they provide ranges from general health to complex illnesses. They observe a potential lung cancer patient's state from the start and are very often called in by other specialists to give them advice and consult them when solving a medical issue. It can be said that an internist cares for the "whole" patient. No matter how small a medical problem is or how common or rare it is, the internist's primary occupation is to prevent and diagnose diseases and cure the patient if possible.[1]

Alongside general internists, there is a subspecialty of internal medicine that is important when it comes to patients suffering from lung cancer. Internists with that subspecialty are pulmonologists. They are concerned with any disease related to the lungs and bronchial tubes, such as asthma, tuberculosis, emphysema, and lung cancer.[2] Pulmonologists help diagnose lung cancer and can provide treatment plans. They are also called pulmonary specialists.[3]

Family Physicians

Doctors who are usually the first to notice lung cancer symptoms are family physicians. They know their patients, take care of their health, and send them to have additional tests done to confirm a potential illness. They also monitor their treatment, help them get through it, and supervise their state after a surgery, chemotherapy, or other medical course. Family physicians usually try to be as involved as possible when it comes to treating their patients, especially if the disease in question is as serious as lung cancer. They can schedule meetings with patients or their family to update them on the results of treatments or surgery. They usually do not get *directly* involved in cancer treatments themselves but can suggest actions or offer advice to patients as well as other doctors. Family physicians provide a detailed medical history of a patient, including prior examinations and blood tests and other potentially relevant information that may help diagnose and determine treatment for lung cancer patients. When a person is suspected of having lung cancer, the family physician sends him or her to specialists for additional tests and treatment.

Patients with insurance can usually choose which doctor they will see from a list of providers during their follow-up, and many choose their family physicians. Many patients regularly see their family physicians during the treatment, but most usually do so afterward during recuperation. It is important to emphasize that those visits are informational.[4] In this way, the family physician can keep up with the patient's state before and after the treatment, and the patient can talk with someone who not only knows cancer and is a professional health care provider but also is a person they have known for a while and trust.

Oncologists

Oncologists are medical doctors who deal with patients suffering from various forms of cancers. They identify malignancies, counsel patients, investigate symptoms and syndromes, and provide treatment with the potential for cure. They (1) explain the disease and stages of the disease to a patient, (2) discuss various treatment options with him or her, (3) offer the best course of treatment, (4) deliver the best possible care, and (5) improve the quality of life. Oncologists must be aware of the medical history of the patient's entire family since some people can be genetically predisposed to cancer, and that history can be crucial in managing patient care.[5]

The three basic types of oncologists are radiation, medical, and surgical. A medical oncologist specializes in chemotherapy cancer treatments. In chemotherapy, drugs are used to exterminate cancer cells. A surgical oncologist is a specialist in the surgical aspects of cancer and performs biopsies, or the removal of a small amount of suspicious tissue for closer inspection under a microscope and the surgical removal of cancer, the surrounding tissue, and, sometimes, nearby lymph nodes, which are small, bean-shaped structures that help deter illness. A radiation oncologist tries to treat cancer with radiation therapy by using high-energy X-rays to destroy lung cancer cells. Other types of oncologists are gynecological and pediatric oncologists. Gynecological oncologists treat gynecological cancers, while pediatric oncologists treat children who are afflicted with cancer.[6]

Another important doctor who can help a lung cancer patient in both inpatient and outpatient settings is a thoracic surgeon.[7] He or she performs surgery in the chest area, such as the heart, lungs, esophagus, or other organs. Some surgical procedures performed by the thoracic surgeon are the following:

- *Bronchoscopy*. Inserting a tube through the nose and into the lungs; needles can also be inserted to obtain biopsy samples.
- *Mediastinoscopy*. Biopsy of the area behind the breastbone for microscopic examination.
- *Posterolateral thoracotomy*. Incision of the chest through which a doctor can reach the lungs or any other relevant organ.
- *Muscle-sparing incision*. A less invasive surgical procedure where a doctor makes small incisions. This does not require cutting the chest muscles.[8]

QUESTIONS FOR PRE- AND POSTSURGERY

Patients affected with lung cancer, especially at the point when they just learn that they have fallen ill, can be confused and discouraged. They often cannot imagine what is going on and are oblivious to some important facts. It is crucial for them to gather as much professional information and advice as possible so that they can confidently approach their disease and treatment. The following are some important questions they should ask before and after the surgery.

Before the Surgery

First, patients should ask the doctor to explain the procedure in simple terms and tell them how they should prepare for the surgery. Since most patients are not medical professionals themselves, there is a strong likelihood they do not know the physiological details of lung cancer. They may not understand all the medical vocabulary, so it is helpful for doctors to explain preparations and procedures in plain, simple terms. It is also vital to know how long the surgery will take, the length of the hospital stay, and whether they will need any assistance when released from hospital care. It is sometimes hard to determine how long a procedure could take, as this varies from patient to patient, depending on his or her overall state of health and the state of the malignant lung cells.

Other important questions to ask concern the portion of lung that will be extricated from the patient's body, and patients should inquire about the risks and benefits of that surgery as well as whether drains, catheters, or intravenous lines will be necessary. *Drip*, or slowly infusing a liquid into the patient one drop at a time, will probably be discontinued as soon as the patient can eat and drink normally. This happens after a couple of days. Drains will be taken out after a week because the fluid from the wound should stop draining around that time.

Should there be a need for a blood transfusion, lung cancer patients can ask if the hospital can store their own blood before the surgery and use that instead of someone else's. It could also be helpful to know if there are any types of treatment that could shrink the tumor before the surgery. Tumor shrinking is usually done by radiation therapy. In general, it can be done before and after the surgery, but if it is done prior and if the patient can endure the surgery, the operation will run more easily and safely with the possibility of better results.

It also essential to investigate whether there are any alternatives to the surgery. One such alternative is *stereotactic body radio-surgery*, a new technology that precisely delivers high doses of radiation to tumors. This method has produced high rates of success. It is performed on patients who are too weak to have conventional surgery, usually the elderly, those with severe lung disease, and others with generally poor health.[9]

Some alternative methods, such as acupuncture, hypnosis, massage therapy, and meditation, may not kill off the disease but can be effective in treating some symptoms, such as anxiety, fatigue, pain, nausea, and shortness of breath. Massage therapy, both an inpatient and an outpatient procedure depending on the clinic, has been found to be helpful for anxiety and pain, as has acupuncture for shortness of breath, nausea, fatigue, and pain.[10]

The type of help needed after lung cancer surgery is also something to ask the doctor about. Nurses and *physiotherapists* (movement and function specialists) will get the patient moving as soon as possible. At first, patients will likely need help moving around. They will also do some breathing and leg exercises with their nurses and physiotherapists to prevent complications, such as blood clots in the legs or chest. Lung cancer sufferers are ready to go home a few week after the surgery, if not earlier, depending on what the surgeon recommends. If patients live alone, they will have a hard time managing everything by themselves. In this case, it is good to make plans with nurses to have them transported home and to have someone check on and help them when needed.

After Surgery

The first thing that comes to mind following surgery is the amount of time the patient will have to stay in the hospital. That depends on the success of the procedure and the patient's overall state of health. The outpatient should ask the physician how long it will take to resume normal activities, such as work, school, gardening, or others. The lung cancer patient who has just undergone surgery should also be careful while driving. Anesthesia and painkillers need to wear off, and the wounds must be healed as well. Seat belts can press on the wound and make it sore. It usually takes about four to six weeks before a patient can drive.

Individuals suffering from lung cancer should also ask about outpatient treatments needed after the surgery and how long they should wait before they can take any other necessary medication.[11] They should ask doctors about the types of painkillers they can take to minimize the pain after the surgery. It is important to take painkillers regularly and in the recommended doses. It sometimes happens that the pain starts weeks or even months after the surgery. This happens because nerve endings that were damaged during the operation have started to grow back. This pain will end when the nerve endings fully recover, and that can take some time.[12]

QUESTIONS FROM DOCTOR TO PATIENT

Doctors need to know the entire medical history of their patients and ask them about any allergies and relevant medical problems so the surgery will be as routine as possible. They also ask about symptoms and their manifestation and medication or treatment received before their first meeting with the patient. Formal caregivers such as physicians have many sessions with the patient where they perform various assessments to prepare the patient for lung cancer surgery. If a doctor asks the right questions, he or she can provide needed therapy or surgery and help that patient get better.

HOSPITAL CARE AND LUNG CANCER

Well-established hospitals have special programs to help patients suffering from lung cancer. They employ a highly professional medical staff and provide high-quality treatments with the best technology available. Those hospitals offer comprehensive care, meaning that they have all the doctors needed on their staff so that the patient need not go to multiple locations to get a diagnosis or treatment. They also offer palliative care specialists who take care of the patient's physical and psychological problems during and after the treatment.

If a hospital has a large number of patients, it might also be in a better financial position; therefore, it can afford the latest technology and do proper research. Such hospitals might have fewer complications during surgeries than might outpatient clinics. It is also possible that such hospitals provide support groups for patients, specifically lung cancer patients. Some hospitals may offer programs that other clinics lack. For example, some clinical trials for lung cancer (chapter 15) may be available in certain institutions but nonexistent in others. Some hospitals even offer alternative treatments, such as acupuncture and massage therapy.[13]

Quality of Hospital Care versus Outcome of Treatment

In general, hospitals that offer more lung cancer treatment options usually have better outcomes than those that offer fewer because they usually are financial stable and can afford more highly qualified and experienced staff.[14] With the different programs and features it offers, a prestigious hospital makes patients feel as comfortable as possible while providing additional venues, such as support groups and alternative treatments. For a patient who suffers from such a terrible disorder as lung cancer, a quality hospital may be a lifesaver.

III

Many Faces of Lung Cancer

9

SQUAMOUS CELL CARCINOMAS AND BRONCHIOALVEOLAR CARCINOMAS

Clinics and doctors are trying to find a cure for lung cancer or, at least, a better way to treat it. Understanding the different types of lung cancer helps in this regard. Earlier phases of cancer, whether referring to squamous cell carcinomas of the lung or other variations, are usually treatable, but it all depends on when people are diagnosed. The more in depth the comprehension of the types of cells and tissues that are at stake, the better the outcome of caregiving. This chapter begins part III by examining two classifications of lung cancer.

NON–SMALL CELL LUNG CANCER

This variation of lung cancer includes the *squamous cell carcinoma* subtype. It is the most common, accounting for 85 percent of lung cancer cases, and it can affect both smokers and nonsmokers by way of secondhand smoke.[1] It has four stages, determined on the basis of the size and location of the tumor as well as how far and how much the cancer cells have metastasized. Stage 1 *non–small cell lung cancer* (NSCLC) has a small tumor (less than three centimeters in size) and shows no sign of metastasizing. Stage 2 tumors are more than three centimeters but stay below seven centimeters. Stage 2 NSCLC is also known as *localized carcinoma*. Cancer cells at this stage have *almost* begun invading nearby structures, such as the bronchi, and causing pneumonia due to infection or partial blockage in the lung. As stage 2 of NSCLC is not fully metastatic or malignant, patients do not necessarily have issues of rapid weight loss and deterioration of health. At this phase of lung cancer, symptoms of NSCLC include coughing, minor *hemoptysis* (coughing of blood), achiness in the upper or lower back, and weakness. Stage 3 NSCLC sufferers have large tumors greater than seven centimeters that have spread farther to areas such as the diaphragm muscle and the chest. In stage 4, tumors have "choked" the lungs, heart, esophagus, trachea, and major blood vessels.[2]

A unique, rare cancer stage in NSCLC is called the occult stage. In this stage, no primary tumor exists, and cancer cells are not found by typical cancer detection methods such as scans. The cancer cells are found only in mucus derived from the lungs and the airways.[3] Occult malignant cancer cells are capable of metastasis and are discovered as a result of metastatic tumors.[4]

The survival rate for NSCLC patients varies, depending on how early the cancer is detected and treated. Stage 1 patients have a nearly 70 percent chance of survival, whereas stage 4 patients have less than a 1 percent chance.[5] NSCLC cells develop mostly like the carcinomas explained in chapter 3. NSCLC adenocarcinomas are located on the periphery of the lungs and are often the cause of scarred lung tissue. NSCLC squamous cell carcinomas grow in the center of the lungs, originating in airways such as the bronchus. It is the type of NSCLC tumor most encountered by males who are past or current smokers. Large cell carcinomas are the most potent of the NSCLC tumors and can develop anywhere in the lung.[6]

SQUAMOUS CELL CARCINOMAS

Squamous cell carcinomas affect the flat, even-surfaced cells of the body forming the skin and the linings of the organs. They are the usual culprits in skin cancer, though they also affect other body parts, including the lungs.[7] Squamous cell carcinomas in the lungs often attack the airways, and smokers in particular are susceptible to this type of tumor, as healthy squamous cells normally handle the repair of cells that have been damaged by external factors, such as tobacco.[8] *Basal cell carcinomas* target the first layer of the skin, making them another culprit for skin cancer. *Transitional cell carcinomas* are found in the lower half of the body, targeting the areas responsible for urinary discharge. This includes the bladder, kidneys, and ureter.[9] At times, there can be a mixture of carcinoma types; such is the case with *adenosquamous carcinomas*. These contain elements of both adenocarcinomas and squamous cell carcinomas and are usually malignant.[10]

Squamous cell lung carcinoma is a classification of lung cancer that is formed from reserve cells located around other cells. This type of cancer is replacing already-injured and damaged cells in the lining of the bronchi. Tumors of this type of carcinoma occur in the center of the lung or in one of the main airway branches, where they can form cavities in the lung so that they can grow larger. Less than 30 percent of all lung cancers can spread through the organism to these specific areas— liver, bones, small intestine, adrenal glands, or even the brain. In the advanced stage of lung cancer, there is a small chance that the patient with this type of diagnosis can be cured. If the cancer is diagnosed in the early stage and removed from the patient, there is a 40 percent chance that the patient will have no larger issues in the next five years. Under the age of 30, there is a better chance for survival.[11]

History

This type of cancer was established as a distinct disorder way back in the 1760s after the advent of tobacco smoking. About 50 years later, in 1810, lung cancer was described in different ways. Autopsies made in 1878 revealed a small percentage of malignant tumors, but by 1900 this number began to rise. Physician Fritz Lickint discovered the connection between tobacco smoking and lung cancer. Decades later, in the 1950s in Britain, the first epidemiological evidence about this connection was published. This led to massive antismoking campaigns in Germany, the United States, and Great Britain. The appearance of lung cancer in the form of squamous cells encouraged experts to find a way to treat this kind of disorder. They started with palliative radiotherapy, then radical radiotherapy was discovered, and finally, in the late 1990s, major advances were made in conventional radical radiotherapy for squamous cell lung carcinomas.[12]

Subtypes

Four kinds of squamous cell carcinomas are recognized today:

- Small cell
- Basaloid
- Papillary
- Clear cell

The most potent of types of cancer can generate the *basaloid* form of cancer and poorly differentiated small cell variants. On the other hand, the papillary type usually appears as superficial endobronchial lesions on the skin, which is less severe than basaloid. Currently, little information exists regarding the prognosis and implications of clear cell lung cancer.

Pathological Squamous Cell Carcinoma Characteristics

Skin color is a significant factor for suffering from squamous cell carcinoma. Fair-skinned and light-complexioned populations are a vulnerable group, as they have the greatest chance of developing this disorder. However, dark-skinned individuals are not immune to squamous cell carcinoma. Tobacco smoking increases the chances of developing squamous cell carcinoma regardless of skin color. Today, people are fond of spending time on the beach. Lack of cautionary information in this regard can be dangerous because longtime exposure to the sun can be a crucial factor in developing squamous cell cancer. This can happen on the certain areas on the body that were burned or exposed to certain types of radiation or chemicals, especially on the nose, neck, arms, shoulders, and other areas that were not even exposed to the sun. [13]

Early manifestations of squamous cell carcinoma can be seen on the skin and might look similar to regular skin damage but in some cases can turn into severe squamous cell carcinoma. Small pink or brown patches appear on the external part of the skin; the medical name for this is *actinic keratosis*. The main symptom that will arise when squamous cell carcinoma has not yet metastasized to other areas of the body is the lesion. In the beginning, such lesions look similar to crusty lesions that are flat; afterward, they become wart-like. In the mouth, they look like wide patches of ulcerations. A horn-like projection can grow out of the lesion regardless of the part of the body the lesion is on or what caused it. Squamous cell carcinoma expands slowly, but chances are high that it will metastasize to the other areas. If there is an early diagnosis of lung cancer, survival rates for squamous cell carcinoma are great.[14]

Staging for Squamous Cell Carcinomas

Modern technology gives people an opportunity to discover this illness in time. Cancer, whether squamous cell lung carcinoma or another form, is a dangerous disease process that poses roadblocks to scientists who are attempting to find an absolute cure for cell malignancy. Proper staging protocols are necessary to evaluate how far the malignant cells have spread and how much a specific tumor has grown. Certain instruments, such as X-ray, positron-emission tomography, biopsies, and physical exams, have crucial roles to play in identifying the stage of squamous cell lung carcinoma in a patient. These imaging tests provide both patient and caregiver with a current understanding of where the stagewise cancerous growth may be. However, noticing the cancer in one region of the body does not confirm that it will remain only in that spot forever. That is why a complete body scan is recommended for full protective screening of the individual suspected of having squamous cell lung carcinoma regardless of the stage the cancer is in.

Modern science utilizes the tumor-node-metastasis (TNM) classification of malignant tumors to rate the growth of squamous cell lung carcinoma. The "T" signifies the size of the tumor and whether it is growing, the "N" represents how much the cancer has spread into the lymph nodes, and the "M" stands for whether the cancer has advanced from the lungs to other organs.

Types of treatment for squamous cell carcinoma include chemotherapy drugs and lasers that are used to treat lip cancers. If the cancer is deep inside an area other than the face, *cryotherapy* (a freezing technique) is an effective solution. Deep cancer might be cut out of the skin. For very deep or larger squamous cell carcinomas, radiation might be used. *Mohs surgery* is a technique used for removing cancer cells layer by layer and looking at each layer under a microscope until the cancer cells have been completely removed.

Squamous Cell Screening Techniques

Specific screening techniques for squamous cell lung carcinomata are used for early-stage lung cancer, when tumorous growths are more likely to be stopped. Screening tests have been carried out on smokers and those in in professions in which exposure to harmful substances is an issue. Chest radiography and sputum examinations are not as effective finding squamous cell lung cancer in preliminary screenings. Although detecting tumors in the earlier stage does not *always* mean that survival rates will be improved, some research has shown that the earlier the tumor is noticed, the better the chances the patient will survive.[15]

Another technology, computed tomography (CT) (chapter 7), can uncover tumors that are still not completely visible on X-ray. CT is used as a screening tool to locate squamous cell carcinomas located in the lungs of high-risk patients. Discovering such cancer at a later stage decreases the chances of survival, the problem here being that CT can discover lung cancer only in the early stages of cell malignancy. CT does not provide any benefit in terms of mortality from squamous cell carcinoma. The will to find a cure for this kind of disease process is ubiquitous, so in 2002 the National Cancer Institute sponsored a research protocol to compare the effectiveness of CT and X-ray scans.[16]

Squamous Cell Carcinoma: State of Research

It can be concluded that squamous cell carcinoma is a dangerous disease process, so research must continue at the clinical level. So far, research clinics and scientists around the world are making some progress addressing the issues of squamous cell carcinoma or are devising the necessary medications. Such research can show only how to *prevent* squamous cell carcinoma of the lungs, not completely cure *all* individuals suffering from lung cancer. Currently, medical centers are making good progress in prevention, early detection, and treatment that can save many lives. Modern research techniques are currently looking for ways to uncover specific DNA changes that affect lung cancer cells. This may lead to detecting squamous cell carcinoma at an earlier stage.

BRONCHIOALVEOLAR CARCINOMAS

Introduction

Bronchioalveolar carcinoma (BAC) is a combination of lung cancer arising in the distal bronchioles or alveoli. The first type of BAC was noticed in France in a clinic that boasted a microscopic description of this type of carcinoma. Historically, BAC was classified as a subtype of pulmonary adenocarcinoma by the World Health Organization. As time passed, this disease process was defined as growth of neoplastic cells along preexisting alveolar structures. That definition of BAC was somewhat retained through the WHO 2004 reclassification, which added *adenomatous hyperplasia*. Japanese scientist Masayuki Noguchi and colleagues observed peripheral adenocarcinoma and separated them into the following six subtypes:[17]

- Subtype A: The BAC is located in a small region and has not spread yet.
- Subtype B: The alveoli (described in chapter 2) collapse.
- Subtype C: Active growth and proliferation of the malignant cells.
- Subtype D: Partially but not strongly differentiated adenocarcinoma.
- Subtype E: Tubular (shaped like a tube) adenocarcinoma.
- Subtype F: Papillary (shaped like a nipple) adenocarcinoma.

Approaches for Treating BAC

BAC is a disease process that is still a mystery to health care professionals and scientists conducting advanced research. It is not known how one specifically contracts this type of lung cancer or what to do to completely prevent it. The best approach might be to simply try to live a healthy lifestyle as much as possible. It is important for parents to start educating their children from the earliest age about lung cancer and, later, BAC if this subtype happens to run in the family. If the parents are smokers, they should be careful about smoking in areas where children are playing or completing their homework. Unfortunately, witnessing a mother holding her newborn in one hand and lighting a cigarette in another is all too common. Even though smokers might say that it is really difficult to quit so as to avoid BAC, quitting smoking is possible at the level of the individual.[18]

Age Groups

While BAC occurs more frequently in older age, no one is completely safe, be they children or the elderly. Children are naturally less inclined to suffer from BAC, perhaps because they have not been exposed as much to the basic or advanced causes of lung cancer (chapter 5). The leading factor causing BAC to affect older sufferers is smoking. Older people who are long-term chain smokers are more likely to experience this disorder, and if one quits, the chances will significantly lessen over time. Younger sufferers who are affected by this type of cancer and nonsmokers suffer from a milder version of BAC, while smokers who are senior citizens have a much greater chance of being diagnosed with this cancer.[19]

Male versus Female Susceptibility

There is a major difference between male and female susceptibility to BAC. One factor that may be obvious at first glance besides smoking is *living environment*. By traditional standards (though it may not be the case as much in modern times), women arguably spend more hours in the kitchen than their male counterparts, and with that they are exposed to fumes and pollutants found in the kitchen air while cooking.[20] With men spending more time outside and at work, they are exposed to stress and greater amounts of environmental pollutants. Nonetheless, clinical experimentation confirms that BAC is more common in young female nonsmokers.[21] In some cases, women on birth control pills are slightly more protected, but if they take the pills over a long period of time, the chances are not reduced but rather amplified. This means that hormones influence the susceptibility of women to BAC, depending on the circumstances.[22]

Characteristics of BAC

The WHO argues that there are eight groups of lung cancer overall:

- Carcinoid tumors
- Small cell carcinoma
- Adenosquamous carcinoma
- Large cell carcinoma
- Squamous cell carcinoma
- Sarcomatoid carcinoma
- Salivary gland-like carcinoma of the lung
- Adenocarcinoma

The *carcinoma* category of cancers in general is vast, meaning that lung carcinomas, whether BACs or other lung carcinomas, have unique characteristics. Four categories are specific histological subtypes of BAC: *lung adenocarcinoma, acinar adenocarcinoma, papillary adenocarcinoma*, and *solid adenocarcinoma with mucin production*. There is also a fifth subtype that could pertain to BAC called *adenocarcinoma with mixed subtypes*.[23]

Screening Techniques for BAC

The screening techniques are almost the same for every type of lung cancer. The two most important are CT and X-ray. When one suspects that one has BAC, the first first thing to do is to see a doctor for screening. At the physician's office, the individual will first have blood drawn, and then be evaluated for specific antibodies. The next step might be to have CT or X-ray screening done. The last step in screening is to conduct a biopsy, which is relatively quick. After the tissue is removed, it is processed and placed under a microscope to see if the patient has the distinctive characteristics of BAC. After that, an expert reads the results and relays the good (or bad) news to the patient. If the patient has this type of cancer, the necessary measures are taken. All in all, screening techniques for BAC have many similarities to the ones already explained for squamous cell carcinomas.[24]

State of Research on BAC

Researchers maintain that BAC is not a well-known type of cancer when speaking of the physiological aspects of the disease process. No one is exactly sure why people get BAC, but it is said that cigarettes and genetics are primarily to blame. Lack of government-backed research funds for clinical researchers is posing problems, and research firms are funding BAC studies on their own. It is hoped that sometime in the near future, governments will (1) become more concerned about the spread of individual types of lung cancers such as BAC and (2) offer further financial support for those looking to make serious advancements in the research field.[25]

10

UNDIFFERENTIATED CARCINOMAS AND ADENOCARCINOMAS OF THE LUNG

The term *differentiation* scientifically refers to when cells become specialized in function. When speaking of differentiation of lung cancer cells in general, there are two main classifications: small cell lung carcinoma and non–small cell lung carcinoma. There are three known subtypes of non–small cell lung carcinoma: squamous cell carcinoma, large cell adenocarcinoma, and large cell undifferentiated carcinoma. Two subtypes of non–small cell lung carcinoma—large cell undifferentiated carcinoma and adenocarcinoma—are discussed in this chapter.

LARGE CELL UNDIFFERENTIATED CARCINOMA

Large cell undifferentiated carcinoma (LCUC) is also called *large cell anaplastic carcinoma* or simply *large cell carcinoma*.[1] It accounts for about 10 to 15 percent of all lung cancer patients and is so named because of the large round appearance of the cells.[2] By the time it is diagnosed, the tumor is already large in relation to other, milder tumors. LCUC is defined as a malignant epithelial tumor that has rather large, prominent nuclei and a generally well-defined cell border with the absence of features of squamous cell carcinoma.[3] LCUC usually starts on the periphery of the lungs, making it prone to develop fluid in the spaces of the lungs. It also grows and spreads faster than any other known types of non–small cell lung carcinoma.[4]

LCUC is strongly associated with smoking, but there are also other factors that contribute to the disease process, such as environmental factors (e.g., asbestos, radon, air pollution, secondhand smoke, and industrial chemicals), work-related hazards (e.g., painter, bartender, and metalworker), and hereditary links.[5]

Subtypes of LCUC

LCUC has five subtypes: *large cell neuroendocrine carcinoma of the lung, basiloid carcinoma, lymphoepithelioma-like carcinoma, clear cell carcinoma*, and *large cell carcinoma having the rhabdoid phenotype*.[6]

Large Cell Neuroendocrine Carcinoma of the Lung

The first subtype discussed here is large cell neuroendocrine carcinoma (LCNEC). It is associated with differentiation in terms of its histological features, including *organoid* (like an organ), *trabecular* (projectory) *growth*, or *rosette* (resembling a rose) formations. LCNEC is relatively large and has more cytoplasm, nucleoli, and structures called *vesicular chromatin* on its nucleus. Furthermore, *necrosis* (cell death due to lack of blood supply) is common in LCNEC, which is also highly fatal and has a poor prognosis. Research has been conducted on treatment for this cancer, but because a small number of patients are affected by this, the effective course of treatment is still undetermined.[7]

Basaloid Carcinoma

This is characterized as a solid nodular pattern with necrosis that bears much resemblance to organic features of LCNEC. Both tumors can be seen in the periphery with nodular nests. Lung carcinoma does not show prominent nucleoli all of the time. Basiloid carcinoma is smaller and more *fusiform* (spindle shaped). Moreover, neuroendocrine markers are negative in basiloid carcinoma, and most basiloid carcinomas are determined to be squamous cell carcinoma or the basiloid variant. Only when basiloid carcinoma lacks squamous differentiation does it justify a large cell carcinoma differentiation.[8]

Lymphoepithelioma-Like Carcinoma

Another subtype is *lymphoepithelioma-like carcinoma* (LELC). Unlike other subtypes of large cell carcinoma, LELC is not associated with smoking but is caused by infection with Epstein-Barr virus, which affects primarily the Asian population. It is characterized as large, with vesicular nuclei together with prominent nucleoli and an indistinct cellular border imparting a syncytial growth pattern. Most significant to this diagnosis is *lymphocyte lymphoplasmacystic infiltrate* around tumor nests and intermingled between tumor cells. The inflammatory population is present in both primary and metastatic sites.[9]

Clear Cell Carcinoma

The fourth subtype is *clear cell carcinoma*. Clear cell carcinoma has cytoplasmic clearing but without squamous or glandular differentiation. Cytoplasmic clearing is most often due to glycogen accumulation.[10]

Large Cell Carcinoma with Rhabdoid Phenotype

Large cell carcinoma with rhabdoid phenotype is an additional subtype of large cell undifferentiated carcinoma. It is characterized as having large eosinophilic cytoplasmic inclusions, with more than 10 percent of the cells exhibiting this morphologic finding.[11]

There are some complexities that arise in practice. For example, a large cell carcinoma with elements of a spindle would place it in the *sarcomatoid carcinoma* class because the spindle is the most recognizable component. A combined large cell neuroendocrine lung carcinoma with spindle or giant cell elements is classified as a large cell carcinoma because the large cell neuroendocrine lung carcinoma component is readily identifiable and *immunohistochemically* (considering the immune system and its relation to tissues and chemicals) confirmable.[12]

Large cell carcinoma tumors that have a neuroendocrine morphology is another area of difficulty because, immunohistochemically, LCNEC is negative for neuroendocrine markers. Although it might be similar to LCNEC, it remains unknown whether this category of tumors is the same as large cell carcinoma or large cell neuroendocrine lung carcinoma.

Stages of LCUC

LCUC has four stages. Stage 1 is a cancer that is confined to the lungs only, and other parts of the body are not yet affected. Stage 2 is a cancer that already involves the lining of the lungs or main bronchus of the lungs or lymph nodes. Stage 3 is a cancer that already involves the adjacent tissues in the lungs. Finally, in stage 4, the cancer has already metastasized to other organs of the body.[13]

Distinguishing Characteristics of LCUC

LCUC is characterized by large, well-demarcated, pink-gray masses with extensive bleeding and cell death. It usually starts on the periphery of the lungs. As the cell is viewed under a microscope, it varies in shape from round to polygonal. Zones of cavitation are also present due to cell death that often accompanies these tumors.

Screening Techniques and New Advances in LCUC

There are various ways to screen for LCUC. First, physical assessment can be used to assess for signs and symptoms related to LCUC, such as a worsening cough or a cough that is continuously present or chest pain that intensifies when accompanied by the following:

- Deep breathing
- Coughing or laughing
- Hoarseness
- Loss of weight and appetite
- Blood in the sputum or rust-colored sputum
- Shortness of breath
- Feeling tired or weak
- Persistent infection
- Wheezing

If the LCUC tumor has already metastasized, bone pain radiates toward the back and hips. The person also experiences yellowish skin and eyes and lymphadenopathy (lumps in the neck or above the collarbone due to the affected lymph node). Risk factors will be assessed as well, such as environmental hazards, occupational risks, and genetic links. After that, imaging tests can be used to detect the presence of tumors in the lungs caused by LCUC. Imaging screening is used to locate the affected area and how far it has spread. Moreover, it can be used to determine the effectiveness of treatment for LCUC and to determine if LCUC has reappeared after treatment. Different imaging studies are chest X-ray, computed tomography (CT) scan, magnetic resonance imaging (MRI), and positron-emission tomography (PET) scan. By way of the imaging results, LCUC can be visualized as tumor in the periphery of the lungs that may progress to the midsection, main bronchus, and *pleura* (chest space).

Aside from imaging tests, observing the lung cells under a microscope can be helpful in screening for LCUC. Sputum, pleural fluid, and suspicious areas in the lungs can be used to analyze the lung cells; however, the most definitive way to confirm LCUC is by detecting suspicious areas in the lungs. This is known as *fine-needle aspiration biopsy*. The tissue from the biopsy will be viewed under a microscope. It usually appears as clusters of round-shaped to polygon-shaped cells. "Dropout zones," or absent clusters in the middle of the specimens due to tissue death, are visible. This could mean that glandular lumen (empty, inner space in the gland) is present.[14]

After the biopsy, special tests will be done to classify the LCUC tumor. The first test that can be done is immunohistochemistry, which analyzes thin slices of samples under a microscope. Certain proteins, such as antibodies, are used to detect the cancer cells in the slide. These proteins adhere only to LCUC cancer cells. Chemicals can also be added to change the color of the cancer cells. In normal adult lung tissue, CK7 and CK18 are parts of type II alveolar pneumocytes and bronchial epithelium. In specimens of LCUC, there are significant levels of CK7 and CK18. Aside from that, about 40 percent of *E-cadherin* protein and 100 percent of *B-catenin* protein are present in patients with LCUC.[15] In normal adult tissue, E-cadherin and B-catenin are proteins usually found on bronchial and bronchiolar epithelium. *Thyroid transcription factor 1* (TTF-1) is also present in LCUC. Keratin is also seen mostly in tissues of LCUC and manifests in about 95 percent of patients with LCUC.[16]

Aside from immunohistochemistry, *mucin* (mucus protein) *staining* is also done to rule out LCUC. Additionally, epidermal growth factor receptor (EFGR) can be used to detect genes in the cell. As far as EFGR is concerned, the K-ras oncogene has been found in 40 percent of patients diagnosed with LCUC.[17] Another point to remember about LCUC is that the process of elimination is used on its diagnosis. When adenocarcinoma, squamous cell carcinoma, and small cell lung carcinoma have been ruled out, LCUC will then be considered.

Proteomics of LCUC of the Lung

Studies on the protein expression of LCUC have been ongoing that employ relatively small amounts of protein. In one study, 42 lung tumors (including LCUC) were used to develop a *histologic* (tissue) *classifier*. These classifiers accurately distinguish the histology of the previously mentioned cases and the additional 14 normal lung tissues. Another study has been completed with 37 lung tumors and 14 normal lung tissues. The histological classifier also was accurate except for one case of LCUC that had been misclassified as adenocarcinoma. This means that LCUC is separable from other groups of non–small cell lung carcinoma but with misclassification of lung adenocarcinoma.[18]

LUNG ADENOCARCINOMAS

Lung adenocarcinoma (LA) affects 40 percent of lung cancer patients.[19] Five years after being diagnosed, less than 10 percent of patient populations survive. However, 35 to 40 percent of patients who have tumors removed during the early stages have a five-year survival rate. Females are usually more affected than males. Approximately 40 percent of female smokers and 30 percent of male smokers are affected. Among other types of lung carcinoma, LA is the most common for young individuals and most commonly seen in nonsmokers. Patients who are under 30 years of age have an 85 percent chance of surviving for five years after contracting the cancer. However, this type of cancer is also common in the smoker demographic as well as in Asian populations.[20]

During the 1980s, LA had the lowest incidence rate among squamous cell carcinoma and small cell lung cancer. According to an autopsy survey performed at the Medical University of Graz, LA accounts for 12 percent of cases, while 35 percent are from squamous cell carcinoma and 25 percent from small cell lung cancer. However, the same survey was also performed during the 1990s; LA had already been considered the most common cause of death, accounting for 37 percent of patients with lung cancer. By 2001, LA increased at an average of 42 percent and became the leading cause of cancer in most industrialized regions.[21]

Smoking causes LA. Although cigarette usage has decreased in industrialized countries, the incidence of patients with lung cancer has increased. This is due to changes in the histological effect of cigarette contents. In 1955, nicotine levels were found to be at 2.7 milligrams and tar at 38 milligrams, while as of 1933, the level of nicotine has been at 1 milligram and tar at 13.5 milligrams, along with the use of "light" cigarettes and the general acceptance of cigarettes with filter tips. The notion that a cigarette is "light" makes the user inhale more deeply and smoke more than normal. Consequently, the peripheral parts of the lungs are exposed to high amounts of carcinogens, perhaps leading to LA. Filters have also greatly contributed to the development of LA. Particulate matter in bound carcinogens is withheld in the filters, but vaporized toxins and carcinogens are delivered to the periphery of the alveoli through the smoke.[22]

Changes in tobacco concentration through time have predisposed smokers to LA. Nitrate content increased in one survey from 0.5 percent to around 1.5 percent, meaning that smokers are more exposed to nitrogen oxide and nitrosamines. Moreover, more intense smoking of low-yield cigarettes increases the incidence of inhaling nitrosamine to two or three times the ordinary. Nitrosamine is a chemical substance capable of triggering LA.[23]

LA is a kind of cancer that inhibits or accelerates the excretion of certain biological substances in the lungs. The growth pattern of this carcinoma usually starts on the periphery, similar to the arrangement of LCUC. Unlike LCUC, LA takes time to spread and grow, making its symptoms develop slowly. At times, it is misdiagnosed as pneumonia or lung collapse.[24]

Like any other type of cancer, the causes of LA are smoking, environmental factors (e.g., asbestos, radon, air pollution, secondhand smoke, and industrial chemicals), work-related hazards (e.g., asbestos worker, painter, bartender, and metalworker), and hereditary links.

LA goes through different stages before progressing to an invasive lung cancer. First is hyperplasia, or an increased number of new cells. Second is metaplasia, which is the degeneration of function in a specialized cell. Third is dysplasia, wherein the cell changes its appearance due to harmful exposure of chemicals in the body. Finally is *carcinoma in situ*, a severe dysplasia confined to the lungs only. Both hyperplasia and metaplasia are reversible, while dysplasia and carcinoma in situ have less chance of regressing and more chance of becoming lung cancer.[25]

Since the most common type of lung cancer is LA, efforts have been made to give it a new classification system. This system is based on clinical, molecular, radiologic, and surgical issues. However, the main basis for the classification system is the histological type of the cancer cell. *Bronchioalveolar carcinoma* and *mixed subtype adenocarcinoma* are terms no longer used by some cancer experts. Meanwhile, *adenocarcinoma in situ* and *minimally invasive carcinoma* have been recently added. Both of these subtypes do not usually secrete mucus and are characterized by layered growths with scaly microscopic coverings.[26]

Distinguishing Characteristics of LA

Professional lung cancer caregivers should be aware that LA is characterized as a solid growth pattern with mucin production or a glandular epithelial malignancy with *acinar* (sac-like), *papillary* (nipple-like), or *tubular* (tube-like) growth patterns. It is usually noted on the outer portion of the lungs with well-circumscribed masses often associated with pleural fibrosis or puckering. LA's cells range from layer, cuboidal, columnar, or polygonal with large vesicular nuclei and prominent nucleoli. On viewing a cut section, LA is gray-white and sometimes lobulated and often has a central scar that might have *anthracotic* (coal-like) pigments. The common signs and symptoms of LA are cough, shortness of breath, wheezing, chest pain, and blood in the sputum.[27]

A Word or Two about LA Symptoms

LA is a non–small cell carcinoma that presents with symptoms on the outer parts of the lungs. Surprisingly, at the benign stage, LA by itself does not reveal any prominent symptoms. Doctors may find various symptoms that can determine the cause of this type of lung cancer. For instance, coughing, wheezing, breathing problems, and weakness are some common symptoms that indicate the onset of LA, threatening the patient in more ways than one. Traditional chemotherapy and radiation techniques restrict the progression of LA symptoms. However, targeted therapy, also known *molecular targeted therapy*, is an innovative medication process that shrinks the limiting symptoms, such as pain. Doctors do this targeted therapeutic process to treat the tumors while avoiding other parts of the body.

Screening Techniques and New Advances in LA

Different screening techniques can be used to detect LA. Screening practices for LCUC and LA are almost the same, but the results may vary. First, physical assessment may be used to detect signs and symptoms that might suggest LA. Second, after the physical assessment, risk factors are also evaluated. Third, screening tests, such as chest X-ray, CT, MRI, and PET scans, can be done to determine the location and the extent of the tumor. Usually, LA is found on the periphery of the lungs and is limited mostly to a single region of the body. Imaging tests can also be used to determine the effectiveness of the treatment and whether the tumor recurred after the treatment.[28] Biopsy by fine-needle aspiration is the definitive way to diagnose LA. Light microscopy can be used to visualize the specimen. Special tests are also considered on screening for LA, such as immunohistochemistry and mucin stain, so that there will be further diagnosis of the tumor. Mucin stain will be positive since LA is characterized as mucus-producing cancer cells.

Immunohistochemistry is a tool used to examine cell growth and the presence of microorganisms in the cell using a microscope. Fluorescent dye, colloidal gold, radioisotope, and color reaction are used to make it more visible. Based on the immunohistochemistry of LA, *TTF-1, CK7, carcinoembryonic antigen, secretory component*, and *B72.3* are gene formations expressed by the tumors of LA.[29] In an immunohistochemical study, 86 LA proteins were analyzed by a nonparametric test, hierarchical clustering, and principal components analysis. It was concluded that squamous cell carcinoma can be distinguished from LA with 98 percent accuracy.[30]

A breakthrough in LA research has been the use of a drug, *crizotinib* (Xalkori), that is specific to the ALK gene found in LA. The drug blocks the abnormal protein found in the ALK gene. Use of this drug has been shown to decrease the size of tumors in about 50 to 60 percent of patients. This is usually taken twice a day. The most common side effects are nausea and vomiting, diarrhea, constipation, swelling, fatigue, and eye problems. Severe side effects include heart rhythm irregularities, low white blood cell count, and inflammation of the lungs.[31]

Proteomics of LA

Studies of protein expression on small cell carcinoma have been analyzed, but the different entities of non–small cell carcinoma have not been further subcategorized because the protein expression between squamous cell carcinoma and LA varies. Different non–small cell carcinomas were included in one study and mentioned in a methods section but were not further separated in a results section. Hence, this study cannot be thoroughly evaluated.[32]

As part of an experiment, 32 protein spots were identified in one of the first two-dimensional *fluorescence differential gel electrophoresis* investigations by a process called principal components analysis. The proteins corresponding to the spots were identified by mass spectrometry and based on an analysis of the 30 or so spots. Cancer cells were categorized into two histologic groups: the *squamous cell carcinoma adenocarcinoma* group and *carcinomas with other types of histology* group. The differential protein for each of these types corresponded very well to the histologic classification. Many proteins, such as surfactant proteins, are peripherally located on the cancer and are spatially expressed, being specific for one or the other group because most LAs arise in peripheral locations.[33]

Another study has been carried out investigating about 50 proteins by *chromatography tandem mass spectrometry*. Twenty-nine of the 50 were unregulated, while the rest were down-regulated. The proteins that were down-regulated have enzymes to control: (1) nutrient absorption by cells such as those of malignant tissues or (2) lung cancer drug metabolism. Most of the TGF beta-induced proteins are involved in such regulation, and these proteins include *tropomyosins, filamins A and B, beta-integrin,* and *ezrin-radixin-moesin.*[34]

To summarize, undifferentiated carcinomas and adenocarcinomas of the lung are more defined in an individual during the later stages of cell malignancy. This chapter explored these two forms of lung cancer, including their characteristics, screening techniques, and new advances in research.

OAT CELL CARCINOMAS AND COMBINED SMALL CELL CARCINOMAS

Oat cell carcinoma (OCC) is a form of small cell lung cancer, and it is termed as such because the malignant cells resemble oats. This type of cancer is caused primarily by smoking and is known for spreading early on. It represents approximately 15 percent of all lung cancers and usually responds well to chemotherapy.[1] As this cancer progresses, it tends to become much more resistant to treatment. This cancer usually begins in the bronchi of the lungs, and early metastasis will usually progress to the brain. The two main stages of this disease are the limited stage and the extensive stage. Unfortunately, at the time of diagnosis, 60 to 70 percent of the people diagnosed with OCC are already in the severe stage.[2]

DISTINGUISHING CHARACTERISTICS OF OCC

Lung cancer occurs when the cells of a lung start to grow uncontrollably. Lung cancer can affect all parts of a lung and is the leading cause of death in the United States, Canada, and China. Of the two main types of lung cancer, small cell lung cancer is the one that accounts for approximately 20 to 25 percent of all lung cancer incidences.[3] OCC is different from other types of lung cancer because it spreads quickly throughout the entire body. It is known to respond well to chemotherapy, which is the process of using medication to destroy the cancer cells, and to radiation therapy, which is the use of high-dose X-rays or some other type of high-energy rays used to destroy the cancer cells. This cancer will usually be associated with specific *paraneoplastic syndromes*, which are an assortment of symptoms that are caused by the substances produced by the tumor and which generally occur at some distance from the tumor itself.

SCREENING TECHNIQUES AND NEW ADVANCES IN OCC RESEARCH

TREATMENT

OCC has been separated into two different *clinico-pathological* stages: the limited stage and the extensive stage. The stage of a patient's cancer is determined by observing the presence of metastases, whether the tumor has expanded from the thorax, and whether the entire tumor burden can be included in a single radiotherapy portal. As a general rule, if the OCC is found only in one lung and in the lymph nodes adjacent to that lung, then that cancer is classified as being in the limited stage. However, if the OCC has spread beyond the mentioned areas, it will be classified as being in the extensive stage.

For OCC identified in the limited stage, a combination of chemotherapy, which will include *cyclophosphamide, cisplatinum, etoposide, paclitaxel, doxorubicin*, and *vincristine*, and chest radiotherapy will be recommended as a treatment method. It has been proven that chest radiotherapy can improve the survival rate for patients suffering from limited-stage OCC. Patients diagnosed with limited-stage OCC who use only chemotherapy have initial response rates to treatment of between 60 and 90 percent, while 45 to 75 percent show signs of a "complete response," which is the disappearance of all signs of the tumor, both radiological and clinical.[4] The problem is that relapse is a common occurrence, and because of this, the median survival rate is between 18 and 24 months.[5]

Since OCC will metastasize early on from the lung in the natural development of the tumor and since nearly always the cancer will respond dramatically to chest radiotherapy and chemotherapy, there is little to no need for surgery. Some recent studies suggest that, by using surgery in the case of small, asymptomatic, node-negative OCC (which can be also understood as a "very limited stage"), the chances of the lung cancer patient's surviving will be improved.[6] This pertains especially to when the surgery occurs prior to chemotherapy. For individuals diagnosed with OCC that is in the extensive stage of development, the standard approach is a combination of chemotherapy and radiotherapy. The role of radiotherapy in this situation is to alleviate symptoms such as bone metastases, dyspnea, or pain from the liver.[7]

The combination chemotherapy is comprised of certain agents, such as *cisplatin, carboplatin, vincristine,* and *cyclophosphamide*. The response rates for this treatment method are high, even for those patients in whom the cancer is extensive; 15 to 30 percent of all the patients subjected to combination chemotherapy have a complete response, while nearly all patients present at least objective responses. However, the responses for OCC patients in the extensive stage usually last for a short period of time.[8]

When complete response to chemotherapy occurs in a patient suffering from OCC, *prophylactic cranial irradiation* (PCI; radiation therapy for the brain) is used to prevent the appearance of brain metastases. Even if the effectiveness of this treatment method is not disputed, it can lead to hair loss and fatigue. PCI provides significant survival benefits for patients; follow-ups on patients who have gone through this treatment method have shown no neurocognitive ill effects. Overall, OCC can respond well to chemotherapy and radiotherapy, but most patients will go through a relapse, and, as such, the survival rate for this type of disease is considerably low.

OCC Prognosis

The median survival for patients diagnosed with limited-stage OCC is 14 to 20 months, and approximately 20 percent of these will live five years or longer. Even if this prognosis seems horrible, the prognosis for patients with extensive-stage OCC is far worse. For these patients, the median survival is 8 to 13 months, and only 1 to 5 percent of all patients diagnosed with this disease process and treated with chemotherapy will live five years or longer.[9]

COMBINED SMALL CELL LUNG CARCINOMAS

Introduction

This type of lung cancer affects smokers, makes up around 15 percent of lung cancer sufferers, and is an aggressive cancer that metastasizes quickly. The two stages of small cell lung carcinomas (SCLC) are the limited stage and the extensive stage. Limited-stage lung cancer tumors are still localized to a particular area of the body, making them easier targets for treatment by chemotherapy or radiation therapy. However, the survival rate for limited-stage lung cancer is low, with only 20 percent living past five years. This is usually the result of relapse following the initial treatment. [10]

Most SCLC incidences are already in the extensive stage by the time the cancer is detected and have already metastasized to different sites. Thus, the survival rate for people in this stage of SCLC is even lower, with less than 1 percent making it past the five-year mark. SCLC is known as small cell undifferentiated carcinoma, as it cannot be determined whether the cells are adenocarcinomas or squamous cell carcinomas. The tumors are so small that they are described as being the size of oat grains. SCLC usually develops in the airways near the central area of the lung and affects only one lung at a time. [11]

Combined SCLC is a multiphasic lung cancer that is diagnosed when a malignant tumor contains a component of OCC and one or more components of non–amall cell lung carcinoma. Non–small cell lung cancer represents approximately 85 percent of all lung cancers and is further divided into squamous cell carcinoma, adenocarcinoma, and large cell carcinoma histology. Combined SCLC is formed by one OCC and one or more non–small cell carcinoma. [12]

Prevalence

Combined SCLC occurs mostly in people between the ages of 50 and 70 years, and the chances of developing this disease process are low for people under 39 years of age. The chances start to rise and grow gradually, peaking for the people who are over 70 years of age. [13]

The risk of developing combined SCLC is higher for men of all ages. In the United States and northern and western Europe, the prevalence of combined SCLC has been slowly decreasing for men, while in southern and eastern Europe, the incidence of developing this disorder in men has increased. Most of the Western countries have had alarming increases for both women and young patients. The chances of developing combined SCLC in the United States are the same for men and women under 39 years, 0.03 percent, or 1 in 3,000. After that age, the chances start to increase for men compared to women, reaching the maximum for those older than 70 years, where the chances are about 7 percent, or 1 in 15, for men and around 4.5 percent, or 1 in 22, for women.[14]

The chances of developing combined SCLC are the same among white women and African American women, but they are higher, about 45 percent, for African American men than for white men. The huge difference in incidence has been attributed by scientists to differences in smoking habits, but there is some new evidence that suggests a difference in susceptibility. Of all the SCLCs, combined SCLC represents approximately 4 to 6 percent, which means that there are about 8,800 to 13,200 new diagnosed cases of this disease each year in the United States alone.[15]

Distinguishing Characteristics of Combined SCLC

The exact mechanisms of all lung cancers are topics that have drawn a lot of interest through the years. The current notion about these subtypes of lung cancers is that they occur from damage done to the genomic DNA, which in turn causes a malignant transformation of at least one *multipotent* (ability to have different characteristics) *cell*. The new cell, which is called a "cancer stem cell," will start dividing uncontrollably, and a tumor will form quickly. Combined SCLC appears to develop from OCC. Because of certain cellular mutations, OCC starts to acquire certain *cytological* (cell-related) *structures* that resemble non–small cell lung cancer, and thus combined SCLC is born.

Some analyses suggest that sometimes non–small cell lung cancer can develop histological and molecular characteristics of OCC, but these analyses are based on specific occurrences rather than on a certain group. Some studies even state that combined SCLC appears by the *field cancerization* of two different cancer cells that are developing adjacent to each other, when one has OCC and the other non–small cell lung cancer.

Regardless of how combined SCLC develops, the manner of progression is based on the same pattern, which is specific to this type of cancer and is different from both OCC and non–small cell lung cancer. The conversion of these two cancers has an influence over the treatment methods that can be used. Combined SCLC can also commonly occur after treating OCC with chemotherapy, probably as the result of the mutations that are brought forth by cytotoxic (disruptive to cells) therapy. The most common types of non–small cell lung carcinoma found in combined SCLC are adenocarcinoma, large cell carcinoma, and squamous cell carcinoma. Sometimes, other combinations occur, including carcinoids, giant cell carcinoma (found in individuals who have gone through radiation therapy), and spindle cell carcinoma. One of the most important tasks for scientists today is to classify the subtypes of combined SCLC based on cancerous development processes in the body.

SCREENING TECHNIQUES AND NEW ADVANCES IN COMBINED SCLC RESEARCH

Treatment

Many clinical trials have been conducted on combined SCLC over the past few decades, and as a result of those tests, some guidelines have been devised on the basis of clinical evidence for treating combined SCLC. The current guidelines suggest that SCLC should be treated the same as OCC, but the guidelines also explain that evidence to support this statement is weak. As such, currently no optimal treatment methods are available for patients suffering from combined SCLC. The current standard of care for all forms of combined SCLC is concurrent chemotherapy combined with thoracic radiation therapy. For past lung cancer sufferers in whom the disease process has disappeared entirely (the complete responders), PCI is sometimes prescribed. Thoracic radiation therapy attempts to increase the chances of entirely eradicating the disease, while PCI tries to eliminate any brain *micrometastases*.

Surgery is only rarely considered as a treatment method for combined SCLC due to the high chances of distant metastases at the moment of diagnosis. Some recent studies suggest that surgery can improve outcomes for people diagnosed with combined SCLC at a very early stage in the tumor's development.[16] Clinical investigations suggest that a resection for residual masses is necessary for patients diagnosed with combined SCLC and that it should happen immediately after the tumor responds completely to chemotherapy and thoracic radiation therapy.[17]

The best combinations of drugs for patients diagnosed with combined SCLC are the ones made of *cisplatin, carboplatin* and *etoposide*, or *irinotecan*. For patients who will not respond to the first line of treatment or who will relapse after going into complete remission, the only agent that has shown some concrete results in increasing the chances of survival is *topotecan*. *Amirubicin* is considered an effective *salvage therapy* (last-resort treatment) in Japan.

Combined SCLC is much more resistant to chemotherapy and thoracic radiation therapy than OCCs are. Even if the reasons that cause these differences in response to treatment are currently unknown, evidence suggests that if a combined SCLC is diagnosed early, the chances of having similar treatment responses as OCC are much higher.

Some new agents have been developed lately with the hopes of treating combined SCLC. These include (1) epidermal growth factor receptors and tyrosine kinase inhibitors, such as *erlotinib* (Tarceva), *gefitinib* (Iressa), and *cetuximab* (Erbitux); (2) inhibitors of vascular endothelial growth factor, such as *bevacizumab* (Avastin); and (3) inhibitors of folate metabolism, such as *pemetrexed* (Alimta).

Clinical trials are attempting to discover new treatment methods for combined SCLC but have been unsuccessful thus far. Some targeted agents have shown some results when dealing with the non–small cell lung carcinoma, and since combined SCLC contains at least one non–small cell lung carcinoma part, these agents might show some results in treating combined SCLC as well.

Epidermal growth factor receptor (EGFR) tyrosine kinase inhibitor drugs have been active against certain mutations of the EGFR gene. These mutations are rare in OCC, and therefore these agents cannot be effective for combined SCLC. Nonetheless, since the incidence of such mutations is considerably higher in combined SCLC, especially in non-smoking women, they can be more effective among the population.

The effects of the vascular endothelial growth factor inhibitors over combined SCLC are still unknown. Some studies suggest that when the inhibitors are combined with other agents, they can improve the chances of survival for patients suffering from this disease, but such studies are not 100 percent conclusive. Combined SCLC seems to express female hormone receptors, such as estrogen or progesterone, in many cases (50 to 57 percent), just like breast carcinomas. It is currently unknown if the growth of combined SCLC can be affected by blocking these receptors.[18]

Prognosis

Combined SCLC is highly lethal, and statistics have shown that the highest five-year patient survival rates occur in the United States. The five-year survival rate for patients diagnosed with combined SCLC in the United States has improved over the years, from 12.5 percent in 1975 to 15.7 percent in 2001. However, this rate is highly dependent on the stage of the disease at diagnosis, being 49 percent for a local disease, 16 percent for a regional disease, and 2 percent for a distant-stage disease.[19]

The current consensus about the prognosis for combined SCLC is that it is determined by the OCC component because the former appears to have the worst long-term projections of all the lung cancer subtypes. Even if the data on this cancer are sparse at best, some studies have shown that survival rates in combined SCLC are even worse than for OCC because of the low response to chemoradiation. Untreated patients suffering from OCC have a median survival rate from four weeks to four months, depending on the stage of the cancer at the time of diagnosis. Some evidence supports the idea that patients suffering from combined SCLC who continue to smoke after diagnosis have a much smaller chance of survival compared to those who quit.[20]

In summary, OCC and combined SCLC are the most dangerous lung cancers and possess the highest mortality rates. The most important factor in determining a patient's survival is the stage in which the cancer subtype is at the moment of diagnosis. While current research in treating both OCC and combined SCLC gives some immediate hope for patients and caregivers (chapter 20), unfortunately the road to finding absolute immunity from these disease processes is rough in the absence of serious intervention.

12

OTHER MANIFESTATIONS OF LUNG CANCER

The face of a disease process such as lung cancer changes over time. With the help of technology and advanced science, medicine has evolved from tracing all possible causes of a medical disorder to all applicable treatments using various methods. The effects and manifestations of disorders are also unraveled, including allied complications. This chapter elaborates on manifestations associated with lung cancer by explaining certain lung cancer–related medical disorders and cancers.

NONCANCEROUS DISORDERS ASSOCIATED WITH LUNG CANCER

Every year, lung cancer affects over 370,000 Americans via some manifestation or another.[1] Poor prognosis stems from late diagnosis of the disease condition originating from delayed health-seeking behaviors. Patients usually display late manifestations, making multiple modality therapies viable options for treatment.

From a compilation of data, lung cancer appeared to be the most common fatal cancer in men and women, at 31 percent and 26 percent, respectively. In 2009, projected mortality figures from lung cancer in the United States amounted to 159,390, with 88,900 men and almost 70,500 women in total, equal to about 30 percent of cancer-related deaths. In 2007, an estimated 1,351,000 deaths due to lung cancer and its related noncancerous disorders were recorded worldwide, with roughly 975,000 and approximately 375,000 in men and women, respectively.[2]

Pneumonia

When lung structures such as alveoli and bronchioles are inflamed due to local irritation brought about by lung cancer, pneumonia manifests. Pneumonia is a common complication of lung cancer. It can be caused by the invasion of pathogens such as bacteria and viruses aggravated by the impaired host defenses of the individual. Common manifestations of pneumonia are fever, general malaise, chest discomfort, and cough with respiratory compromise. Without proper treatment, sepsis may occur. The upper airway structures were designed to prevent potential infectious particles from reaching the sterile lower respiratory tract. Usually, pneumonia arises from the body's normal flora in patients whose resistance has been altered due to an acute or a chronic condition. A tumor in the lung parenchyma, principally when the tumor closes a bronchial tube, causes inflammation and infection and can extend beyond the blockage, affecting alveoli and bronchioles. This inflammatory reaction renders exudates that interfere with the exchange of oxygen and carbon dioxide in the peripheral airways. Because of this, a *ventilation-perfusion* (breathing vs. blood flow) mismatch results. With the presence of infection, white blood cells migrate to the alveoli and fill the normally air-containing spaces, resulting in further occlusion of the airways. Pus and other drainage may be contained in the peripheral airways, and blockage may lead to solidified tissues (consolidation), a common finding on chest X-rays. Pneumonia is usually treated with antibiotics based on the results of culture and sensitivity tests, whether or not the causative agent is viral or bacterial. Supportive treatment may also be ordered initially, including oxygen therapy and chest physiotherapy to facilitate mucus elimination.[3]

Pleural Effusion

Not a primary disease itself but a complication of maladies such as heart failure, tuberculosis, pneumonia, pulmonary infections, nephritic syndrome, and pulmonary embolisms, among others, *pleural effusion* is the accumulation of fluid in the pleural space. The most common malignancy associated with pleural effusion is bronchogenic carcinoma, or a tumor arising from the bronchi. Around 5 to 15 milliliters of fluid is normally present in the pleural space, serving as a lubricant that enables movement of the surfaces of the pleura without friction. Fluid may accumulate in the pleural space to the point that it is clinically evident and may produce signs and symptoms of pathologic significance. The effusion may be clear, purulent, or bloody, depending on the nature of its occurrence. Clear fluid may be identified as transudates or exudates. Transudates result from imbalances in the hydrostatic or oncotic pressures involved in the formation and absorption of pleural fluid. Generally, this indicates that the pleural membranes are not diseased, such as those with heart failure. Exudates, on the other hand, result from inflammation by bacterial products or neoplasms involving the pleural space, such as is the case with lung cancer.[4]

The manifestations of such complications root from the underlying disease itself. For malignant effusions, it may result in shortness of breath and coughing. A small pleural effusion may result in acute or minimal shortness of breath, while a large pleural effusion may present with shortness of breath and lead to acute respiratory distress. On assessment, the patient may present decreased or absent breath sounds, decreased *fremitus*, and a dull, flat sound when percussed.

Achieving relief from pleural effusion requires eliminating the primary cause, such as exudate fluid, and treatment for malignant neoplasm should be instituted. In lung cancer patients with plural effusion, the objectives of care are directed to preventing the reaccumulation of fluid and relieving discomfort and respiratory distress. Thoracentesis (explained in chapter 7) is a primary treatment that may also be considered a screening procedure for pleural effusion.

Superior Vena Cava Syndrome

Superior vena cava syndrome (SVCS) is an obstruction in the flow of blood through the superior vena cava and is usually manifested by patients with underlying cell malignancies in the chest; 70 percent of the cases are stem from lung cancers, particularly adenocarcinomas. Additionally, 5 to 10 percent of patients with right-sided malignant thoracic mass lesions have developed the syndrome. In one survey, around 4 percent of almost 5,000 patients with lung cancer developed SVCS wherein 80 percent of cases involved the right lung.[5] The prognosis of lung cancer patients experiencing SVCS related to a malignant process depends on the history of the tumor itself. Manifestations of SVCS, such as laryngeal and cerebral edema, are signs of a poor prognosis and are life threatening. In addition, there is a greater occurrence of SVCS in males because this group has a greater incidence of developing lung cancer.[6]

The superior vena cava is a large vein situated in the upper chest and is responsible for collecting blood from the head and arms and directing it to the right atrium. Being a vein, it is composed of a thin wall and is under little pressure, causing it to be easily compressed by outside structures. Abnormalities in the central structures of the chest, such as the heart, trachea, esophagus, and aorta or vena cava, can cause compression or obstruction of the superior vena cava. More often than not, obstruction of the superior vena cava is caused by neoplastic invasion, causing extrinsic pressure by a tumor mass against its wall. Cancer or tumors located in the upper lobe of the right lung or in the mediastinum can cause compression of the vena cava, resulting in this condition. As the compression intensifies, symptoms such as shortness of breath and swelling of the arms and face begin to manifest. This results from congestion of the systemic circulation and facilitates blood return to the heart, resulting in limited newly oxygenated cells that normally meet the metabolic needs of the lungs. Consequences may also include distention of neck veins, shortness of breath, and chest pain. Diagnostics include an order for chest radiography, computed tomography (CT) scan, and magnetic resonance imaging (MRI). Chest radiography may reveal a widened mediastinum or a mass in the right side of the chest.[7]

Like all other complications, SVCS is treated when the underlying cause is eliminated. Measures are taken to relieve symptoms, often to gain improvement in well-being, such as elevation of the head of the bed and supplemental oxygen. Corticosteroids and diuretics are ordered in the event of laryngeal or cerebral edemas, which are life-threatening signs of the condition. To eliminate the underlying disease, such as that of a neoplasm, radiotherapy is indicated as the initial treatment to relieve obstruction and compression. Chemotherapy could also be instituted. Clinical evidence has shown that patients achieved complete relief of SVCS symptoms within just a couple weeks of institution of chemotherapy alone, combined with radiation, or with radiation alone.[8]

Horner's Syndrome

Scientific research also confirms that lung abscess can cause Horner's syndrome, and therefore it is important to know that opportunistic lung cancer can arise in the resulting, weakened lung.[9] When an interruption of the sympathetic nerve supply to the eye results, a classic triad of *miosis* (constricted pupils), *ptosis* (partial drooping of eyelids), and *an-hidrosis* (loss of facial sweating) occurs, collectively termed *Horner's syndrome*. In some countries, such as France, this is referred to as Bernard-Horner syndrome. It can be a defect at birth, acquired, or purely genetic with an autosomal dominant trait. Lesions that interfere with *preganglionic* (anatomically located before nerve bundles) fibers through the upper thorax commonly cause the syndrome. Preganglionic Horner's syndrome is a complication of a serious pathologic disorder, such as lung cancer, and results from cell malignancy. Postganglionic Horner's syndrome usually results from benign conditions.[10] The causes of Horner's syndrome can be classified further into first-order, second-order, or third-order neuron lesions; however, this discussion focuses on second-order lesions that result in the development of the syndrome, including tumors in the apex of the lung referred to as Pancoast tumors; 45 to 50 percent of these cases consist of squamous cell carcinomas, while the remaining are either adenocarcinomas or undifferentiated large cell carcinomas. Because the tumor is localized in the apex of the lung, it invades the lower part of the brachial plexus, vertebrae, subclavian vessels, or stellate ganglion. Manifestations of Pancoast tumors include shoulder pain radiating to the side of the arm and hand; 30 percent of Pancoast cases report Horner's syndrome as a complication.[11]

It is important to assess the patient for recent procedures that may have caused neurologic damage, such as chest, neck, and *otolaryngologic* (ear, nose, and throat) procedures. In addition, several drugs may cause signs and symptoms similar to those of the syndrome, such as antipsychotics and oral contraceptives. It is also important to measure the papillary diameter and the reactivity of the pupils to light and their accommodation thereof during physical examination. Other abnormalities, such as nystagmus (uncontrolled eye movement), facial swelling, *lymphadenopathy* (disease of the lymph nodes), and vesicular eruptions, must be observed and reported immediately to the physician. Imaging studies, such as a chest radiography, must be obtained, as the most common cause of Horner's syndrome is bronchogenic carcinoma.

For better visualization and further testing, MRI or ultrasound may also be performed. To treat Horner's syndrome, the underlying cause should be treated entirely first. Medical studies confirm that Horner's can be caused by lung abscesses with or without lung cancer, but if a bronchogenic carcinoma is identified as the underlying cause, it should be treated first, depending on its severity.[12] It may be removed by surgery, which is commonly done to most tumors. The earlier the detection, the greater the chances for long-term survival. Also, it is important to be critical in assessing the patient's condition to commence appropriate referral to specialists. Treating the condition would be a collaborative effort between the pulmonology, neurology, and oncology specialties.[13]

TRUE RELATIONSHIP

Knowing the Connection between Cancers

It is essential for the lung cancer patient and caregiver to know the connection between different types of cancer. Cancers originating from the lung and bronchus made up the top 10 cancers in 2009, having a rate of nearly 65 out of 100,000 for both males and females and across all races in the United States. Prostate cancer remains the most frequent. Other types included in this list are breast, colorectal, and urinary bladder cancers and melanoma of the skin.[14]

Because the development of lung cancer takes a certain amount of time before symptoms become noticeable, health care providers have always emphasized primary prevention regarding diet, physical activity, and the avoidance of carcinogenic substances. Because of the delay of obvious manifestations, lung cancers can be diagnosed only when they have developed into a more advanced stage or when the tumor cells have metastasized to other parts of the body. If the metastasis is too widespread, multiple organ systems may become affected, producing common symptoms, such as pain, malaise, and, more often than not, side effects of the body's compensatory mechanisms. It is thus important to know the different types of cancers, as health care providers can anticipate which symptoms commonly appear with each type and which immediate and proper interventions should be undertaken. This also provides them with the information on which organ systems or body parts each type of cell malignancy metastasizes to based on the surrounding tissue and the incidence of complications. For example, tumor cells in the lungs or bronchus can invade the surrounding structures, commonly the bone, brain, and adrenal glands, resulting in cancer of these organ systems. The health care team can anticipate and therefore prevent further complications.

Before unraveling the different types of cancer that can originate from the lungs, one must understand the concepts of invasion, metastasis, and angiogenesis, which are mechanisms by which cancer cells spread. Understanding the staging and grading system of tumors and malignancies also allows a better understanding along the course of this reading and the extent of the spread. Malignancies have a characteristic of allowing the spread of cancerous cells from one organ to another through invasion or metastasis. Invasion or metastasis can be attributed to (1) circulatory patterns and (2) the unique affinity of certain malignant cells to bind to molecules in specific body tissue.

Process of Invasion

Invasion refers to the growth of the primary tumor into the surrounding host tissues, commonly due to mechanical pressure exerted by rapidly proliferating neoplasms that result in finger-like projections toward surrounding tissues and *interstitial* (between tissues) spaces. These cancer cells adhere less and may wander off the primary tumor, invading structures near them. They are also thought to produce certain enzymes that destroy the vascular membranes of structural tissues, a process that further facilitates invasion of malignant cells.

Detailed Expansion: Metastasis

Metastasis is the term used to describe the spread of cancer cells not only to surrounding host tissues but also to distant sites through the direct spread to body cavities or through the lymphatic and blood circulation. Growing tumors or those that penetrate body cavities may shake off cells or emboli that travel within the body cavity and start new growth on the surfaces of other organs. Through lymphatic spread, cancer cells can enter the lymphatic circulation. Tumor cells or emboli through the interstitial fluid enter the lymph channels. On accessing the lymphatic circulation, malignant cells either lodge in the lymph nodes or pass between lymphatic and venous circulation. Metastasis can also be accomplished through *hematogenous spread*, wherein malignant lung cells are dispersed through the blood. Dissemination through the blood depends also on the vascularity of the tumor. Because of the turbulence of arterial circulation, insufficient oxygenation, or impairment in the body's immune system, few malignant cells can survive this kind of spread. Those cancer cells that do spread are able to attach to endothelium and gather platelets, or fibrin and clotting factors that serve as a seal to prevent differentiation of the immune system. The endothelium then retracts, allowing the cancer cells to enter basement membranes and produce strong enzymes of the lysosome (chapter 1) responsible for destroying surrounding body tissues and permitting invasion and implantation.

To sustain growth and provide for nutrients and oxygen, cancer cells surfacing from or leading to lung cancer have a unique ability to induce the growth of new capillaries from the host tissue, appropriately termed *angiogenesis*. It is through this that tumor *emboli* (clots) have a great possibility of entering the systemic circulation and traveling to distant sites, such as the lungs.[15]

Staging and Grading

Staging refers to the determination of the size of the tumor and the existence of metastasis. The tumor-node-metastasis system (chapter 9) is commonly utilized for staging the invasion of cancers associated with lung cancer. Grading refers to the classification of tumor cells and is used to determine the tumor's tissue of origin and the degree to which functionality and histological characteristics are retained. Samples are obtained through cytology, biopsy, or surgical excision. Grade I tumors are well differentiated and are highly similar in their original structure and function. In contrast, grade IV tumors are poorly differentiated, or undifferentiated, and may require more aggressive treatment and produce less responsive results.

CANCERS ASSOCIATED WITH LUNG CANCER

Bone Cancer

The human body is made up of 206 bones of different shapes and functions. The three basic types of cells in bones are osteoblasts, osteocytes, and osteoclasts. The bone marrow is a vascular tissue located in the shaft of long bones and in flat bones. The long bones are shaped similar to rods or shafts with rounded ends called *epiphyses*. A tough, elastic, avascular tissue encloses the end of the long bones to serve as a cushion. Short bones consist of *cancellous* (spongy) *bone* covered by a layer of compact bone. Flat bones are sites of *hematopoiesis*, or the formation of new blood cells. Located in the sternum, ilium, vertebrae, and ribs of adults is the red bone marrow, responsible for producing blood components, such as red blood cells, white blood cells, and platelets. Bone tissues receive a rich supply of blood and are dynamic, undergoing constant turnover throughout the life span. When an individual reaches early adulthood, the process of remodeling occurs to maintain bone structure and function. Every 10 years, there is complete skeletal turnover through simultaneous *bone resorption* (removal of old bone) and *osteogenesis* (creation of new bone). Physical activity and good dietary habits to ensure adequate calcium intake are essential for the bone health of a lung cancer patient.[16]

An estimated 30 to 40 percent of patients with advanced lung cancer has an incidence of bone metastasis. An autopsy study found out that in roughly 50 percent of the cases of bone metastases, the lungs were the primary site. In a recent retrospective review, 24 percent revealed incidence of skeletal metastasis out of 435 patients with non–small cell lung cancer—most of this detected at the time of initial staging.[17]

Because of the dysregulation of the remodeling process of the bone, tumor cells stimulate osteoclast activity, leading to bone resorption. With this, the bone matrix releases cytokines (chapter 1) that further stimulate the growth of the tumor. Spread to the bones is usually asymptomatic, and symptoms of metastasis to the bone are the first

manifestation of malignancy, with an estimated 80 percent of lung cancer patients suffering from bone pain either at presentation or at some
point in the course of the disease. This has a great impact on mobility,
thus also affecting the individual's quality of life.[18]

As supportive treatment, one of the priorities for bone cancers includes pain management. Pharmacologic interventions for pain relief
vary from (1) nonsteroidal anti-inflammatory drugs to (2) narcotic anal-
gesics, (3) corticosteroids, (4) tricyclic antidepressants, (5) anticonvul-
sants, and (6) *neuroleptics* as deemed appropriate by the health care
provider. As a result of the pathologic condition, fractures may also
result; thus, it is also important to implement interventions to ensure
the safety of patients. This can be done through the direct assistance of
nurses or nursing aides, the use of assistive devices, or general interventions for safety, such as the use of side rails. Radiation therapy remains
the most common treatment for painful bone metastases. Surgical
intervention for the root cause of the pathologic complication is still the
mainstay treatment of bone cell malignancy associated with lung cancer.[19]

Brain Cancer

A neuron is the basic functioning unit of the brain. A single neuron is
composed of a dendrite, a cell body, and an axon, which are together
designed to (1) transmit impulses to and from the brain to the lungs and
(2) contribute to total functioning of the human body. The human brain
weighs nearly 1,400 grams and is divided into three major areas: the
cerebrum, the cerebellum, and the brain stem. The cerebrum consists
of the two hemispheres: the left and the right. It is further divided into
the frontal, temporal, parietal, and occipital lobes. It is important to
note which lobe is primarily affected, as each lobe has a specific relationship with the rest of the body and its functioning. The frontal lobe,
for example, is responsible for concentration, abstract thought, information storage or memory, and motor function. It affects the lung cancer
sufferer's motor speech as well as personality and affect. The parietal
lobe is responsible mostly for sensory functions, including awareness of
the body in space. This lobe concerns auditory reception. The occipital
lobe has key roles in the visual functioning of the lung cancer patient.
The cerebrum also includes the following:

- Corpus callosum, which serves as a bridge between the two hemispheres and allows transmission of one hemisphere to another
- Basal ganglia, responsible for the control of fine motor movements
- Hypothalamus, which has an important role in hormone secretion, appetite control, the sleep–wake cycle, and often emotional behaviors
- Pituitary gland for hormonal regulation

The brain stem serves as a neurological pathway that can be obstructed by lung cancer that has progressed to a severe stage. It is composed of the midbrain, pons, and medulla oblongata and includes sensory and motor pathways. The medulla oblongata contains motor fibers that connect the brain to the spinal cord, while portions of the pons also regulate blood pressure, the heart, and respiration. The cranial nerves also play a role in connecting these structures. The cerebellum has both excitatory and inhibitory actions and contributes greatly to the control of movement, balance, and orientation in space. It is responsible for processing input from other areas of the brain.

The clear, colorless fluid produced and circulated around the brain and spinal cord is called *cerebrospinal fluid.* This is important in immune and metabolic functions, both of which are necessary in the quest for healthier lungs. A blood–brain barrier is also present, serving to protect the brain from most substances that circulate in the blood plasma, such as dyes and medications, especially antibiotics. This can be disrupted by trauma and cerebral edema, among other factors.[20]

Neurologic deficits manifested by lung cancer patients are thought to be a result of metastasis to the brain. It was observed that metastasis from small cell lung cancer commonly involves the brain wherein about 10 percent of lung cancer patients manifest signs and symptoms spreading to the head and an estimated 40 to 50 percent will develop brain metastasis at some point during the progression of the disorder. Approximately 30 percent of non–small cell lung cancer patients develop brain metastases.[21]

Metastasis to the head can be due to (1) separation of the tumor from the primary site, which could be the lung, and (2) spread through the bloodstream or lymphatic system. The brain's microenvironment plays a significant role in the progression of lung cancer cells in the brain, resulting in a high incidence of metastases to the central nervous system. Neurologically anomalous expressions of metastasis originate from an autoimmune process wherein the primary tumor, such as that of lung cancer, produces substances similar to those normally produced by the nervous system. This leads to the production of *autoantibodies* (special proteins created by the immune system) that cross-react with neuronal *antigens* (foreign substances), thereby damaging normal, healthy tissues. This results in inflammation and swelling, placing pressure on specific structures of the lung cancer patient's brain. The signs and symptoms of lung cancer metastasis to the brain depends greatly on which structure(s) is affected, the extent of tumor spread, and the general health status of the individual. Common manifestations of neurologic disturbances are due to increased intracranial pressure, such as headache, or disturbances specific to certain areas of the brain, such as focal weakness, mental disturbances, ataxia and problems with gait, aphasia or speech difficulty, and visual and sensory disturbances, among others. To detect the structures affected and the extent of brain damage resulting indirectly from lung cancer, imaging studies are ordered, particularly MRI or CT scans. The MRI is preferred, as it is able to detect small lesions that cannot be seen in a CT scan. With the data acquired from these imaging studies, together with physical examination and history taking, prompt treatment is instituted to prevent further damage. Palliative care is also provided, aiming to reduce symptoms rather than cure the disease itself. The initial management is to reverse increased *intracranial pressure* (pressure in the head), commonly with the use of corticosteroids that reduce edema. Antiseizure medications are also given as prophylaxis, and treatment of the primary tumor remains an essential part of the management of a brain tumor in a lung cancer patient.[22]

Whole-brain radiation therapy is also recommended for metastases originating from small cell lung cancer. Patients initially have a good response to whole-brain radiation therapy, but the recurrence and progression of the intracranial disease develops most of the time; thus, external beam radiation therapy and brachytherapy are also considered alternative treatments. Chemotherapy could also be instituted together with whole-brain radiation therapy. Surgery of tumor and lesions in the brain is generally not recommended, as this approach may lead to further complications and even death. The prognosis of patients with brain metastases remains poor despite new approaches and years of research-based interventions.[23]

Lung Cancer and the Adrenal Glands

The adrenal glands play a major role in the autonomic nervous system of the individual with lung cancer. Stimulation of the preganglionic nerve fibers travels directly to the adrenal medulla, causing the release of catecholamine hormones, such as norepinephrine and epinephrine. These regulate metabolic pathways that promote the breakdown of stored energy to meet metabolic demands. They play a significant role in the fight-or-flight response. Hormones secreted by the adrenal cortex are vital to life, including glucocorticoids, mineralocorticoids, and androgens, which help the body adapt to all kinds of stress. Glucocorticoids are influential in glucose metabolism, resulting in increased blood glucose levels that can be used as energy sources, especially in stressful situations. These also have an anti-inflammatory response useful in the management of tissue injury. Mineralocorticoids are influential in fluid and electrolyte balance. These act primarily in the renal tubules and lead to increased sodium ion absorption in exchange for the excretion of potassium or hydrogen. These are helpful in blood pressure regulation and sodium balance for the lung cancer patient.[24]

The adrenal glands, which are vascular organs, can be a site of metastasis of primary tumors, especially on surrounding structures, such as the lungs, breast, and colon. Cushing's syndrome can be a manifestation of metastasis to the adrenal cortex wherein steroid hormones are produced excessively. Tumors present in the adrenal medulla produce excessive amounts of *catecholamines* (specialized nervous system hormones), resulting in signs and symptoms such as flushing, elevated blood pressure, and palpitations. Metastasis from primary lung cancer can occur in the adrenal gland. Unilateral adrenal metastases are seen commonly; however, up to 10 percent of lung cancer patients have bilateral adrenal metastases. Between 2 and 3 percent of unilateral adrenal metastases occur in the initial presentation of non–small cell lung cancer. As a result of metastasis, disruption of the structure and function of the adrenal occurs.[25]

Like all other tumors, diagnosis of adrenal masses related to lung cancer can be made through laboratory tests. Most important, imaging studies are ordered to evaluate the extent of damage and identify appropriate treatment. Radiography can be ordered initially, but this provides a limited visualization, and large masses in the adrenal glands can be indistinguishable from renal masses. CT scan and MRI remain the two most reliable imaging studies ordered for diagnostic evaluation. Systemic treatment is an option that is most frequently opted for in treating metastasis to the adrenal glands. Management of pain through pharmacologic and nonpharmacologic means is instituted for comfort. Early identification of lesions is vital, and surgical resection remains the primary intervention, as this increases the chances of survival. This can be done through aggressive surgical removal of the cancer through *adrenalectomy*, or the removal of one or more of the adrenal glands. There is a good chance that some of the surrounding tissues around the affected area will require removal as well. If adrenalectomy is not possible, combination chemotherapy should be instituted as treatment but is not a guarantee of a good prognosis. Studies have shown that *stereotactic body radiation treatment* increases control of the tumor and could be an alternative intervention or be used combination with surgery. It has proven to be a safe and feasible technique with minimal acute side effects.[26]

Liver Cancer

The liver is a vital organ located behind the ribs in the upper right portion of the abdominal cavity. It serves several functions, including glucose metabolism, ammonia conversion, protein and fat metabolism, vitamin and iron storage, drug metabolism, bile formation, and bilirubin excretion. Of the more than 1,000 lung cancer patients diagnosed between October 1976 and May 2002, 62 (almost 6 percent) of the patients studied had liver metastasis.[27] The incidence of liver metastasis was nearly 18 percent in small cell lung cancer patients, whereas the incidence in non–small cell lung cancer patients was roughly 4 percent. Like all other metastases of lung cancer, spread to the liver is initially asymptomatic and may manifest only when extensive damage already exists to the secondary site or when diagnosed through imaging studies such as CT and MRI. Common signs and symptoms include right upper quadrant pain, body malaise, nausea, and jaundice. The latter is a result of obstruction to the bile ducts, causing a yellowish discoloration of the eyes and often the sclera.[28]

Imaging studies persist as the most reliable diagnostic tests to confirm the presence of liver cancers associated with lung cell malignancy. Abdominal ultrasound could also be performed. To institute appropriate treatment, medical practitioners may also order a liver biopsy. The goal of treating liver metastases is palliative care (chapter 17), which focuses on alleviating symptoms rather than curing the disease itself. A combination therapy of surgery, chemotherapy, and radiation is helpful for liver cancer but does not promise much in slowing or curing lung cancer that has spread to the liver.

IV

Resolutions

13

INITIAL APPROACHES TO LUNG CANCER

Cancers of the lung and other organs are among the most difficult disorders to initially approach. This is often because of a lack of solid early-stage symptoms that can alert one that one is sick so that appropriate measures can be taken to prevent the further expansion of the cancerous growth throughout the body or, in the case of lung cancer, throughout the respiratory system.

REASON WHY THERE IS NO FINAL CURE FOR CANCERS

Currently, lung cancer is responsible for a third of all cancer deaths and is one of the most common cancer diagnoses in the world. It is a very difficult, dangerous disease to treat. While there are indeed viable treatments for many cancers, there is no one absolute treatment for any one cancer.[1] Treatment often depends on the type of cancer, the location, the stage of the cancer, and other health factors of patient. Some cancers caught early still can't be cured, and some detected later can sometimes be treated well enough that a patient reaches remission. There is no guarantee that cancer will not come back. However, some approaches can lengthen a patient's life and even bring some quality to that patient's life even if his or her time is limited.

There are many speculations as to why no absolute cure for cancer or a certain method for dealing with the disease process still exists. Most such speculation revolves around the fact that the disorder itself is elusive and hard to diagnose early—and that is when the treatment is the easiest. The symptoms sometimes can be mistaken for the symptoms of other clinical disorders, which can then lead to a completely wrong treatment or a delayed diagnosis.[2] Cancer is, by nature, a tough disease process to spot because its cells have some similarities to normal tissue cells, and that causes the immune system to miss anything malignant until it is already too late and the tumor has already spread throughout the lungs, causing severe damage to the patient's respiratory system.[3] That is what makes curing cancer—and diagnosing it in the first place—an extremely difficult task. Some types of cancer can form in the lungs alone, not to mention all the other cancer types that can form elsewhere in the body.[4] Because of this, finding a cure for each and every type of lung cancer is difficult, as scientists need to focus on each different cancerous cell separately and devise a way to counteract it before focusing on another cancer type.[5] This is also what makes finding an absolute cure for cancer so difficult and why there is still not one available to the public.

Ethical issues are also concerns in the initial approaches to lung-related oncology. People involved in oncological practice need to deal with ethical questions and dilemmas, usually regarding end-of-life care, that are relative to the patient's personality, culture, family life, and spiritual beliefs. These issues may include (1) what facts to provide the patient about disease prognosis, (2) consideration of clinical trials for terminal illness, (3) the withdrawal of active treatment, and (4) do-not-resuscitate orders.

STEPS TO TAKE WHEN CANCER IS INITIALLY SUSPECTED

Unfortunately, there are no solid, surefire symptoms that point directly at lung cancer (or any other type of cancer for the matter).[6] However, some symptoms, if investigated in time, may lead to the early diagnosis of the disease process. Such symptoms include persistent coughing with blood in the sputum, chest pain, weight loss, or shortness of breath.[7] Normally, such things should be reported to the patient's caregiver immediately because, even if they are not symptoms of lung cancer, they are still abnormalities in the body's physiological behavior. That is the first thing to do when someone suspects that he or she has lung cancer—talk to a physician so that another investigative step can be taken to identify whether the symptoms are indeed those of lung cancer. It is also wise to provide the physician with a full medical history. This is helpful because it can help the doctor determine whether the patient's symptoms are those of lung cancer or some other disease that may be common in the patient's family because, as mentioned previously, lung cancer can cause symptoms that are also the symptoms of several other diseases.[8]

Tests and scanning procedures (chapter 7) to confirm or deny those suspicions can be undertaken when lung cancer is initially suspected. There are many such tests and procedures one can participate in: some of them are more invasive and dangerous, while others are as simple and easy as coughing in a cup and then submitting it to be examined under a microscope.

To some extent, symptoms of lung cancer are similar to other disorders and therefore pave the road for an initial suspicion of lung cancer. For instance, constant aching in the body, obstructed inhalation, and squeamishness are symptoms that appear in both pneumonia and lung cancer. Patients also experience a harsh vibration in the lungs. With a stethoscope, doctors can hear the embedded growling sound coming from the lungs.

Clinical researchers believe that a single sign or symptom is not enough for proper diagnosis.[9] Therefore, when a potential patient or informal caregiver initially believes that lung cancer is present, he or she should consult with a physician who is attentative enough to find a group of symptoms to identify the disease process. A patient initially suspecting lung cancer must therefore be cooperative and should reveal his or her problems to the doctor as soon as possible.

WHAT TO DO IN A CANCER-RELATED EMERGENCY

The term *cancer-related emergency* can be perceived in several different ways: either as an emergency where the patient is told that he or she has cancer or as an emergency where the patient suffers from immediate complications caused by cancer in the body. First, it is vital that the person to whom the bad news of lung cancer is delivered be provided with enough time to digest the diagnosis and then to ask questions relative to the type of cancer, whether it has spread, what treatment options are available, and what his or her prognosis might be. It is a good idea, too, to have a family member or friend present during such discussions with doctors so that notes can be taken and all questions can be covered. It is difficult to maintain composure when such a diagnosis is rendered, so having support available will help. Asking about treatments and what benefits and risks they bring is something that should be done as well.[10] Asking such questions is vital, as it is important that the patient know the benefits and risks, just as it is for the doctor to know the same.[11]

Second, things can be "a bit more complicated" since there are many cancer-related emergencies and complications that may occur, whether speaking in relation to lung cancer or other cell malignancy.[12] Some of those complications include *cardiac tamponade* (mechanical compression of the heart, which limits its functions), *spinal cord compression* (which can cause severe spinal cord damage), and *hypercalcemia* (excessive amounts of calcium in the blood). Each of those complications has its own symptoms and treatments.[13] All are treatable if diagnosed in time but can also cause severe damage to the body, which can also worsen the cancer patient's condition even more. In such an emergency, the attending physician should be contacted immediately and allowed to (1) diagnose the condition promptly and (2) assess why the patient may have contracted such a medical disorder in the first place.

Whenever cancer is the diagnosis, it is important for the patient and his or her family and friends to develop an action plan for approaching the disease and its treatment. In the early stages, questions may revolve around treatment and prognosis. Later, different questions will emerge.

14

NATURAL AND NONPHARMACOLOGICAL LUNG CANCER APPROACHES

The word *natural* exists when something is not artificial and is simply produced by nature. The term *nonpharmacological* refers to therapy that does not make the use of prescription drugs.[1] When it comes to lung cancer treatments, these two terms fall under the umbrella of complementary and alternative medicine (CAM). According to the National Center for Complementary and Alternative Medicine, CAM is really a broad field that includes diverse medical and health care systems, practices, and products that are not considered a part of conventional medicine. This chapter is an examination of CAM and the role it plays in modern-day resolutions for lung cancer.

NATURAL APPROACHES: BENEFITS AND DRAWBACKS

CAM for lung cancer refers to methods and treatments that are not yet practiced in standard medical care.[2] Complementary medical treatments and products are those used alongside conventional treatments or standard practice,[3] while alternative treatments are those used *in place of* standard practice.[4]

Complementary and integrative practices are typically grouped into five categories, according to the National Institutes of Health.[5] These categories are (1) ancient medical systems, which include traditional

Chinese medicine, acupuncture, and Ayurvedic medicine; (2) mind–body methods, which include yoga, meditation, and hypnosis; (3) nutritional methods, which make use of herbs, diets, and supplements; (4) pharmacologic and biologic treatments, which prescribe drugs, herbal medicine, and other products that are not yet generally accepted as cancer treatments; and (5) energy therapies, such as magnetic field therapy.[6]

In a sense, alternative approaches for lung and other types of cancers forgo best practice altogether and make use almost entirely of diet regimens and herbal medicine. Popular examples are as follows:

- Gerson regimen: an organic, vegetarian diet that includes a strict schedule for drinking fruit and vegetable juices
- Macrobiotic diet: a low-fat, vegetarian diet that includes large amounts of complex carbohydrates
- Sun's soup: a mix of select vegetables that are blended, boiled, then freeze-dried, supposedly stimulating the immune system and containing anticancer properties
- Botanicals such as ginseng and green tea, which are also manufactured into pills, liquids, and powders and used as anticancer medicine[7]

When to Go Natural

Although their safety and efficacy are still being determined, the use of CAM methods is steadily increasing.[8] It is worthwhile for lung cancer patients looking into using CAM treatments to consult with their professional caregivers first instead of taking the counsel of friends and family, as is often the case.[9] Studies also show that CAM users, though not dissatisfied with standard practice, find the use of alternative treatments more in line with their personal beliefs and philosophies on life.[10] There are also factors associated with the use of CAM treatments that further urge patients to try it out. These are increased psychosocial stress, being given a less hopeful prognosis, having the feeling of "nothing to lose," and age and gender (i.e., younger versus older or women more than men).[11]

Whatever the reason for choosing CAM, each method has its own effect, especially when paired with standard medical treatments, and thus such methods not always appropriate for every lung cancer sufferer. In order to determine when a particular approach is appropriate, it is necessary to first identify what the treatment can do, how it interacts with standard therapy, and how it affects the lung cancer patient's body. Complementary treatments, for example, are not specific to a particular kind of cancer. Instead, they are used to address general symptoms experienced across different cancer diagnoses since most of these symptoms are a result of treatments rather than the initial diagnosis itself.[12] For example, nausea and vomiting are common side effects of chemotherapy.

Alternative treatments, on the other hand, are completely discouraged by health care professionals when treating lung cancer. Studies show that these treatments are usually invasive and biologically active, meaning that they may have unintended consequences. In most cases, they are found to be unproven or disproved and instead cause further harm to the lung cancer patient.[13]

Effects of Natural Approaches on the Patient

Many studies show several complementary treatments in a good light. A couple of treatments in particular, paired with conventional methods, produced significant results in alleviating cancer symptoms. One such treatment is acupuncture. Acupuncture is typically defined as the process of stimulation using an apparatus, such as *moxibustion* or cone burning, cupping, acupressure, and (most fittingly) needling on certain regions of the body known to be pressure points. In lung cancer, its main use is for symptom management. It is commonly used to treat symptoms such as pain, chemotherapy-induced nausea and vomiting, side effects of radiation therapy, as well as other factors that affect the lung cancer patient's quality of life, such as weight loss, anxiety, and depression, among others.[14] It is highly recommended for pain control, especially when side effects from more conventional methods are too significant or when lessening pain medication becomes a goal.[15] Currently, the efficacy of acupuncture for pain after chest surgery is being studied. In addition, mind–body methods such as massage therapy are also highly recommended for managing anxiety, mood disturbance, and chronic pain, but great care must be taken when performing it near cancer lesions or on patients who just underwent operation.[16]

Another approach that has produced dramatic results is herbal medicine and vitamins integrated with conventional methods. A study showed a dramatic survival rate for stage 3 and stage 4 lung cancer patients who underwent this treatment long term versus those who took it short term and those who continued with conventional methods alone.[17] When it comes to alternative medical treatments, however, results are not as positive. Saint-John's-wort is a plant used as herbal treatment for cancer that was found to make conventional treatments less effective.[18] Meanwhile, macrobiotic diets resulted in further complications for cancer patients caused by weight loss and the diet's restrictive nature.[19] Although using Sun's soup (naturally processed selected vegetables) showed positive effects in studies, the studies themselves were flawed. Therefore, additional research is needed before this treatment becomes a viable alternative solution.[20]

CHANGING THE LOCATION OF LUNG CANCER PATIENT

Geography's Role in Natural Approaches

Physical surroundings have a substantial impact on a person's susceptibility to any kind of clinical disorder. Lung cancer is perhaps the most common ailment directly caused and affected by physical surroundings. Almost all of the top causes of lung cancer can be attributed to a person's environment rather than genetic predisposition. Sometimes not even lifestyle modifications can help, as in the case of lung cancer sufferers who have never smoked in their life. As explained earlier, top causes of cancer are smoking, exposure to radon gas, and exposure to environmental tobacco smoke or secondhand smoke—the latter two being the leading cause of cancer for nonsmokers.[21] All three of these can be found both indoors and outdoors, thus making exposure and subsequent risks higher.

In the United States, some areas are more prone to certain factors over others. For instance, potential indoor radon levels are found to be highest in northern and northeastern states, followed by the West and Midwest, with the southeastern regions having the lowest potential radon count.[22] As such, state and local governments of these areas are urged by the U.S. Environmental Protection Agency to implement radon-resistant building codes. For residents of these high-risk areas, especially those already living with lung cancer, it is important to have homes tested to ensure the least possible exposure and be able to take necessary action in preventing further damage that can be caused by radon gas.[23]

Geography and culture also seem to play major parts in lung cancer incidence and morbidity rates in the United States. A recent study shows an increase in death rates among middle-aged women from southern and midwestern states.[24] The study attributed this to the states' cultural views on smoking, few antismoking laws, and low cigarette taxes.[25] On the other hand, California—the first state to implement a tobacco control program, the first state to have a statewide smoking ban in the workplace, and a state that generally has aggressive tobacco control policies—has steadily decreasing lung cancer death rates among all age groups, ethnicities, and genders.[26]

Hot, Cold, and Clean Air

Weather and climate also have a significant effect on health. Cold air and hot, humid weather are known triggers for breathing problems.[27] Based on a discussion by lung cancer patients online, this can be a major concern, especially for those in the more advanced stages suffering from dyspnea or shortness of breath or those who just underwent major procedures, such as chemotherapy, radiation therapy, and surgery, and still have scarring on the lungs.[28] Air-conditioning and breathing masks are advised to regulate air temperature going into the lungs.[29] Nonetheless, in cases where a patient lives in a climate with extreme weather changes, masks are not enough, and relocation is considered. Doctors say, though, that not any one state or city is best for alleviating breathing problems; reactions to weather and climate are very individualized and vary from person to person. For instance, while some experience better breathing in a more humid climate, others fare better when it is slightly cold. If a lung cancer patient wants to consider relocation, it is advised that he or she does it first on a trial basis to see if the general climate improves this condition.[30]

When it comes to air cleanliness, however, the ideal for all individuals suffering from lung cancer is one and the same: the cleaner the better. Because the disease process could have been caused by some form of air pollution in the first place, it is crucial that further exposure to high levels of polluted air be abated. Again, geography plays a huge part in this in the United States, where some cities have appreciably cleaner air than others. Based on a study by the American Lung Association, the top five cities with the cleanest air are St. George (Utah), Espanola (New Mexico), Cheyenne (Wyoming), Prescott (Arizona), and Farmington (New Mexico).[31] These cities were found to have the lowest levels of year-round particle pollution.[32] The top five cities with the most polluted air, meanwhile, are all found in California: Bakersfield–Delano, Merced, Fresno–Madera, Hanford–Corcoran, and Los Angeles.[33] These cities were found to have unhealthy levels of ozone and high levels of particle pollution.[34] Particle pollution refers to the fixation of very minute solid and liquid particles in the air. The smaller the particles, the more dangerous they become because they get trapped in the lungs and can even be absorbed into the bloodstream.[35] Long-term exposure to high levels of particle pollution decreases lung function[36] and accordingly shortens life expectancy.[37] On the other hand, studies do show that approximately four months can be added to a person's life expectancy due to cleaner air.[38]

On Traveling

As part of a natural and nonpharmacological approach to lung cancer, patients and caregivers should consider certain factors when traveling, first and most importantly, whether traveling is an option at all. It is best for lung cancer patients to consult with their physicians first before making travel plans, especially when what they have in mind involves long distances, foreign countries, and plane rides. Flying is a major travel concern for lung cancer patients. Different symptoms produce different health risks and thus require different kinds of provisions. For instance, the degree of lung damage a patient is suffering can determine how safe it is for him or her to fly. Any degree of *lobular collapse* (when a single lobe of a lung recedes) can become aggravated by lower air pressures and can result in complete lung collapse, also known as *pneumothorax*.[39] Because the air is so much thinner at high altitudes, blood oxygen levels drop, and for people with lung conditions who already have lower levels of blood oxygen, a further drop can be very risky.[40] Air pressure and oxygen levels also cause vomiting and nausea.[41]

Another concern is *deep vein thrombosis* (DVT), which has high incidence rates in lung cancer patients.[42] DVT is a condition where a clot forms in a deep vein. This is usually caused by long periods of immobility or inactivity due to cramped plane space. Although DVT itself causes only discomfort, danger comes when a clot breaks off and flows to the lungs. The resultant material is called a *pulmonary embolus*, and it can cause severe injury or death.[43]

Other factors lung cancer patients might want to think about when traveling are (1) travel insurance; (2) their airline's capacity to accommodate their health needs, such as onboard assistance and oxygen if needs arise; (3) in-flight medical preparations; (4) the services and facilities they could take advantage of at their destination in case of emergency, such as hospitals and doctors; (5) extra medications; and (6) their own overall fitness.[44]

"NATURE" AT ITS BEST

Botanicals and Supplements: How They Work

Herbal medicine, or botanicals, makes use of plants and plant extracts to heal ailments. Some common types of herbal medicine are Chinese (Oriental), Indian (Ayurvedic), and Western (conventional). They may come in the form of topical creams, tablets or capsules, tinctures, or just plain *raw*.[45] These are usually taken to help counteract the side effects of cancer treatments, to alleviate symptoms of cancer, or in an attempt to treat cancer itself.[46]

The names of a couple of plants and herbs consistently appear in relation to botanicals for lung cancer. These are ginseng, green tea, Saint-John's-wort, and *quercetin*.[47] Studies found that ginseng inhibits tumor growth in cancer and has the ability to protect radiation-exposed lymphocytes. It is taken mainly for cancer prevention, as it boosts the immune system and contains antioxidants.[48] However, it is not advised for breast cancer patients, as it may stimulate the growth of breast cancer cells.[49] Another herb used to prevent cancer is green tea. When it is steamed at high temperatures, it produces molecules called *polyphenols*. These are believed to prevent inflammation, protect the cartilage, lessen joint degeneration, and help kill cancerous lung cells as well as stop them from growing.[50] Most tests conducted on the efficacy of green tea for lung cancer have been in trials, and few clinical studies show decisive positive results.[51] This remedy (green tea) is normally taken to help with depression, and lung cancer patients may turn to it for the same reason.[52] Saint-John's-wort is proven to interact with cancer drugs—such as *irinotecan*, *docetaxel*, and *imatinib*—making the three less effective.[53]

Quercetin is part of a plant pigment class known as *flavonoid*, which is what give fruits and vegetables their color. Flavonoids are known antioxidants. In animal testing, quercetin shows the ability to inhibit cancer cells in tumors. Although studies so far show the potency of quercetin in treating lung cancer, more conclusive research is still needed.[54]

Diet and Lung Cancer

Scientific evidence demonstrates that a high-fat diet is linked to lung cancer.[55] Conversely, nutrition is one neglected aspect affecting lung cancer patients facing malnourishment, and changes in eating habits can add up to fatigue and loss of energy. A well-balanced diet needs to be strictly followed even if fluctuations to nutrient levels occur. The benefits of a good nutrition plan will aid in coping with treatment side effects and allow for a faster recovery. The body's defenses benefit from proper nutrition in order to fight infection in all stages of the disease. All efforts should be focused on consuming a variety of healthy foods along with a supervised routine of physical activity to strengthen muscles and compensate for the damage caused by lung cancer management. Should the patient suffer from lack of appetite associated with nausea, it might be wise to take the following pointers into consideration:

- Before treatment, consume light meals and drinking plenty of liquids.
- After treatment, drink small amounts of liquid.
- Avoid foods that upset the stomach.
- Have frequent snacks rather than large meals.
- Eat slowly and chew well.

Nausea and vomiting induced by chemotherapy are some of the most disturbing symptoms experienced, but fortunately the incidence of such problems can be predicted beforehand by monitoring side effects and prescribing medicine prior to each round of treatment. Anxiety-alleviating medication can be prescribed to prevent anticipatory nausea. Vomiting can be avoided by noting the following:

- For cases of ceaseless vomiting, taking small sips of liquid and repeating that several times a day
- Introducing solid food into the digestive system gradually
- Getting back to normal dieting as soon as possible while avoiding fried and fatty food
- Avoiding constipation by eating fiber from bread, whole grain, pasta, fruit, and vegetables
- Having apples, prunes, or pear juice
- Drinking plenty of liquids to help digestion
- Getting some light exercise
- Eating several smaller meals throughout the day
- Eating potassium-rich foods, such as bananas, potatoes, and peaches
- Avoiding spicy greasy food, gravies, and sauces
- Avoiding unnecessary dairy products
- Avoiding citrus and chocolate

Weight loss is a symptom that may progress during the course of the disease and make the respiratory patient become anxious and self-conscious about his or her physical appearance. Poor appetite, mouth sores, difficulty swallowing, cough, shortness of breath, depression, sore mouth, and esophagitis all contribute to weight loss and should be carefully managed by the health care team. Should the weight loss be significant, the appetite must be stimulated with the use of medications such as *dexamethasone*, *megestrol*, and *prednisone*. It is important not to increase the intake of fat and instead consume foods rich in vitamins, minerals, carbohydrates, and proteins. Lung cancer may cause muscle loss, which can be improved by a healthy diet and, in more formidable cases, through the administration of anabolic steroids.

Great nutrition also helps in dealing with cancer-related stress. Due to treatments and medications, it may be difficult to maintain proper nutrition if patients have side effects such as loss of appetite or nausea and vomiting. A healthy diet can boost the lung cancer patient's strength, which is especially needed during treatment cycles. In general, nutritionists recommend that cancer patients eat a wide variety of healthy foods and drink plenty of liquids. People with cancer are often advised to increase their protein and fat intake. Protein intake is important during treatment since proteins provide the building blocks for repairing normal tissues that have been injured as a side effect of therapy. Proteins are also essential for healing after lung cancer surgery.[56]

The patient may speak with their caregiver to customize his or her diet to include supplements. The doctor can advise the patient about diet; he or she may also refer the patient to a dietitian or nutritionist for dietary questions and needs. The diet may be adjusted several times during the course of the illness, depending on where the patient is with the treatments and what symptoms he or she is experiencing. Although it is believed that diets high in fruits and vegetables reduce the risk of cancer, the efficacy has actually been disproved.[57] Significant risk reduction applies only for lung and bladder cancer and only for a fruit-rich diet.[58] Even then, the results may also be attributed to lifestyle factors, such as smoking habits, alcohol intake, and physical activity.[59]

Another diet regimen is called the macrobiotic diet, consisting mainly of eating whole grains and cooked vegetables and avoiding the toxins that come from meats, dairy products, and oily food.[60] It has resulted in more complications in some patients because of the weight loss it may cause.[61] Its earlier versions were thought to be so restrictive that it caused malnutrition and, in some cases, death in the patients practicing it.[62] Although its proponents endorse it as a viable alternative treatment to conventional medicine, studies show that these claims are unfounded. Neither does this diet have any proven benefits as a complementary treatment to standard practices.[63]

A well-balanced diet is recommended for those already undergoing cancer treatments. Despite loss of appetite caused by some treatments, continuing to eat is a must to get adequate nutrition. Certain foods also lessen side effects and can ease the discomforts that come with treatment. Freshness and cleanliness also become a concern for the lung cancer patient since the immune system is already weak, and a little food contamination can escalate into something much worse.[64]

A Cautionary Word or Two about Diets

Antioxidant vitamins are not definitely proved to have a 100 percent protective role, though some evidence shows vitamin C and E have some benefits.[65] In some cases, supplemental (not dietary) antioxidant intake may in fact increase the cancer risk in smokers. Three independent trials among the high-risk population groups, including smokers and persons subject to asbestos exposure (*Beta-Carotene and Retinol Efficacy Trial*, *ABC Cancer Prevention Study*, and *Physicians' Health Study*), have concluded that there is no protective effect of beta-carotene, retinol, and *alpha-tocopherol* intake.[66] Moreover, the results pointed to an increased mortality rate among participants taking supplements. Dietary habits, particularly the intake of saturated fats, may also represent lung cancer risk factors. The risk rises as a result of eating red meat, dairy products and saturated fats, lipids in general, and cholesterol.[67]

EXERCISE FOR APPROACHING LUNG CANCER NATURALLY

What Exercise Does

Following a regular fitness routine positively affects a lung cancer sufferer's physiology. Studies show that exercising improves cardiorespiratory function; increases levels of high-density lipoprotein, or "good" cholesterol; improves blood pressure and bone density; decreases insulin need; and improves the body's glucose tolerance. Exercise also positively affects the lung cancer sufferer's psychological well-being.[68]

According to investigators, the beneficial effect of the higher physical activity is associated with improvement in pulmonary function and ventilation in active compared to inactive individuals. The improved lung efficiency might reduce the time that cancer-causing substances spend in the lung as well as lower their concentration. A positive consequence of regular exercise is also attaining a body weight that is within healthy limits.[69]

Solid clinical research demonstrates a boost in physiological effect for lung cancer patients who exercise.[70] With exercise, the body works more efficiently. A better *cardiorespiratory* (heart and lung) function means that oxygen is being absorbed into the bloodstream and being transported to working muscles with more productivity. Here, the oxygen is used in the metabolic processing of energy. Better flow of oxygen in the blood (an already-diminished function in lung cancer) helps make a person feel less winded or out of breath. This makes him or her more capable of performing tasks that those who never perform exercise would normally find challenging, such as climbing the stairs or taking long walks uphill.[71] Improved glucose tolerance results in the body's ability to better handle sugars broken down from food or glucose. This means that the glucose levels in the body are just right and are more efficiently used for energy or converted into fat, which happens to be the body's store of energy.[72] Basically, exercise improves the body's functionality, making it more efficient when performing fundamental processes.

Exercises for Survivors

For lung cancer survivors, preventing cancer from recurring becomes a primary goal. Recent studies show that exercise plays a significant part in this as well. Not only does exercise help prevent lung cancer, but it also helps keep cancer from coming back. Moreover, a higher level of physical activity reduces the risk of recurrence, but it also helps in longer survival after cancer diagnosis. This is largely due to exercise keeping the patient's body lean, the muscles strong, and the weight in check. Exercise also improves functionality in organs, especially the lungs, and it helps make various physiological processes more efficient.[73]

Best Exercise for Lung Cancer Patients

While the benefits of exercise for cancer in general have been widely studied, research specific to lung cancer is still not as abundant. Unlike breast or prostate cancer, lung cancer is not often discovered early and has higher mortality rates, making studies on the benefits of exercise scarce. Initial studies investigate the effects of aerobic exercises for lung cancer patients.[74] Weight training or resistance training has also been looked into.[75]

These kinds of exercises target two things in lung cancer patients. Aerobic-based training involves exercises that increase heart rate and lung function. Examples are walking, jogging, and swimming. This is geared to improving a patient's lung capacity and breathing. Improved lung functionality then translates into coping better during treatments. Another issue addressed by exercise is the high level of fatigue patients experience after treatment. Because of extreme tiredness, lung cancer patients have the tendency to not move much, unfortunately letting their muscles waste away. Moderate weight training or resistance training makes use of weights to condition muscles and keep them strong. It also helps with lung function.[76]

Studies on the effects of various types of exercises, especially aerobic-based exercises, resistance training, and walking, have been performed. Peak oxygen consumption, perhaps the most telling factor of cardiorespiratory fitness, is a result of these exercises. It was found to abate treatment-related symptoms and to help improve the patient's general quality of life.[77]

Although studies show that aerobic training is helpful to lung cancer patients, improvements are only moderate at best. This could be due to poor oxygen delivery in some patients who participate in aerobic training in poorly ventilated areas as well as muscle weakness and deconditioning from the lack of physical activity in relation to other, more strenuous forms of exercise. Resistance training, meanwhile, has positive effects on patients. Apart from improving muscle function and strength, it also improves a patient's oxygen consumption. However, just like aerobic exercises, its improvements are only moderate. Researchers believe that a combination of aerobic and resistance training may be best in improving a patient's oxygen consumption and lung functionality. The combined exercises will result in better oxygen delivery and processing in the body and more muscle strength, leading to higher muscle endurance, less fatigue, and stronger lungs overall.[78] One study documented the effects of exercise on lung cancer patients by using the *incremental shuttle walk test* and the *endurance shuttle walk test*. On completion, there was significant improvement in the patients' ability to perform the tests. However, no significant improvements in quality of life were reported.[79]

Making the Right Choice

There are two types of exercises that clinical researchers are looking into for lung cancer patients.[80] The first is aerobics. The term *aerobics* literally means "with oxygen." These are exercises that elevate lung function and heart rate, where breathing regulates the amount of oxygen muscles receive in order to help them burn energy.[81] Common aerobic exercises are walking, jogging, swimming, and biking.[82] Aerobics is helpful to lung cancer patients because it improves cardiorespiratory fitness, elevates lung capacity, and helps make cardiovascular processes more efficient.[83]

A category of exercise commonly prescribed for lung cancer patients is resistance training or weight training. Resistance training refers to exercises that put the muscles against an external force or resistance, with the goal of increasing their strength, mass, or endurance. Resistance can be anything ranging from weights, body weight, or any other object that causes the muscles to contract.[84] Although it does not really make huge improvements in fitness for healthy adults, it is beneficial to lung cancer patients because it helps strengthen and condition muscles that may have been weakened by treatments and its symptoms.[85]

When to Exercise

Although lung cancer may be restrictive in terms of physical activities, studies show that exercise during treatment can be beneficial to patients; it may even be more effective at this stage than after treatment.[86] Through research conducted in the United States, two groups of patients were given exercise programs involving aerobic training, resistance training, and a nutritional regimen. One group underwent the program while attaining treatment, while the other group underwent it after treatment. Although symptoms of fatigue and dyspnea improved for both groups, the score for those who exercised during treatment was far more significant than the other group.[87]

There is no single-best, ubiquitously advised routine for all lung cancer patients. One study conducted by Duke University researchers used individualized routines for its participants and found their adherence rates very significant.[88] In the end, lung cancer experts say that it is not the routine that is most important; rather, it is getting up and starting something, even for just short periods or for minimal regimens.[89]

Physical Activity and Lung Cancer Demographics

The National Cancer Institute defines physical activity as body movement caused by the musculoskeletal system or, more specifically, by the skeletal muscles. It is a component of "energy balance," which refers to how weight, diet, and physical activity influence health, including the risk of lung cancer. A significant number of studies have been done all over the world regarding the effects of physical activity on cancer risk, prevention, abatement of symptoms during treatment, and even mortality rates after undergoing treatment. Although gender-specific studies record different rates of cancer risk between men and women in relation to the amount of physical activity and its intensity, most studies show that physical activity plays a major part in reducing cancer risk.[90]

In an experiment involving men aged 40 to 59, the intensity of physical activity revealed an inverse relation to cancer risk. It was found that risk was significantly reduced only in men who engaged in moderately vigorous or vigorous activities; men who engaged in no, light, or light to moderate activities did not experience this benefit.[91] When it comes to women, high levels of physical activity reduce the risk of lung cancer as well. Studies show that risks are significantly reduced among current smokers and former smokers who engage in physical activity. However, there is no significant difference in women who never smoked.[92] The relationship between age, physical activity, and cancer risk has not been as widely considered. Lung cancer incidence is highest among people aged 70 and above and lowest among people aged 40 and below.[93]

SURGICAL RESECTION, CRYOTHERAPY, AND LASER THERAPY AS NONPHARMACOLOGICAL APPROACHES

Surgical Resection

Surgical resection is usually the treatment of choice for patients in the early stages of the non–small cell lung cancer described in chapter 9.[94] This means that the cancer is still of a controllable size and has not yet spread further in the lungs or to other parts of the body.[95] In this scenario, surgical resection may be the first kind of treatment prescribed. It may also be received by patients after chemotherapy or radiation therapy has shrunken down the tumor. Undergoing this procedure usually depends on the size of the cancer, its position in the lung, and whether it has spread to the opposite lung or other parts of the chest or is very near the heart, windpipes, esophagus, or major blood vessels.[96] It is not performed on patients with small cell lung cancer because this type of cancer has usually spread by the time it is diagnosed and thus cannot be treated with surgery alone.[97]

There are several methods of surgical resection. One is the *wedge resection*. This procedure removes a wedge-shaped section from a lobe in the lung, including healthy tissues surrounding the tumor. Another is a *segmentectomy*, or segment resection, which removes a larger portion from the lobe than a wedge resection. These two procedures are usually preferred when doctors think that the cancer has been diagnosed early and is only in a small region of the lung. These are also preferred when doctors think that *lobectomy* (removal of a whole lobe) could impair the patient's breathing and lung functionality. This is the most common type of surgery for lung cancer and is recommended when the cancer is situated in only one section of the lung. Finally, there is *pneumonectomy*—a nonpharmacological technique that removes an entire lung. This is recommended when the cancer has spread in either the two lobes of the left lung or the three lobes of the right. The size and location of the tumor, as well as the patient's lung functionality, usually determine which method is most appropriate.[98] Studies show that although overall survival rates for lung cancer patients are quite low, a common factor for survivors is surgical resection, thus making it a viable and effective first treatment.[99]

Cryotherapy

Cryotherapy or cryosurgery is a procedure where cancer cells are destroyed through freezing. This method is used to treat patients with advanced lung cancer, where surgery is no longer a viable or effective option.[100] Cryotherapy makes use of liquid nitrogen or argon gas that flows through a thin, insulated tube.[101] The medical personnel then puts a probe, called a *cryoprobe*, on the tumor and freezes the cells.

The process can be repeated a couple of times in one area, letting the frozen tissue thaw just enough to remove the cryoprobe, before moving on to freeze the next affected area. Once the procedure is completed and the entire area has been treated, the frozen tissue is extracted using forceps or the cryoprobe itself. [102]

Cryotherapy has common side effects. It causes pain in the treatment area and will require patients who underwent it to go on painkillers for a couple of days. It may also result in coughing up blood or bleeding as well as coughing up tumor tissues right after therapy, difficulty breathing, or a change in heartbeat. One rare side effect of this treatment, on the other hand, is the development of a *fistula*. A fistula is a bridge in the lungs joining the air passage and the *esophagus* (food pipe). [103] Other, more extreme complications include *pneumothorax* (lung collapse), pulmonary infection, and pleural effusion, or the accumulation of excess fluid surrounding the lungs. [104]

Studies on the effects of cryotherapy on lung cancer patients generally show it in good light. A clinical study conducted in China resulted in considerable survival rates spanning one to three years. In vitro studies also show that cryotherapy of lung cancer cells helps improve the immune system in triggering anticancer responses. [105] This procedure also helps abate lung cancer symptoms, such as coughing and dyspnea, or shortness of breath. [106]

Laser Therapy

Laser therapy is a kind of treatment that makes use of laser beams, or narrow beams of high-intensity light, to kill cancer cells. [107] The word *laser* actually stands for "Light Amplification by Stimulated Emission of Radiation." Unlike regular light, laser has a specific wavelength and can be focused into a narrow beam. This beam is so powerful that it has the ability to cut through steel. Because of its power and precision, laser is a great tool for surgery. [108] In cancer, lasers are normally used to shrink or destroy tumors. They are most commonly used on cancers on the surface of the body or on the lining of internal organs. They are also sometimes used to relieve symptoms such as bleeding and obstruction. [109] In lung cancer therapy, lasers are administered with the use of a thin, lighted tube called an endoscope. It contains optical fibers that transmit light and is used to look at tissues inside the body. It is then inserted through an opening and then aimed to cut or destroy a tumor.[110]

There are three types of lasers used in lung cancer treatments. Carbon dioxide laser can cut tissues without causing much bleeding when its light energy changes to heat. It is usually used to treat superficial cancers, where going into deeper layers of the body is not needed. Another variety of laser is the *argon* (an element) *type*. Like carbon dioxide, it cannot penetrate deep into tissues and is used in treating superficial cancers. It is also commonly used in photodynamic therapy, a type of laser therapy that makes use of light-sensitive drugs to kill cancer cells. Finally, there is neodymium:-yttrium-aluminum-garnet (Nd:YAG). Unlike the previous two types, this laser can penetrate deep into lung tissues. It is applied with the use of an endoscope into areas of the body that are more difficult to reach.[111]

There are also two types of laser therapy. First is *laser-induced interstitial thermotherapy*. This procedure makes use of heat to shrink and kill tumors containing cancer cells. Another type of therapy is photodynamic therapy. In this method, a drug classified as a *photosynthesizing* agent is injected into the patient's bloodstream. This drug stays longer on cancer cells than it does on normal cells. A certain kind of light is then shined on the drug, causing a chemical reaction that eradicates lung cancer cells.[112]

Like all other methods, laser therapy has its "pros and cons." It is more precise than the usual surgical tools, such as scalpels. It is also less intrusive on the body. These result in faster healing time and shorter operation time; it can even be as fast as an outpatient (chapter 8) procedure. Nevertheless, only a few doctors and nurses specialize in laser therapy for lung cancer. Equipment is also bulky, costly, and not yet streamlined, making this method comparatively expensive. The effects of laser may also not last long, meaning that it has to be repeated to reach its maximum efficacy.[113]

In the end, one must understand that although the road to treating lung cancer may be long and arduous, it is not lacking in natural and nonpharmacological options and partial means to become well. Patients have a choice the whole way on how to handle themselves using alternative means, from lifestyle changes to location to levels of fitness, before even reaching the critical decisions of which conventional treatment method to take. More and more ways to cure cell malignancy and to cope with treatments are emerging. With studies reporting positive re-sults, patients are being offered a wider selection of techniques that will help them to deal better with lung cancer.

15

PHARMACOLOGICAL LUNG CANCER APPROACHES

The magnitude of lung cancer in the world today has pushed forward the efforts of diagnosis into opening new alternatives for treatment, especially in the field of *pharmacology* (in this case, conventional medication). With the diligent efforts made by today's best medical teams, knowledge regarding the dynamics of pharmacological lung cancer approaches has been broadened. This has paved the way for the introduction of various drug-related treatment options, all of which have been geared to eliminating unhealthy and malignant cells in the lung cancer patient's body. These pharmacological lung cancer approaches, including other related aspects, are addressed in this chapter.

LUNG CANCER PRESCRIPTION TREATMENTS: BENEFITS AND DRAWBACKS

Benefits

In modern times, advances in medicine have made certain types of complex pharmacological treatments more effective in the treatment of cancer. Several prescription treatments for lung cancer have been proven to have beneficial effects, and many patients have shown great chances of recovery through prescription treatment. It is important to remember that the effect of the type of prescription treatment on the patient depends on the severity of the lung cancer itself.

Moreover, the effectiveness of a particular prescription treatment may vary according to the biological nature of the patient or the severity of his or her lung cancer condition. Prescription treatments have been shown to slow the growth of cancer cells. Such drug treatments may provide long-term positive results, depending on the severity of the cancer.[1]

The pharmacological approach also prevents patients from undergoing any form of drastic surgical operations that might lead to radical changes in the body, such as surgical removal of the mass or major incisions. Moreover, patients and their caregivers can read about the various medications and their trials to determine their side effects, their efficacy, and any other risks or benefits that taking such drugs may entail. Also, various types of drugs that work in different ways may be available, so patients and doctors together can decide which might work best.

While chapter 14 promotes the use of natural treatments, one must understand that alternative treatments for lung cancer, such as acupuncture or herbal treatments, *according to some standards*, lack the proper scientific study to back up their effectiveness. Most evidence for their effectiveness is anecdotal—from patients and doctors who have seen positive effects but have not conducted research on overall effectiveness. Moreover, these alternative treatments have been found to relieve only the symptoms of lung cancer and do not directly cure the cancer. By comparison, pharmacological treatment provides a higher survival rate compared to alternative options.[2]

Drawbacks

Due to the relatively high potency of the drugs administered in treating lung cancer, the patient should be ready for an onslaught of side effects traceable to the conventional prescription drug. These unpleasant side effects, which include nausea, vomiting, or lack of energy, may then result in susceptibility to infection and problems in blood clotting. For obvious reasons, side effects can be scary to a lung cancer patient, as they might include loss of hair, mouth sores, mental fogginess, disorientation, and even diarrhea or constipation for patients undergoing chemotherapy sessions. The seriousness of the side effects can vary, but even mild symptoms can cause concern and should be discussed with a doctor.

Although chemotherapy remains an important part in the treatment of lung cancer, it cannot by itself be considered a cure. Each patient and each doctor team should weigh the benefits of chemotherapy before embarking on what can be a grueling treatment approach. In addition, the cost of chemotherapy can be high. Based on a statistic on the total expense incurred for lung cancer patients administering prescription treatment, an initial treatment cost could be around $26,000.[3] This does not include the maintenance cost per year, which is at least $11,300.[4] Considering the current rate of inflation, this figure will probably almost double. This is also why most patients might prefer alternative methods.[5]

Despite the efficacy of these pharmacological treatment methods for lung cancer, there are some long-term side effects to be seriously considered. In some instances, side effects brought about by these pharmacological approaches may not appear for months or years after treatment has been done. These long-term effects may include kidney problems, nerve damage, or even heart problems. Despite the effectiveness of the drug, its level of toxicity should be seriously considered, as that may cause adverse damage to the individual suffering from lung cancer.

NATURE OF PRESCRIPTION LUNG CANCER DRUGS

The following sections discuss various lung cancer drugs and their corresponding indications, mechanisms of action, and side effects. One should note that the potency of each of these drugs varies in each person and the severity of the lung cancer malignancy. Therefore, it is imperative that any lung cancer patient, after having undergone the necessary test screenings and examinations, consult with his or her doctor about the appropriate prescription treatment option based on several vital factors. These factors include the overall health condition of the patient and also the cancer condition, especially its type and stage. Due to its complexity on several fronts, treatment for lung cancer might include one drug or a combination of several pharmacological drugs. For clarity's sake, the various prescription lung cancer medications are dealt with here according to the two main classifications of lung cancer: non–small cell lung cancer and small cell lung cancer.

PRESCRIPTION TREATMENTS FOR NON–SMALL CELL LUNG CANCER

Gefitinib

Gefitinib is a chemotherapy agent used for the treatment of non–small cell lung cancer that may be advanced in a local area of the body or metastasized throughout some portions of certain organs. This medication may also be used for other lung-related conditions as prescribed by the doctor. It specifically functions by blocking a protein enzyme in the body called *tyrosine kinase*, which immobilizes pathogens or corrects any functional system that is not working properly. Gefitinib thus helps prevent cancer cells from spreading to other areas and from growing en masse. Because gefitinib is a chemotherapy agent, side effects may include weight loss, vomiting, blurred visions, mouth sores, diarrhea, acne, nausea, and general weakness. Severe effects may include tightness in the chest, dizziness, yellowing of the skin or eyes, and swelling of any part of the body. These effects may be caused by allergic reactions to the drug.[6]

Erlotinib

Erlotinib is usually used for treating late stages of lung cancer that is already advanced or metastasized to other areas of the body. The medication is taken after a prior chemotherapy session has failed or has not worked in the body. Like gefitinib, it is a tyrosine kinase inhibitor, and thus the side effects of gefitinib are the same as those of erlotinib. Erlotinib is an improved version of gefitinib, as lung cancer patients have reacted more positively with erlotinib than they have with the previous drug.[7]

Bevacizumab

Bevacizumab is indicated for treating advanced cases of lung cancer. In addition, it is used to treat other types of cancer, such as rectal, brain, or kidney cancer. It may also be utilized as treatment for other conditions as per a doctor's prescription. This drug contains monoclonal antibody, which works by blocking the *vascular endothelial growth factor*, which is responsible primarily for the stimulation of angiogenesis, defined in chapter 2. The drug suppresses the development of new blood vessels in the tumor, thus slowing or halting the spread of cancer cells. Adverse effects from administering this drug include general weakness, hypertension, abdominal pain, damaged skin, vomiting, fatigue, constipation, and discomfort in the abdominal area. It may also cause various adverse chemical reactions to the body.[8]

Paclitaxel

Paclitaxel is also a chemotherapy agent that is indicated for the treatment of non–small cell lung cancer. It is also indicated for the treatment of other cancers, such as breast cancer and others as determined by the physician. Like the previously mentioned drugs, paclitaxel is a chemotherapeutic medicine. It is considered a mitotic inhibitor, meaning that it stops mitosis (cell division) in the body, thus disrupting the growth and spread of malignant cells. The most persistent side effects brought about by this drug are cough, hair loss, joint and muscle pain, mouth sores, vomiting, and general weakness. Other side effects may include numbness as well as severe allergic reactions.[9]

Protein-Bound Paclitaxel

This type of paclitaxel is indicated for the treatment of non–small cell lung cancer and breast cancer. It is also considered as an aid for ovarian cancer, head-related cancers, and even Kaposi's sarcoma, a virus-associated tumor. Protein-bound paclitaxel is a cytoskeletal type of chemotherapy drug that functions to stop the further development of *tubulin*, a protein in the cell responsible for the growth of mitosis, hence suppressing the development of cancer cells originating from the respiratory system. Side effects of taking paclitaxel may range from minor to serious conditions, such as nausea, constipation, diarrhea, discoloration of the nails and skin, hair loss, general weakness, numbness, jaundice, unexplained bleeding, and even seizures.

Pemetrexed

Pemetrexed is another type of chemotherapy drug in the class of *folate antimetabolites* (iron-based substances that interfere with cellular metabolism). It is indicated for the treatment of certain non–small cell lung cancer and is also used to treat *pleural mesothelioma* (chapter 4). Chemically, its composition is similar to that of folic acid, which works by restraining certain enzymes in the formation of RNA and DNA. Both are vital in the continued existence of both cancerous and normal cells. Side effects of this drug include diarrhea, skin rash, constipation, nausea, vomiting, mental and physical fatigue, and mouth ulcers.[10]

Cisplatin

Cisplatin is indicated for the treatment of small cell lung cancer, ovarian cancer, and other sarcomas and carcinomas. It is also used to counter cancers of the ovaries, testes, and bladder. It functions as a more developed *alkylating agent* wherein it binds with DNA, thus affecting its replication and stopping the spread of cancer cells. It also binds with mitochondrial cells, thereby hindering its development. This drug may sometimes bring about kidney-related problems and allergic reactions. Common side effects include vomiting, extraordinary tiredness, fever, palpitation, unexplained bruises and sores, diarrhea, and even constipation.[11]

Porfimer

Porfimer is used for non–small cell lung cancer and esophageal cancer's symptoms or other esophagus-related conditions. To be effective, this drug should be exposed to laser light so that it can properly bind to cancerous cells. Porfimer is an antineoplastic, which inhibits the growth of neoplastic cells that are normally a part of lung tumor, thus stopping the development of cancer. The administration of this drug can bring about harsh allergic reactions, trouble sleeping, fever, general and mental fatigue, loss of appetite, diarrhea, swelling, and even weight loss.[12]

Vinorelbine

Vinorelbine is indicated for the treatment of advanced non–small cell lung cancer through either a combination or a single agent. It can also be used as a treatment for breast cancer that has already metastasized after a failure of the primary chemotherapy session. Vinorelbine is a type of *vinca alkaloid*, a semisynthetic that binds to tubulin and stops the progress of microtubule formation, inhibiting the continuous growth of cancer cells. The drug stops the process of cell mitosis, thereby preventing cancer cells from dispersing. Vinorelbine has various adverse side effects, including chest pain, back pain, dizziness, fatigue, skin color discoloration, shortness of breath, headache, muscle weakness, hypersensitivity, nausea, and even hearing defects.[13]

Methotrexate

Methotrexate is also a chemotherapy drug that can be administered alone or through a combination of other chemotherapy drugs. It is indicated for the treatment of various cancers, including both small and non–small cell lung cancer, breast cancer, leukemia, and head- and neck-related cancers. It is also used as an indication for psoriasis in its severe stages and even rheumatoid arthritis. Generally, it has a cytotoxic function that inhibits growth during the DNA and RNA synthesis of cells in the body. The drug is amply toxic to the process of cell division and thereby causes the death of malignant tumor cells. It produces a number of side effects, including dizziness, ulcers, vomiting, stomatitis, low white blood cell count, nausea, bleeding, skin discoloration, and kidney-related diseases.[14]

Capecitabine

Capecitabine is indicated for the treatment of non–small cell lung cancers and some other types of rectal cancers, breast cancers, and colon cancers. It works by impeding the creation of proteins in the body necessary for the proliferation and development of cancer cells. On the basis of its function, it is an *antimetabolite* (blocks metabolism). However, its administration should be carefully monitored, as it may cause excessive bleeding, especially when taken with *anticoagulative* (anticlotting) agents. It may also cause peeling of the skin with redness, skin tenderness, vomiting and nausea, pain throughout the body, and irritation in the eyes.

Cyclophosphamide

Cyclophosphamide is also a chemotherapy drug that is used for the treatment of non–small cell lung cancers, ovarian cancers, lymphoma, immune system–related diseases, and other disorders and conditions as prescribed by the doctor. Like porfimer, it is an antineoplastic that hinders the growth of neoplastic cells. It has severe side effects, such as hair loss, suppression of bone marrow, kidney-related diseases, darkening of the skin and nails, vomiting and nausea, severe stomachache, and other side effects that may be brought about by a chemotherapy drug.[15]

Crizotinib

Crizotinib is indicated primarily for the treatment of non–small cell lung cancer that may have metastasized or advanced locally. It may also be used to treat other conditions and diseases as may be advised by a professional caregiver, such as a doctor. It inhibits tyrosine kinases, which are also responsible for the survival of the tumors and ultimately hinder the reproduction of malignant cells all throughout the body. Side effects on taking this drug include fatigue, skin rashes, abdominal pain, edema, dizziness, various infections in the upper respiratory tract, severe abdominal pain, and general weakness.[16]

Docetaxel

Docetaxel has the same indications as the previous drugs and is used for treatment of non–small cell lung cancer and even breast cancer that may have metastasized or advanced locally. It is also an antineoplastic agent that inhibits the proper development of RNA and DNA in the cell caused by the developmental restraint of tubulin. This is responsible for the cell growth and development of cancer cells in the body. Severe side effects include various infections, skin rashes, nail and skin discoloration, fever, nausea and dizziness, diarrhea, hair loss, liver-related diseases, and low white blood cell count, which may be considered fatal to the lung cancer sufferer.[17]

Amifostine

Amifostine is used as treatment for non–small cell lung cancers. It is also used to lessen damage to the kidney from a chemotherapy-induced session, particularly using the drug cisplatin. It may also be used to lessen the side effects brought about by radiation treatment. As opposed to other cytotoxic drug agents, amifostine is a *cytoprotective* (protects cells) *agent* that removes the toxins in platinum and alkylating agents in the cell. It also detoxifies free radicals—cancer cells included. The effect is the acceleration of the reparative function of the DNA. However, adverse effects are also noted, including vomiting, nausea, skin rashes, mouth sores, chest pains, severe tiredness, and, in rare cases, loss of consciousness.[18]

Cetuximab

Cetuximab is indicated for the treatment of non–small cell lung cancers. It may also be used for the treatment of certain types of colorectoral, head-related, and neck-related cancers. In certain cases, it may be used in other conditions as prescribed by a doctor. Like bevacizumab, this pharmacological substance contains monoclonal antibody, which works by binding itself to certain growth factor receptors responsible mainly for the cell division in the body. Since certain cancers cause rapid cell division through these receptors, cetuximab deactivates this receptor's ability to cause the cell to divide, thus stopping the further development of cancer cells. Side effects of taking cetuximab are loss of appetite, *xeroderma* (dry skin), unexplained general and mental weakness, mouth sores, nausea and vomiting, indigestion, and certain allergic reactions.[19]

Gemcitabine

Gemcitabine is indicated for the treatment of non–small cell lung cancers as well as ovarian, pancreatic, and even breast cancers. Depending on the doctor's prescription, it may also be used to treat other sicknesses and conditions. This drug is also an antimetabolite that inhibits DNA synthesis by affecting *polymerase* and *ribonucleotide reductase*, enzymes generally responsible for the development of cancer cells. It has also its adverse side effects, including blood in the urine, fever, loss of appetite, hair loss, general weakness, discoloration of the skin, flu-like symptoms, difficulty urinating, and other mild to severe allergic reactions.[20]

PRESCRIPTION TREATMENTS FOR SMALL CELL LUNG CANCER

Topotecan

Topotecan is indicated for the treatment of small cell lung cancer, certain types of cancers of the ovary, and other cervical cancers. This may also be used if the patient has not responded positively with other chemotherapy drugs. Topotecan is also an antineoplastic agent that inhibits the proper development of RNA and DNA in the cell caused by the developmental restraint of tubulin, which, in turn, is responsible for the cell growth and development of cancer cells in the body. The intake of topotecan brings about mild side effects, such as hair loss, general tiredness, vomiting, and nausea, and severe side effects, such as shortness of breath, unexplained bleeding, flu-like symptoms, and burning sensation on urinating.[21]

Etoposide

Etoposide is indicated for the treatment of small cell lung cancer and other cancers related to testicular tumors. It may also be used with other chemotherapy drugs as may be prescribed by a doctor. It is also an antineoplastic agent that specifically targets the inhibition of cell mitosis, therefore hindering the proliferation of cancer cells. Possible side effects include loss of appetite, skin and nail discoloration, fever, cough, unexplained bruises, and bleeding in any part of the body. Often, etoposide causes the lung cancer patient to be more susceptible to infections and diseases.[22]

TAKING SIDE EFFECTS OF PHARMACOLOGICAL DRUGS SERIOUSLY

Once a lung cancer patient takes a pharmacological approach, aside from the malignant or cancerous cells, his or her healthy cells may also be affected by these drugs. That is why one should seriously consider taking this route. Although some pharmacological drugs may cause only minor side effects that may not be a serious concern, others present serious health care issues that need to be discussed with a health care provider. Thus, it is wise that these side effects, whether serious or minor, be properly and carefully gauged to determine if the drug's benefit outweigh the risks. Is it worth undergoing the aggravation brought about by these side effects in exchange for the treatment that the drug promises? Is it more burdensome to experience these side effects rather than endure and accept the risk of not receiving the treatment?

The next section covers the undercurrents of side effects brought about by pharmacological drugs and, more importantly, the value that these side effects hold to unlock treatment potential.

Frequent Topics about Lung Cancer Drugs' Side Effects

One must (1) be well aware of why side effects exist in parallel with the prescription treatment and (2) understand the nature of these side effects on different lung cancer patients. The following is a list that patients and caregivers might want to become familiar with.

Side effects may or may not be a consequence of the administering of a particular drug.

A lung cancer patient may experience certain symptoms or signs that may be confused as the primary side effect of the drug but that may be related to some other condition. In certain cases, signs and symptoms may appear as triggered by the occurrence of the cancer itself and not due to the side effects brought about by taking the drug.

Side effects can either be immediate, long term, late, or permanent.

It is a misconception that side effects are always temporary or immediate and that they go away after treatment or after the body has adjusted to the administration of the drug. There are other types of side effects that are long term, persisting months after the patient has taken the drug. Moreover, some side effects appear late and then remain for days or weeks after one has taken the drug. In certain cases, side effects can be permanent, depending on how the patient reacts to the drug.

One should anticipate the occurrence of these side effects.

Certain signs and symptoms brought about by these lung cancer pharmacological medications can be detected earlier after proper consultation with a doctor. One must be able to find a means to alleviate certain minor side effects that are somewhat tolerable, such as vomiting or skin rashes. However, both the patient and the caregiver must know what to do once major side effects are experienced. The lung cancer sufferer needs to have a health care provider ready at all times or at least have easy access to the nearest hospital or clinic.

Unexpected side effects may occur, and there are predicted side effects that are more common.

Some side effects may result from the body's chemical reaction to the drug and are unexpected. This is normal. However, more commonly than not, predicted side effects are more prevalent since most if not all of the side effects can be anticipated on the basis of the drug's mechanism of action in the body. Since certain drugs affect a certain hormone or protein in the body, side effects brought about by these cases can be foreseen.

Side effects may be different for each lung cancer patient.

Side effects are not absolute, but this varies, depending on the patient, his or her lung cancer severity, drug dosage, and the duration of the treatment. Other factors can be considered, such as the current condition of the patient and the individual's tolerance to the drug.[23]

Understanding the Side Effects of Lung Cancer Pharmacological Treatments

Below are the more common side effects of various lung cancer drugs. Although these side effects persist, this sometimes shows simply that the drugs are pharmacologically working as they should.

Bleeding

Medical research confirms that lung cancer causes bleeding in other organs.[24] Irregular bleeding also occurs because certain anticancer drugs may bring about a low platelet count. In addition, some drugs are severe anticoagulants, resulting in this particular side effect. Bleeding may be relieved through blood transfusions, but other remedies, such as *colony-stimulating factors*, will alleviate a low platelet count. To help prevent or minimize this, the lung cancer patient may be advised to avoid any strenuous activities.[25]

Anemia

Some anticancer drugs may affect the accumulation of cells in the bone marrow, resulting in *anemia* (deficiency of red blood cells). This may be unavoidable considering the drug's mechanism of action. Anemia is relieved through blood transfusions, among other techniques, such as getting enough rest, a healthy eating lifestyle, and limiting more strenuous activities.[26]

Low White Blood Cell Count

The main function of white blood cells is to prevent infections from entering the body. However, since anticancer drugs suppress the development and growth of malignant cells, they also wipe out healthy white blood cells that fight sickness. To lessen the condition associated with this side effect, the patient can wash his or her hands often to avoid infection that may not be well fought off when white blood cells are low and take other precautionary, hygiene measures. Moreover, avoiding crowds is preferred to avoid viral infections.[27]

Fatigue

This is the most common side effect brought about by anticancer drugs. This may be considered normal and can be tolerable in some cases through good nutrition, proper stress management, and a caring support group. Proper management of fatigue, on the other hand, should be done by taking frequent naps, drinking plenty of water, and other natural approaches described in the preceding chapter.[28]

Gastrointestinal Problems

The function of most anticancer drugs is to diminish or stop the cells from continuously dividing. Since the cells in the gastrointestinal region, such as the esophagus, stomach, intestines, and mouth, usually go through rapid renewal, they are more likely to be affected by gastrointestinal issues. This may be alleviated through a doctor's prescription for other medications that may counteract these effects.[29]

Constipation

This normally occurs among lung cancer patients who have a history of constipation, which is only aggravated by the administration of a lung cancer drug. Patients who have low fiber intake are also more vulnerable to this side effect. In some cases, patients who are taking other pharmacological substances for pain from lung cancer symptoms may experience constipation. To help with this, one should drink plenty of water and increase fiber intake while consulting with a health care team as to the which fibrous fruits to eat, as some food items may be prohibited during treatment. The doctor may even suggest that the patient take a laxative or another medicine that will soften bowel movements.

Vomiting and Nausea

Normally, the severity of vomiting and nausea varies among lung cancer patients. Moreover, not all anticancer drugs produce this side effect. Some anticancer drugs that directly affect the gastrointestinal tract may be associated with nausea and vomiting. Should this happen, doctors usually prescribe antiemetic drugs.

Malfunction of or Damage to Vital Organs

These are considered among the serious if not fatal side effects brought about by anticancer drugs. Disease of the heart may occur when chemotherapy drugs are utilized with other forms of lung cancer therapy. Symptoms showing the occurrence of related side effects may include swelling of the hands or feet or irregular heartbeat. This should immediately be presented to the health care provider. Kidney disorders may also result from lung cancer drugs. Since the main function of the kidney is to expel toxins from the body in the form of urine, the level of toxicity brought about by these drugs might impair the function of this organ. Signs of damage to the kidney may also include puffiness, pain in the lower back, and change in the color of the patient's urine and the frequency of urination. In most cases, the liver may be greatly affected by the use of anti–lung tumor medications. Patients with a history of liver problems are sometimes encouraged by their physician to minimize the dosage of the drugs that they are taking. Most anticancer drugs get excreted in the *bile* (chapter 3) or are processed in the liver, and certain chemicals in these drugs may be considered harmful. It is recommended that doctors acquire regular blood samples from their patients to determine the current status of liver function.

Hair Loss

Certain anticancer drugs impede the usual development and the increase of cells in the hair follicle area, causing loss of hair in lung cancer patients. However, this is temporary, and the normal growth of hair may continue after the stoppage or the reduction of treatment.[30] Indeed, undergoing lung cancer treatment is arduous, but trying to muddle through with these side effects is a difficult ordeal for many. Pharmacological anticancer approaches, particularly the traditional chemotherapies, work by killing cells that grow and divide rapidly but may destroy healthy hair cells.[31]

NEW BREAKTHROUGHS IN PHARMACOLOGICAL LUNG CANCER DRUGS

On the brighter side, newer methods have been recently proposed to develop a less harmful effect on lung cancer patients. Although it may take years before a certain protein formulation is forwarded from laboratory test tubes to the pharmacy, some researchers have devised some new, nonconventional strategies to combat lung cancer.

Drug That Inhibits Rac-1 Protein

On the basis of information published in an academic journal, a team of scientists from the University of Hawaii discovered and developed an anticancer drug named *BP-1-102*, which inhibits a protein responsible for the growth of certain types of cancer, lung cancer being among those at the top of the list. The protein involved here is named *Stat3*, which, when inhibited by BP-1-102, stops its normal function of generating cancer cells. Moreover, the function of Rac-1 is primarily to boost the molecular cycle of lung tumors (particularly their development and proliferation), and the protein Stat3 actively interacts with Rac-1. The aim of Rac-1 is to create a fresh anticancer drug that is particularly focused on Stat3, which will eradicate tumor formations found mainly in non–small cell lung cancers. The scientists and pharmaceutical agents who are involved with developing this drug are hopeful that it will better combat lung cell malignancy.[32]

Monoclonal Antibodies Combating Cancer Cells Only

A team of clinical investigators at the University of California has found a monoclonal antibody, known as *HB22.7*, that targets a protein complex named *CD22*. The latter is expressed profusely in lung cancer cells. This discovery was nothing short of a miracle, as this test was being done expressly for the treatment of non-Hodgkin's lymphoma. Accordingly, this exciting discovery could bring forth a new method of therapeutic treatment. An initial laboratory test successfully reduced the size of a lung tumor after the administration of HB22.7. Researchers are currently perfecting this drug, so it might soon be introduced to the lung cancer patient population.[33]

Drug That Inhibits the Myc Protein Complex

A biomedical research center named Vall d'Hebron Institute of Oncology, which is composed of renowned principal investigators, scientists, and physicians, has found initial success being able to eradicate cancerous tumors in laboratory rats by inhibiting a certain protein named *Myc*, which functions as a developing agent in many types of tumors, including those of the lung. A more promising result was also noted in that this type of drug has not demonstrated many side effects. A study has shown that the inhibition of Myc is a viable target for the introduction of a newer, better pharmacological drug designed to treat lung cancers and other forms of cancer. Moreover, as per their initial preclinical mouse model, the treatment using this approach was determined to lack any side effects. There is still much work to do before the drug finds its way into therapy, but a big step has been taken to its introduction as a viable and approved anti–lung cancer drug.[34]

CLINICAL TRIALS FOR LUNG CANCER

A fair amount of pharmacological clinical trials are being done by many individuals and organizations throughout the world. Trials are the link between the lung cancer treatment option and the laboratory. Since doctors are choosing candidates for experiments more carefully, the possibility of obtaining positive results is growing with each passing year.[35] Finding a clinical trial is a matter of speaking to a doctor who may already be involved in clinical trials him- or herself or may assist in locating one. It is advisable to ask for a second opinion to be assured that it is a decision that can prove beneficial for the patient.

During a clinical trial, the lung cancer patient may be closely observed and constantly be asked to fill out forms as a way of actively involving him or her with the clinical trial offering the service. While there are downsides of clinical trials (e.g., worsening of the lung cancer patient's condition, unintended side effects, or lack of results), it is important to understand potential benefits, such as those that follow:

- Participants get premium-grade cancer treatment.
- Participants may quit at any time if stipulated by their agreement.

- The trials make participants part of cancer research that may work well.
- New promising treatments are obtained and legalized only in this way.
- Frequent checkups for free.
- The trials empower lung cancer patients to keep fighting the disease process.

Insurance companies usually pay for clinical trials, and in many cases the referring doctor is the one who contacts these companies and arranges all the paperwork to save time.

Indeed, the absolute cure for cancer is still elusive. Despite numerous studies and clinical tests done to find the perfect treatment for lung cancer, researchers, scientists, and the top caregivers still clamor for that faultless pharmacological approach worthy to be considered the cure for cancer. It is true that some lung cancer patients might attest that they have been cured through the use of medications, but that depends on how they define the word *cure*. For the purpose of this book, cancer cure refers to completely removing malignant cells and thus eliminating any possibility of the return of such cell groups.

Proper acclaim and recognition should be given to the field of pharmacology, which has put forth extreme efforts in prolonging the life of the lung cancer patient and improving his or her quality of life. Currently, studies are becoming more focused on targeting the killing of malignant and cancerous cells while sparing normal and healthy cells, thereby reducing the risks involved in the side effects of standard pharmacological therapy. There is hope that better and better treatments will become available and that curing lung cancer will become a reality someday.

16

ADDRESSING THE MENTAL ASPECTS OF LUNG CANCER

Lung cancer is a difficult form of cell malignancy to deal with for the implications, location, and changes brought to patients and their caregivers. Its late detection only makes matters worse. Psychologically, it can be traumatizing to receive this kind of diagnosis, as cancer can be fatal. Of course, physical treatment is necessary to address the disease, but early mental intervention is also necessary to help alleviate the psychological and emotional symptoms a cancer patient will face.[1]

The aftermath of a lung cancer diagnosis triggers a series of negative emotions and mental states that may turn counterproductive to treatment. This chapter aims to provide an overview of the mental and behavioral disorders often associated with a cancer diagnosis and their consequences as well as measures to be taken by the lung cancer patient and caregiver.

MENTAL AND BEHAVIORAL ASPECTS ARISING FROM LUNG CANCER

Stress

Psychological stress alone is not the cause of cancer, but if it lasts for a long period of time, it may affect a person's coping abilities (chapter 18) and overall health. People who are better able to cope with stress have a better quality of life while they are being tended to for lung cancer. It is normal for a person to experience psychological stress at some point in his or her life. People who experience it often, on a daily basis, or over a longer period of time may also develop physical health problems. Stress can be caused by daily responsibilities, by routine events, and maybe even by more unusual events, such as trauma or illness in a patient or a close family member. When people feel that they have lost control over the changes that lung cancer provokes, they are in distress. There is even some evidence that extreme distress is associated with poorer clinical outcomes. Clinical guidelines are available to help doctors and nurses to assess levels of stress and to assist with managing it.[2]

The lung cancer patient's body will respond to physical, mental, or emotional pressure by releasing stress hormones, such as epinephrine and norepinephrine. This increases blood pressure, speeds up the heart rate, and raises blood sugar levels out of physiological necessity. These changes give a person greater strength and speed in order to help him or her escape a perceived threat. Research has shown that people who experience persistent stress manifest side effects such as fertility problems, digestive problems, urinary problems, and a weakened immune system. Chronic stress also leaves people more vulnerable to viral infections, such as the flu or the common cold, and to regular headaches, sleep troubles, depression, and anxiety.[3]

Stress is known to be behind a number of physical health problems, though a direct link to cancer has not been established. Some studies have shown a connection between numerous psychological factors and an increased risk of developing cancer.[4] Obvious connections between psychological stress and cancer can manifest themselves in several ways. For example, people under loads of stress may acquire certain behaviors, such as overeating, smoking, or drinking alcohol, all which can increase the risk for lung cancer in the long run. Someone who has a relative afflicted with malignant cell growth may be exposed to a higher risk of cancer because of a potentially shared, inherited risk factor and not directly because of the mental stress suffered as a by-product of lung cancer diagnosis.[5]

People afflicted with lung cancer may find the emotional, social, and physical effects of the disease to be stressful. Some try to address their stress-related issues with risky behaviors, such as drinking alcohol or smoking, while others become more sedentary. The chances are that these approaches will not work. On the contrary, those who better manage emotional stress using methods such as relaxation and stress management techniques have shown enhanced results, such as lower levels of depression, anxiety, and symptoms related to the cancer and its treatment. Nonetheless, there is no sufficient evidence that successful management of psychological stress can improve lung cancer survival by 100 percent. Results from experimental studies do, however, argue that psychological stress can increase the chances of other tumors' ability to grow and spread.[6] Some experiments have shown that when mice carrying human tumors were kept enclosed or isolated from other mice, creating stressful conditions, they had a greater chance for tumor growth and development.[7] In other experiments, scientists transplanted tumors into the mammary fat pads of mice. When the mice were put under constant stress, there was a much greater chance of metastasis to the lungs and lymph nodes as opposed to mice that were not intentionally placed under duress. Experiments in mouse (and also in human) cancer cells grown in laboratories prove that the stress hormone norepinephrine, which is a part of the body's *fight-or-flight* response system, may encourage tumor angiogenesis and metastasis.

Data suggest that people can regress and show a sense of helplessness or hopelessness when stress becomes overwhelming. This kind of response is correlated with higher rates of death, although the cause for this outcome is unclear. It might be that people who feel hopeless or helpless may unfortunately find themselves to have the following characteristics:[8]

- They do not take any kind of action against the mental stress.
- They do not feel the need to seek treatment when they become ill.
- They give up prematurely or fail to stick to a potentially helpful therapy.
- They engage in unsafe behaviors such as illicit drug use.
- They refuse to maintain a healthy lifestyle, resulting in premature death.

Some organizations recommend that all cancer patients be screened for severe stress early in the stage of treatment. They also recommend rescreening at precise points during the course of care. There are a variety of screening tools available to medical providers—such as a questionnaire or a selective stress scale—to find out if patients need clinical support with managing their emotions or other common concerns. Patients who show mild to strong distress are usually referred to adequate resources, such as a social worker, a clinical health psychologist, a chaplain, or a psychiatrist. Stress management at the personal level, particularly at home, is discussed further in the upcoming chapter.[9]

Posttraumatic Issues from Diagnosis and Treatment

Posttraumatic stress disorder (PTSD) is an extreme psychophysiological response to a painful event. In the context of lung cancer, the diagnosis as well as the risk of dying may cause PTSD to occur at any stage of the disease process. Another possible variation of PTSD related to cancer is the time frame when this traumatic reality begins. Cancer-induced PTSD can be considered bidirectionally traumatic in terms of past and future: reminiscences of a happier past contrasted with a traumatic future and the fear of existing one day and not existing the next. The fact that the culprit is not external but internal and keeps growing and killing healthy cells is another source of traumatizing thoughts that lead to PTSD.[10]

Lung cancer survivors are not safe either, as the fear of disease recurrence, harsh treatments, medication side effects, doctor appointments, and procedures may also cause PTSD to occur. PTSD in turn leads to the following mental symptoms:

- Avoidance of referring to cancer in conversations
- Avoidance of places that remind the lung cancer sufferer of a negative experience
- Difficulty remembering experiences with the disease process
- Lack of interest in activities that would otherwise be enjoyable
- Feeling detached from other people
- False perceptions of a curtailed future with unfinished business left
- Marked anxiety
- Sleep problems caused by bad dreams and nightmares about the condition

- Bad temper
- Numb emotions
- Lack of concentration

Adjustment Disorder

This is characterized by considerable amounts of distress experienced after exposure to stressors or following traumatic life events.[11] Experts in 2006 classified *adjustment disorder* as short term and stress triggered, and scientists have agreed that it is in fact a stress syndrome.[12] The nature of lung cancer and its treatment unfortunately allows for stress to occur throughout the process. Adjustment disorder can negatively impact a person's ability to function in his or her social and occupational environments. As a result, there is an increased dissatisfaction with the ongoing treatment that causes the patient to postpone, end, or completely give up on the lung cancer management. An individual suffering from lung cancer may also refuse to search for treatment altogether.[13]

With adjustment disorder, lung cancer patients could experience anything ranging from fluctuating periods of sadness, anger, despair, uncertainty about the future, guilt, fear of death, and aversion to the possibility of becoming a burden to family members and society. The intensity varies individually, depending on age, culture, personality traits, strengths, weaknesses, gender, experience, and importance assigned to the stressors that initially activated the emotion.[14]

Adjustment disorder may happen at any point during the course of lung cancer treatment and should be given high priority. Interventions have been shown to be very effective in improving psychosocial functioning, perception in quality of life, overall psychological responses, lower morbidity, treatment effectiveness, and fewer relapses.[15]

Depression

Depression, which is present in at least 8 percent of lung cancer cases, is defined as an illness that brings about feelings of sadness and detachment from life. It accounts for the majority of cases of mental disorders reported by mental professionals and affects twice as many women than men.[16] Depression may cause people to experience physical as well as psychological disturbances that cause severe impairment and disability.[17] The most common symptoms of depression found in lung cancer patients are depressive mood, general loss of interest, weight gain or loss, insomnia, lack of response, fatigue, diminished libido, delusions of worthlessness, guilt about being sick (particularly in those who have been heavy smokers), and recurrent thoughts about suicide and end of life. According to a study, depressive disorders are common and persistent in lung cancer patients, being more severe in those with more serious symptoms and physical limitations.[18] The highest incidence has been found in patients in the advanced stages, in older patients, and in those with short survival expectancy.[19] Depression is also more prominent immediately after diagnosis of lung cancer than at the later phases of treatment.[20]

There are several studies that have found a strong association between a higher risk of mortality and depression both before and during treatment.[21] There is also evidence from a study conducted in Japan involving over 1,000 participants that symptoms of depression in lung cancer patients, before the start of treatment, can be mistaken for the clinical symptoms of the disease process.[22] Despite different conclusions and findings, the common ground for all studies is that once the symptoms of lung cancer and depression are assessed by a multidisciplinary medical team, the recovery process returns to its fullest potential and "the sooner the better" to avoid the ultimate consequence of major depressive illness: suicide.[23]

Signs of depression in a lung cancer sufferer may include the following:

- Feeling helpless or hopeless or that life itself has no meaning
- Showing no interest in family, friends, hobbies, or things that the person used to enjoy doing
- Losing appetite
- Feeling irritable, testy, and grouchy at all times
- Not being able to expunge certain thoughts from the mind
- Crying for longer periods or many times each day
- Thinking about hurting themselves or even suicidal thoughts
- Feeling "wired," having bad thoughts, or experiencing panic attacks

- Having problems with their sleep such as insomnia, nightmares, or *hypersomnia* (excessive sleepiness)

Depression is treatable with medicine, but it is important for the doctor to know if the patient is manifesting one or more of the signs listed above. Solutions beside medicine can include talking about the feeling with a psychologist or a counselor or joining a support group.

Suicide

Suicide among cancer patients is more common than in any other segment of the population and usually happens during the first year after diagnosis in such cancers as lung, pancreas, head, neck, and prostate. A major study in Sweden showed that the probability was 13 times higher during the first week following the diagnosis.[24] The usual late detection of lung cancer, as well as the dismal prognosis accompanied by debilitating symptoms, encourages patients to try to find ways to end their lives and stop the pain and suffering. Furthermore, the highest rates of suicide are found in males with respiratory cancers.[25]

Suicide is also a major consequence of severe, undetected, untreated depression among older males, which is why it is so important to stop the progression of depressive disorders as soon as possible. Suicidal tendencies have been observed in patients with more severe symptoms and impairment in their physical and social environments.[26]

The harboring of thoughts about committing suicide is known as *suicidal ideation*. This happens especially in the advanced stages of cancers, such as lung cancer. It is characterized by an impending desire for a hastened death that, in the mind of the patient, must occur before nature takes its course.[27]

A person suffering from lung cancer may (1) have a passive desire to die without an exit plan or (2) be willing to actively ask for assistance in ending life. *Physician-assisted suicide* (PAS) is a practice that involves the removal of medication or life support equipment to bring about "natural" death sooner than expected. PAS remains controversial and has been legalized only in the state of Oregon through the Oregon Death with Dignity Act, passed via legislation in the late 1990s. Euthanasia, which is still legal in the Netherlands, is performed with the lung cancer patient's prior consent through the administration of lethal doses of medication.[28] PAS is also called *passive euthanasia*. One of the most widely publicized cases of euthanasia took place in the United States with a notorious doctor who claimed to have helped 130 people with terminal illnesses end their lives between 1990 and 1998.[29]

Anxiety

Roughly 44 percent of patients with cancer have reported some anxiety, and 23 percent have experienced significant episodes.[30] Anxiety can be classified as a *psychobiological* reaction to danger that mobilizes the whole body to diminish exposure to threats.[31] This response causes the individual to act in different ways according to the situation. Anger, fear, courage, strength, speed, fainting, and freezing are some of the reactions someone can experience while going through a period of anxiety. Anxiety can be adaptive or maladaptive. Adaptive anxiety refers to a focused reaction that effectively alleviates the unpleasant situation. Maladaptive anxiety, on the other hand, happens when the emotions caused by a certain real or imaginary threat become a misperception that unnecessarily affects the person, impairing his or her ability to properly discern and function mentally.

When it comes to lung cancer, patients could feel anxious about the following:

- Onset of unpleasant symptoms
- Financial hardship
- Anticipated fear of high cancer markers for tests
- Treatment complications
- Diminished physical stamina
- Prognosis
- Relapse after remission
- Concerns with physical appearance
- Loss of mobility[32]

Solid research confirms the presence of anxiety in lung cancer patients before and after diagnosis.[33] It is therefore necessary for patients and caregivers to realize the widely accepted causes of anxiety, many of which are as follows:[34]

- Atypical metabolic states, including but not limited to hypoxia, lung embolus, sepsis, abnormal blood sugar levels, coronary blockages, pneumonia, and heart conditions.
- Hormone-secreting tumors, such as adenomas and carcinomas in the thyroid and parathyroid glands.
- Drugs commonly known to produce anxiety: *corticosteroids* (steroid hormones), *antihistamines* (anti-allergics), *antiemetics* (anti-vomit drugs), *benzodiazepines* (drugs that slow down the nervous system), *bronchodilators* (drugs that increase diameter of the airways), and *thyroxine* (thyroid gland hormone).
- Withdrawal symptoms from strong medication, alcohol, and tobacco.
- Phobias: extreme fear and anxiety about something or someone. Lung cancer patients generally develop *needle phobia*, a fear of wounds or blood, and *claustrophobia*, an irrational fear of being trapped in an enclosed space. These phobias severely complicate treatment of respiratory cancers.
- Panic disorder: an uncontrollable period of anxiety that is marked by shortness of breath, light-headedness, dizziness, fear of impending heart attack, nausea, trembling, and fainting. Panic attacks in the lung cancer sufferer happen without warning and quickly gain intensity and last for a few minutes, but the discomfort can last for several hours.
- Generalized anxiety disorder is an excessive and unrealistic worry about one or more life situations that is difficult to manage by the lung cancer sufferer on his own. It may cause motor disturbances such as tension, uneasiness, and tiredness. Shortness of breath, palpitations, irritability, dizziness, and sweating are also reported physical symptoms.
- Obsessive-compulsive disorder: This is characterized by obsessions and compulsions that are intrusive thoughts that cloud a person's mind. It can provoke an anxious individual suffering from lung cancer to perform illogical actions or rituals to help calm distress. Obsessive-compulsive disorder may negatively affect the individual's daily activities. For instance, lung cancer patients with obsessive-compulsive disorder repeatedly wash their hands, fearing infection or relapses.

Delirium

Patients with advanced lung cancer who are hospitalized are at greater risk of delirium, a serious neuropsychiatric condition that disturbs cognition, consciousness, and perception. In most scenarios, it requires immediate medical attention, for it may be an indication of a potential life-threatening situation, such as organ failure, damaging side effects from medication (chapter 15), or severe infection. Given the seriousness of delirium, clinicians must be prepared to diagnose and rapidly intervene before it endangers a patient's life. Older lung cancer sufferers are more prone to develop delirium, which occurs in roughly 50 percent of postoperative patients.[35]

The symptoms of delirium include irritability, restlessness, anxiety, insomnia, distractibility, depression, anger, euphoria, hallucinations, delusions, disorientation, memory impairment, language disturbance (*dysnomia*), and the inability to write (*dysgraphia*). Neurological effects include tremors, myoclonus, incoherent speech, and muscle tone changes. Another consequence of delirium is a well-known reversal of the sleep–wake cycle in the terminally ill. The result is that pain management becomes more challenging as the previously mentioned reversal interferes with detection and treatment. For instance, agitation mistaken for severe pain can lead to an improper administration of opioids, and being a lung cancer sufferer does not make matters any better.[36]

Guilt

A great sense of guilt can be mentally experienced by lung cancer patients, as they may feel worthless and like a burden to their family and society. Unfortunately, many of them would rather die than continue to live in such conditions. Patients are also overcome by guilt from not having quit smoking while there was still time. Other patients feel guilty about the fact that they are still smoking even though they have been diagnosed with lung cancer and the window of opportunity for a possible recovery is rapidly shutting. A study conducted to assess the degrees of guilt and shame in non–small cell lung cancer patients found that smoking-related cancer is tied to higher levels of guilt and shame than other types of cancer.[37]

Prescription Pain Medication Addiction and Alcohol Usage

It is reported that approximately 50 percent of lung cancer sufferers experience pain during the course of treatment and particularly advanced stages.[38] Pain from lung cancer is attributable to several sources, including the following:

- Pressing of nerves, bones, and *pleura* (lung lining) by tumors
- Coughing
- Chemotherapy sores
- Surgical incisions
- Headaches and joint pain

Lung cancer can induce substance abuse and addiction from the heavy use of opium derivatives inasmuch as pain management is an indispensable component of overall mental well-being. Tolerance and physical dependency are phenomena that may lead not only to substance abuse but also to addiction and overdose. Tolerance materializes as the need to increase the dose of pain medication to keep the same effect, but it is not an automatic cause of addiction for lung cancer patients. Physical dependency, on the other hand, triggers withdrawal symptoms on decrease of medication dose, putting a patient of any medical disorder at risk of addiction. The use of pain medication quadrupled from 573,000 users in 1990 to 2.5 million in 2002, exceeding illegal drugs such as marijuana and cocaine.[39]

Alcohol abuse in cancer populations has been the subject of few studies, but there is evidence that links alcohol to low income and unemployment. This phenomenon may be underestimated in major cancer centers. A study on the subject suggested that in spite of multiple hospital admissions caused by alcoholism in terminal patients, only one-third had this recorded in their medical history.[40]

Somatoform Disorders

Lung cancer patients can be afflicted by somatoform disorders, and ironically those patients with a better prognosis are at an increased risk. Somatoform disorders involve the creation of physical symptoms that lack an organic origin or explanation. These symptoms might baffle health care professionals trying to find the right approach to lung cancer and somatoform disorder concurrently. Oncologists should be able to recognize and differentiate between somatic symptoms and somatoform disorder effects. Such disorders can be classified as follows:

- Somatization disorder: This involves a series of recurrent inexplicable symptoms that start in adulthood and continue for about two years. Patients visit several doctors becoming avid users of the health care system.
- Hypochondrial disorder: The lung cancer patient is preoccupied about having illnesses and disorders despite the doctor's assurance that no disease is present.
- Somatoform pain disorder: The patient experiences pain for more than six months, thereby rendering the disorder as chronic or long term.
- Conversion disorder: This is characterized by motor symptoms, such as seizures, paralysis, and speech and vision problems.
- Body dysmorphic disorder: A persistent worry clouds the mind of the patient about his or her body being deformed or diseased in some way or another.

Personality Disorders

Solid clinical evidence proves that personality disorders are associated with cancers such as those of the lung.[41] Lung cancer patients can take on new personality traits as a response to the disease process. The personality traits mostly seen in oncological settings are as follows:

- Schizoid: Socially detached with feelings of uselessness and shame
- Avoidant: Inhibited and inadequate; greatly affected by negative criticism
- Paranoid: Someone who distrusts everyone
- Dependent: Indecisive and submissive with a tremendous need to be taken care of; fears being alone
- Histrionic: Extremely emotional and attention hungry
- Borderline: Unstable with a marked impulsivity and intense sensitivity to rejection
- Passive-aggressive: Resentful, self-critical, hostile, and defiant

- Obsessive compulsive: Perfectionist, showing excessive preoccupation with orderliness
- Antisocial: Someone who disregards and disrespects others
- Depressive: Overly self-critical with a marked sense of pessimism

PSYCHOLOGICAL ISSUES FOR THE FAMILY

While the next chapter discusses the roles of family members in approaching lung cancer at home, it is essential to now review the *mental aspects* of family members of lung cancer sufferers. In essence, families represent the first line of psychological defense against lung cancer. A situation where a family member is suffering from a deadly disease directly affects its core, creating an imbalance between normal family life and family life dealing with cancer. Even when the diagnosis has been made early and the prognosis is good, the fact that a form of cancer afflicts a family member brings about a lot of fear, uncertainty, worry, foiled future plans, and despair.

Respiratory cancer by itself represents not a single source of stress for a family but rather an array of multiple psychosocial transitions. These transitions, which are internal and invisible to even other family members, make them try to look for answers that may explain their misfortune. All this is part of a destabilization process that hits even the most well-off. The recovery process is known as *restabilization* and initially involves the efforts that need to be made to accommodate themselves to the mentally affected family member. New communication strategies are made and new objectives drawn, but *stuck points* make their appearance at this stage. Stuck points, as their name suggests, are issues where families get stranded, turning their support for a lung cancer patient into a daily struggle with no easy answers or solutions on hand. An example of a stuck point is when a child with a parent or parents diagnosed with cancer has to be supported and family members do not exactly know how to start dealing with the situation. All this can help make or break, bring together and consolidate, or separate and destroy, a family.

The spouse of a patient with lung cancer is considered in health care circles as the primary caregiver.[42] Unfortunately, the needs of the sufferer may increase over time and begin to require professional attention, and the primary caregiver may not be enough to meet even the most basic needs. This causes a mentally straining situation known as caregiver burden. Caregiver burden is reported to provoke stress, health problems, desperation, and despair mostly in women because, as mentioned previously, lung cancer is more common in men than in women.

LIVING WITH LUNG CANCER AND TRYING TO STAY HAPPY

One of the first things lung cancer patients need to know is that they are not alone; there are many people willing to provide help and support at all times. Lung cancer does not mean death; the fact is that many people survive it, and that is a piece of great news. Lung cancer patients usually have more supportive care needs than people with other cancers. It is important to improve the chances for these patients through early intervention in order to allow them to take an active role in their journey to healing. It is essential to consider daily activities as an aspect that, if handled correctly, will bring happiness and fulfillment to the lung cancer sufferer as well as a better quality of life.

The psychological aspect goes hand in hand with the physical aspect, which is why the correct management of physical symptoms will greatly ease the psychological effects of lung cancer. This approach places the patient at center stage and makes him or her the most important member of the health care team. Communication channels must be open at all times to ensure that symptoms and side effects are properly handled, which makes it easier to assess the patient's mental state. The goal of the team is to provide the best possible plan to promote emotional and physical well-being by controlling symptoms and treating side effects.

Pain management remains crucial when it comes to trying to live happily despite suffering from lung cancer, but to obtain the best results, the patient must keep in close communication with his or her doctor. Since every human being has different characteristics, there may be various attempts before a strategy works to effectively relieve the mental and physical anguish from lung cancer. It may take weeks, but once that happens, things will dramatically improve for the sufferer.

Sleep as an Approach to a Happy Mind

Sleep issues are another essential area to be reckoned with. Special emphasis must be placed on insomnia—a sleep disorder that prevents a patient from getting a good night's rest. Lung cancer patients generally suffer from poor or inadequate rest as well as repeated awakenings that can lead to fatigue and psychological symptoms. If a patient is experiencing sleep problems, he or she must consult with a health care professional. Some additional insights follow:[43]

- Planning activities for the whole day and not just part of it
- Eating healthy and avoiding skipping meals
- Drinking plenty of liquids to keep the body hydrated
- Getting other people to help with house chores, shopping, child care and driving
- Working from home during the first weeks of treatment
- Light exercise and avoidance of engaging in other activities if not directed by a doctor
- Relaxation to eliminate stress through meditation, relaxing music, and reading books
- Cessation of caffeine consumption to avoid insomnia

Breathing exercises and relaxation should also be a part of the psychological arsenal, as both help alleviate sleep problems. Furthermore, lung cancer patients must surround themselves with positive people that create great energy to keep them going. Relaxation is the key to success preventing and easing sleep issues. A plethora of resources are available to that end, and most of them are easy to find and affordable.

Emotion and Happiness

For lung cancer patients, learning to accept their feelings no matter what is a good start. They should take things one step at a time and avoid self-blame and self-criticism. If possible, the causes of their un-happiness should be identified and addressed. When a lung cancer patient is feeling overwhelmed, it is good practice to focus on people and good things that brings them happiness. They should also try to keep their sense of humor, as laughter is a good way to relieve stress. It helps if they keep their focus on what needs to be done immediately, but it is also important to set priorities. They should think about what matters most to them and spend most of their time doing it.

Exercise, for instance, is a great means of staying happy and emotionally healthy. The belief that a patient should always go to bed to recover is not so true, and a series of trials published in *The Lancet* showed that patients experienced no improvement when they were sent to bed to treat their conditions.[44] Researchers at Yale University also found that bed rest can be disastrous for people 70 years and older.[45] As a matter of fact, exercise can slow down the division of cancer cells for people who exercise at least an average of four hours per week.[46] Even more dramatic: physical activity that includes household chores can help keep cancer at bay, according to a large European study.[47] Lung cancer patients can benefit from exercise because once they stop smoking, their lung capacity improves, and that paves the way for a gradually increasing active lifestyle. There is a wide array of physical activities to help patients mentally cope with lung cancer and stay emotionally sound.

All in all, the patient must be placed at the center of the health care team's efforts, thereby making him or her an active participant in the decisions concerning the treatment plan. Depression and delirium must be detected and cared for due to their dangerous, debilitating, and disabling nature. Pain management of the lung cancer patient, whether speaking of mental or physical pain, is a major psychological component of lung cancer treatment and must be treated as a high priority. Quitting smoking is as important as pain management because treatments fail or succeed depending on the individual. People who continue smoking have already given up, and they express that anger and hopelessness through feelings of guilt and shame.

Nonetheless, there are options to cope with lung cancer psychologically as well as alternatives to find better treatments and possibly a cure through clinical trials. Concerning people who survive lung cancer and even those coming from late detection, their will to fight makes a big difference in the end. In light of the mental aspects of this disease process, it is important to keep will, desire, and determination from waning over time and to ask for help when help is needed.

V

Homestretch

17

LUNG CANCER AT HOME

Coping with lung cancer is a challenge that no person should have to face alone. Any cancer diagnosis causes considerable emotional reactions, and the thought of living with lung cancer can be overwhelming. When a person is told that he or she has cancer, the diagnosis affects not only the patient but also his or her family and everyone close by. Maintaining strong relationships with family and friends at home may help the lung cancer sufferer's emotional well-being. This chapter further discusses the role of family members of lung cancer patients and ways to deal with issues that these patients endure within the household.

IMPORTANCE OF A DUAL APPROACH: AT HOME AND THE DOCTOR'S OFFICE

Home as a Starting Point

In the days or weeks after the diagnosis, the person will face difficult tasks, such as (1) coming to terms with the news, (2) telling the immediate family about the news, and (3) deciding when, what, and how to tell others. Dealing with the news is strenuous at the onset. A lung cancer patient has to worry about his or her physical, emotional, and financial situations—both personally and from a family standpoint. Most people may experience shock, disbelief, fear, sadness, confusion, helplessness, and worry about the future. These feelings are normal and justified. The patient could be preoccupied with questions such as "Am I going to die?," "Why did this happen to me?," "What happens now?," or "How will my family react to the news?"[1]

Telling family or loved ones that a person has lung cancer is difficult. The sooner a person can tell one's family about the cancer, the sooner everyone will be able to adjust to life at home. People diagnosed with lung cancer should talk about their concerns with their family and friends, though this may sometimes be difficult at the start since they may feel as if others do not completely understand what they are going through. At times, a family member or friend may even avoid talking about the condition because they do not know what to say or are afraid to say something insensitive. In these cases, the patient should reach out to family and friends so that they can get a better understanding of his or her experience.[2]

For lung cancer patients with children and grandchildren, it is equally difficult to tell them the news. Parents always want to protect their children, and likewise they may not opt to tell their children the news. Hiding the sickness is usually not in the children's best interest. Children can sense when something is wrong, especially when they develop a strong bond with other family members after living at home for so long. It is recommended for parents with very young children to be honest, but it is also important to give them information that is appropriate for their age and level of understanding. It is best to answer children's questions about the lung cancer consistently and honestly. Another recommendation is to have a professional talk with the children. A professional who is an expert in child mentality may help in addressing potential problems early on. Young children see their parents as their source of safety, and hence they fear losing their parents. When a child asks if his or her parent is going to die, it is important to be truthful and focus on the present, such as what the doctors are doing to prolong the parent's life and what the likelihood of a recovery might be. It is essential to keep in mind that children love their parents and will want to help them in any way they can.[3]

Parents of the lung cancer patient are also likely to be deeply affected by the news. Just like how one feels responsible for one's children, a person's parents feel responsible for their children's welfare. Sometimes, the parents may wonder whether the disorder is their fault or whether they could have done something to prevent it from happening. They may feel guilt, and they may have the tendency to revert to treating their adult children as if the latter were youngsters.

Aside from immediate family living at the lung cancer sufferer's home, other people in the patient's life need to be informed about the illness. *What*, *when*, and *how* to tell others about the cancer is a decision that needs to be carefully planned. It may include one's siblings; extended family, such as uncles, aunts, and cousins; and even close friends, employees, or coworkers. Breaking the news in a group setting can take some of the pressure off. If giving the news in person is difficult, writing letters may be a helpful option. This may lead to developing or deepening relationships with these people, who can be a great source of support for the lung cancer patient. Family plays an essential role in coping with lung cancer. When the cancer was diagnosed, the family's own personal journey with lung cancer also began. Having open communication and accepting the love and support of loved ones are important in dealing with lung cancer at home.

Lung Cancer: From Home to the Doctor's Office

Throughout a patient's cancer treatment, the oncologist is one of the most important people who will support the patient. The lung cancer patient should feel comfortable talking with the doctor and asking questions about the illness both at home and elsewhere. After a cancer diagnosis, the patient is encouraged to start learning about the disease and its treatment. This can be done by asking doctors or reading factual information from reliable sources. During the initial visits to the oncologist or pulmonologist, some information or medical terminology may confuse the patient. It is recommended that the lung cancer sufferer ask the doctor to explain any medical term(s) that he or she is having a tough time understanding. Ideally, both the doctor and the patient should be open in exchanging information so that they can work together in making treatment decisions.

A lung cancer patient will usually start gathering information about his or her cancer and the available treatment options. Other tasks that need to be completed may include making appointments, getting test results, and collecting records. It is wise to be organized, as this helps the patient gain control and to make well-informed decisions. For the most part, management of the cancer care involves organizing all the information. Some of the specifics include gathering information about lung cancer types and the action plan, taking notes during appointments with doctors, and writing down the latter's contact information, along with noting any information about the appropriate hospitals and insurance companies.

A patient may also request to work with the doctor to develop a personalized cancer care plan so that home therapy schedules do not conflict with outpatient clinical care. A personalized plan serves as a one-stop reference for information relating to the patient's treatment and care. The plan will include the initial approaches (chapter 13) and a list of home-based therapies to reinforce the medical treatments, possible side effects, and symptoms to watch out for. After severe treatment (e.g., surgical resection), the care plan may be updated to include information on (1) any medicines the patient is continuing to take, (2) any ongoing medical issues that need to be addressed, and (3) when to return for checkups. The following is a basic outline for a personalized care plan that originates from home:[4]

- What treatment was provided and whether it will conflict with home-based approaches
- Treatment purpose (cancer treatment, bone strengthener, ease breathing, and so on)
- How often to take medications at home
- How to store lung cancer medications at home
- When and where to go for treatments
- Reactions to look out for
- Whether follow-ups needed
- Follow-up date(s)

Exploring and understanding the types of care available also help the patient and doctor develop a personalized treatment plan that takes into account the individual's needs, goals, and preferences. The usual care options are the standard treatment, clinical trials, palliative care, and hospice care.[5]

Standard (pharmacological) treatment is the current and most effective treatment available for malignant cells in the patient's lung. It focuses mainly on controlling the disease process at the physiological level. Some people with advanced cancer opt to stop receiving standard treatment since it causes unpleasant or harmful side effects, and remaining at home with a sedentary lifestyle will not improve that situation much.

A clinical trial is a highly controlled research study involving people who choose to participate. Clinical trials test new drugs and treatments to determine if they are safe, effective, and possibly better than the standard treatment. Participation in a trial should be considered early in the course of treatment and not as a last resort since serious cases of lung cancer may require that the patient remain at home unless absolutely necessary.

Palliative Care

Palliative care is initiated to improve quality of life, and home is obviously where life is the most situated for a lung cancer patient. *Palliative* comes from the word *palliate*, which means to devise comfort levels by treating and relieving symptoms of an illness. The treatment is also called supportive care. It helps people with different stages of cancer live as happily and comfortably as possible for weeks, months, or years. This is especially important to remember here because "home" is where most people are expected to live comfortably. Moreover, palliative care addresses the physical, spiritual, emotional, and practical needs of the patient. Palliative care also provides support for the patient's family, friends, and caregivers.

Hospice or home care is a palliative approach that is provided to patients who are expected to live six months or less. The goal of hospice care is to help patients who are no longer receiving disease-directed treatment and their families to cope with the physical and emotional effects of dying. It focuses on compassionate care that provides the highest quality of life possible. Hospice care can take place at home or in a specialized center or facility.

It is not entirely the doctor's responsibility to make the patient feel at ease at home since the former obviously does not live in with the patient. The patient should initiate the communication and talk honestly with the doctor about how to deal with lung cancer within the confines of house. Some tips to build a good relationship with the oncologist include openly discussing the patient's lifestyle, talking about symptoms that could warrant phone calls to the office, and writing down questions between appointments and then asking the physician for answers. It is important to build a strong partnership and trust with the doctor throughout the cancer treatment, as this leads to a clear understanding of the diagnosis and treatment options and also gives the lung cancer patient confidence in the decision-making process even while away from the doctor's office and at the place where he or she has spent (or will spend) most of his or her life: at home.

ROLE OF THE FAMILY MEMBERS AND OTHERS

Talking Openly

The involvement of family members is important in ensuring treatment compliance, continuity of cancer care, and support for the patient. *Family* can mean close relatives, spouses, life partners, primary caregivers, and important friends. During the crisis of cancer, challenges are plenty, and home is where the family functions best in making critical decisions. Furthermore, a family's beliefs about cancer and the meanings attached to those beliefs may affect how a family responds to a cancer diagnosis.[6] Some examples follow:

- Some families believe that illness is an emotional or a mental weakness. This belief may prevent family members from being able to support one another.
- If cancer led to death in a family over generations, the family may believe that cancer always leads to death.
- Some families believe that if their family member with cancer is optimistic and positive, the cancer may be cured; cancer will return if that member is pessimistic. This belief can place a huge burden on the lung cancer sufferer.
- Unresolved family issues at home, such as blame, shame, or guilt, can also strongly affect views of cancer's cause or cure.[7]

Roles of Spouses or Partners

Lung cancer can be just as scary for the spouse or partner as it is for the patient. Partners should always talk openly about the changes and limitations that they may experience. Hiding the truth and becoming over-protective is not encouraged, as there will be plenty of changes as the family's struggle against cancer continues. A change that could occur between partners is the switching of roles wherein a partner may become the new head of the family and assume control. A husband or wife may take over and assume primary responsibility for the family, and it might be difficult for the husband or wife who is accustomed to being in charge to switch to a dependent role due to medical disorder. It is important to note that this kind of change (from head to dependent) greatly affects a person's self-esteem at home and elsewhere. He or she may experience frustration when left out of decision making. Conversely, partners who used to depend on their significant other may experience trouble taking charge and being the care provider. The cancer patient may also feel guilty about being a burden to his or her family members.[8] It is highly encouraged that partners talk about the matter and figure out what setup will make both of them comfortable. It is best to take the time to sit down and listen to one another's concerns at home.

Lung cancer has a strong effect on marriages and long-term partnerships. Some people may not tell their partners because they want to avoid upsetting them. They consider hiding it as a way to protect their partners from the pain. This is not the best option, as there is always the need to help and support each other in any way possible. Telling a person's partner that he or she has lung cancer will depend on the relationship at hand. Home is where such intimate and personal news is most often shared initially, and the following are a few things that should be considered when telling a partner about the cancer:[9]

- Privacy: Talking with a partner in a private place may make it easier to break the news. In a quiet, private room at home, emotions can be let out freely.
- Time: The couple should try to select a time when both of them are available, such as when neither of them is too busy to be called away. This will allow freedom to talk about the situation and be together for as long as possible.

- Emotional and mental preparedness: The individual with lung cancer should be prepared for the possibility of a strong emotional reaction, especially if the diagnosis was unexpected. The news is so full of impact that it affects the partner (patient) deeply, and his or her immediate reaction may be strong. Denial or a refusal to believe the diagnosis is a common initial reaction, and it may be better to go through this frustration at home rather than in public.
- Understanding the difficulty of the situation: The partners should be aware of the fact that the situation (severe lung cancer) is going to be very difficult. Both will need one another's support and understanding.
- Decision making and care planning: This should be shared with the patient, who would want to feel independent and in control. The family should let the patient share in decision making or make the decisions as much as possible. They should also avoid making decisions without consulting the person with lung cancer. It would be better to work together as a team when creating plans with which everyone is comfortable.
- Honesty: Although it can be difficult, being open and honest about one's feelings certainly helps. Truthfulness is really the only way to make others understand the situation better, and there is no better place to begin the truth about a lung cancer diagnosis than at home.

The usual reaction is that both partners may experience depression, anxiety, anger, and hopelessness. For many people, living at home without their partner is painful. Some partners may seek support from local groups for personal, psychological, or spiritual assistance. For other couples, facing the difficulties of cancer together while spending time at home tends to strengthen their relationship. Facing the many challenges over the coming months makes their bond stronger than before. It is best for a couple to handle the situation in whichever way works best for them. It is also important to note that some changes may occur in the couple's roles and other familial relationships. This may include changes in responsibilities, needs, intimacy, and the future plans of the immediate family.

Formulating a plan or strategy together can be initiated by simply jotting down tasks or chores and discussing who should assume responsibility for each. The cancer patient may need additional help in doing his or her daily tasks, such as cleaning, doing yard work, cooking, or shopping for groceries. A patient may often be left feeling tired or in pain because of the illness itself or following treatments such as chemotherapy or radiation. Moreover, cancer treatments such as surgeries require time to recover from and may leave the patient feeling extremely fatigued. Depending on how the patient's body copes with treatments, he or she might need to take time off work. In these cases, the spouse or perhaps another relative could take over the responsibilities. There are instances when the lung cancer patient needs to cease working completely, and there is added pressure on the partner to compensate financially by working extra hours. All the responsibilities may become too overwhelming for a single person alone and can cause frustration in the household. Hence, accepting outside help from other family members or friends is encouraged.

In addition to the change in roles between partners, sexuality and intimacy are also affected by the cancer diagnosis. A long-term side effect of treatment for cancer patients, be it for lung or other cancer, is sexual dysfunction that may be accompanied by depression and other physical and emotional issues. Cancer and its treatment affect how people feel about themselves and their bodies and how they relate intimately to their spouses or significant others. Most lung cancer patients struggle with shortness of breath, but overall many cancer patients consider fatigue, hair loss, body image, and discomfort as limitations for sexual enjoyment. Both partners usually feel anxious about this matter and are often reluctant to talk about it, and being stranded in a home environment does not make things any better in this regard. If a couple finds it uncomfortable or awkward to discuss sexuality, there is always help available from therapists, counselors, or even doctors. They can provide guidance and give suggestions for managing and maintaining sexual intimacy.

As spouses and partners, sharing information and making decisions together about treatment options is equally important. They need to visit and talk to the doctor together and learn about symptoms, available treatment options, and possible side effects. If the spouse or partner goes with the patient to the doctor, he or she can also ask questions to better understand the disease process and to help take care of the patient emotionally and physically. Spending time together is important, but just because one member of the couple has cancer does not mean he or she has to spend every minute with the other. Each person needs to set aside some time for him- or herself. The spouse or partner may use his or her personal time to enjoy hobbies, such as reading, or just leaving the house to do errands, visit friends, or simply take a walk.

Role of Children

If there are young children at home, the parent may be worried about how the children will respond to the lung cancer diagnosis. How a child reacts to upsetting news often depends on how the adults are handling it. It presents a unique challenge for parents to explain the bad news. Sometimes, if children are not given honest answers, they tend to imagine worse situations. In handling children, it is best to share small bits of information over time and keep the answers suitable to their age and level of understanding. The lung cancer patient should try to use vocabulary they already know or is easy to understand. For instance, *medicine* can be said instead of *chemotherapy* or *doctor* in place of *pulmonologist*. There are illustrated children's books about cancer that could be used to help explain the situation to a child. It is also recommended that the patient inform other adults in their children's lives about their condition, such as teachers, coaches, and guidance counselors, since these people might be able to listen to and answer the children's questions. It is also important to constantly reassure children that they will always be cared for and that they are loved.

For households with teenagers, a lung cancer diagnosis might cause adolescents to "act out." Their behavior may change as they adjust to the situation. They are already dealing with physical changes and emotional issues, especially the desire to be independent. They may become depressed, get into trouble at school, or get involved with a negative group of peers. It is recommended that parents encourage their teens to stay involved in school activities, church, or even the community. They may also seek expert help if needed through a social worker or teacher. This provides the teen with support that is outside his or her home.

If the lung cancer patient has grown children, it will be easier to tell the latter about the cancer diagnosis. They will still be affected by the news and may feel upset, but it is important to tell them about the type of cancer and its treatment plan so that they can also get involved. If the adult children live near the parents' house, they can always help with home chores or could accompany their parents during treatments when appropriate. They may also help in financial matters by helping to pay their parent's health or hospital bills. As is the case with a spouse, children can also go with the patient on doctor appointments to ask questions and take part in decision making regarding treatment options. These activities will strengthen the parent–child bond and help the children mature and bear the experience. The following are some suggestions that can help in managing and adjusting to the relationship and role changes within the family:

- There should be one person in charge of giving medical updates. It can be tiring to explain the cancer diagnosis to every member of the family. There should be one member of the family who can serve as the "go-to" person for medical information and updates. This person may also assign other tasks to other family members who live in the same household. [10]
- Proper expectations about the relationship changes should be set. Some family members or friends may not be able to provide the support that the patient expects. Some friends or family members may distance themselves and avoid talking about the cancer for fear of "saying something wrong" or making a statement that may be upsetting. Others could be surprisingly supportive and caring throughout the endeavor.
- The patient should take the lead in talking. Again, some people may avoid talking about the matter simply because they do not know what to say. The sufferer should advise family or friends whether it is okay for them to talk about the cancer. He or she should talk openly and tell friends that help may be needed at times. This is not a sign of weakness.

Role of Friends and Other Adult Members of Society

Even though friends don't usually live at home with the individual suffering from lung cancer, they are still a great source of support. The effect of cancer on the friends' relationship depends on the closeness between themselves and the patient. Like family members, friends may feel shocked, upset, angry, depressed, and afraid on hearing the news. This does not mean that the patient gets to spend less time with his or her peers. The patient can always get support from friends and should let them help whenever needed. Asking for simple favors, such as taking children to and from school, can help immensely, especially if the patient is not feeling well. As a friend, he or she could accompany the patient to doctor visits or run simple errands. Patients should accept offers of help from friends who visit the house often. Below are tips and guidelines for supporting a friend with lung cancer: [11]

- Close friends should not be afraid to ask questions. If the family is not sure how their loved one wants to deal with his or her lung cancer, they should not hesitate to ask. It is best not to assume that the patient cannot handle an honest talk about his or her experience. They should also consider that the cancer patient may want to be treated as normally as possible. Open and honest communication will help each family member feel better.
- Friends should become good listeners, and telling a lung cancer patient how the latter should think and feel is not advisable. Friends should be sensitive to and acknowledge the patient's feelings. They should allow for sadness and empathize with any uncomfortable feelings from the patient. There may be times when the patient does not want to talk at all, and simply being there can make him or her feel cared for. It is also recommended to avoid mentioning phrases such as "I know how you feel," "You need to talk," "I feel hopeless," "I do not know how you are planning to manage this," "I am sure you will be fine," or "How long do you have?" Instead, it would be best to provide statements such as "I am sorry this has happened to you," "I care about you," or "If you ever feel like talking, I am always here to listen." If one is unsure of what to say, simply saying so and staying honest is better.
- Friends should be more understanding and comforting. Lung cancer patients who spend most of their time at home are often under stress, both physical and emotional. They cannot be expected to always be cheerful and positive. They may suffer fatigue and loss of energy after treatments. They may have difficulty concentrating and remembering. Sometimes, they may become depressed, and it is best to give them space occasionally and to try

not to take things personally. The family should always remind the patient that he or she is needed and loved. They should not hesitate to make plans for the future, as this will give the patient something positive to look forward to. .

- Friends are encouraged to offer practical help. Any assistance with daily chores or tasks is valuable. The cancer patient's needs may change occasionally, so it is important to be flexible with their plans. The following are some tasks they might need help with:

  - Grocery shopping and picking up of prescriptions
  - Cooking dinner or ordering takeout food
  - Talking about interests and hobbies or other topics that are unrelated to cancer
  - Babysitting children and taking them to and from school
  - Doing simple chores around the house, such as taking care of plants, taking out the trash, getting the mail, or even taking care of pets
  - Driving the patient to a doctor's appointment
  - Keeping the patient company during the doctor's appointment or during a treatment session

Lung Cancer–Related Stress at Home

Researchers believe that stress plays a role in cancer survival.[12] They have found that stress is correlated with poorer survival rates. It cannot be denied that stress in patients with lung cancer is a human response to illness.[13] Patients with lung cancer tend to experience psychological and biologic stressors that may be caused by delayed cancer diagnosis, symptom management issues, and social stigmatization of the illness.[14] Managing lung cancer–related stress at home involves techniques and practices that generally promote overall health and better quality of life. The following are recommendations on how to deal with lung cancer–related stress at home.

A common way to manage stress is to discover activities or practices that increase the patient's coping abilities. Ordinary activities, such as reading books, watching television, playing games, or listening to music, can help the lung cancer patient relax. Some people with lung cancer find that yoga helps relieve discomfort associated with the spread of a cancer from one organ to another. Meditation and muscle relaxation, both of which can be accomplished at home, can also help. The patient could also try to find pleasant diversions from stress, such as spending time on hobbies, or treating him- or herself to something new, such as an outfit, a pet, a gadget, or even a car if cost is not an issue. Parents or grandparents with cancer can enjoy playtime with their children or grandchildren. A simple walk alone or with someone in a setting the patient enjoys is also a good way to relax.

The Cancer Treatment Centers of America formed a mind–body program to help lung cancer patients and their families cope with stress through various techniques and practices.[15] Some of these practices, such as guided imagery, can be completed at home. Guided imagery is a relaxation technique that teaches patients to use positive mental images to manage stress and physical discomfort. It can help the patient handle pain and anxiety. Deep-breathing exercise can also be a form of relaxation and a stress-relieving technique. Laughter therapy can also reduce stress and balance the patient's blood pressure at home. Reiki is a technique of Japanese origin that is commonly called *palm healing*. It helps restore the body's equilibrium, strengthens the ability to heal, and increases peace of mind. Qigong, which means *life energy cultivation*, is another technique that is taught. It is a practice of aligning breath and movement to improve the immune system and lymph circulation—both important for cancer patients.

Staying Physically Active at Home

Taking part in physical activities or regular exercise can help the patient feel better overall. Although it may not seem to make sense, physical exercise is a great treatment for fatigue brought about by lung cancer. Studies have shown that people with cancer who exercise regularly feel less tired and have more energy.[16] Weight-bearing activities, such as something as simple as walking, can help strengthen bones, which is important if the patient has lung cancer that has spread. The patient can choose a physical activity that he or she enjoys the most and practice it daily. Sometimes, the exercise might cause discomfort or pain. If this happens, the patient can modify the exercise into a form that the body can tolerate.

Lung Cancer and Rest

Since home is where people generally rest the most, it is appropriate to discuss *rest* in this chapter. Sleep disturbances are common among people with cancer, and lung cancer is no exception. One reason is that fatigue related to cancer and its treatment leads people to take frequent naps during the day, making it difficult to sleep at night.[17] A recommendation for patients is that they can still set aside time in the day to rest or take naps, but it must be limited to 20 to 30 minutes each. They should also avoid napping in the late afternoon or early evening. The doctor may review and change the medications if he or she thinks the lung cancer drug has side effects or contributes to the sleeping problem. He or she may also recommend a medication to help the patient fall and stay asleep.

LUNG CANCER: FROM HOME TO SUPPORT RESOURCES

Many resources beyond family exist to support both the lung cancer patient and his or her caregivers at home. These support groups include counselors, patient navigators, and social workers who can give the best help learning about resources and securing financial assistance. Counselors can help families overcome denial of the cancer diagnosis, address grief issues, and serve as a consultant to other professionals on the health care team. They can help educate children about cancer and help them work through feelings and concerns that arise specifically at home but that are absent when the patient is elsewhere. Patient navigators help people manage the maze of clinics, doctor's offices, hospitals, outpatient centers, and insurance and payment systems. Almost all major cancer hospitals in the United States have patient navigators, and ideally the patient navigators speak the preferred language of the patient and family. Cancer centers without patient navigators might have social workers who can assist lung cancer patients. The most expensive part of cancer treatment is the medication(s) used for chemotherapy.[18]

Pharmaceutical companies have patient assistance programs that provide for medical assistance at home. Government programs, such as Medicare and Social Security, and nongovernmental organizations, such as CancerCare and the American Cancer Society, can also help patients who spend most of their time at home receive all forms of support.

To summarize, home-based approaches versus those at professional clinics are widely varied. This chapter has explored this variation by explaining the roles of family and friends in the lung cancer patient's life.

18

FINDING MOTIVATION AS A LUNG CANCER PATIENT

A cancer diagnosis can be devastating. The diagnosis immediately moves the person from a land of *wellness* to a box of *cancer*. Patients often report feeling isolated and overwhelmed on hearing a cancer diagnosis. Once the news is absorbed, the battle begins. When a person starts to battle lung cancer, he or she will pick up the pieces of control and take lung cancer bit by bit until the disease process looks and feels much less overwhelming. As the field of medicine is progressing, more treatment options are becoming available for people with advanced lung cancer, and that in turn can eventually strengthen one's ability to find motivation to either persevere with treatment or know when to give up and enjoy as many remaining days as one might have. Moreover, it is important for a lung cancer patient to rely on his or her inner strength and to never give up hope.

In the journey to find motivation, it is essential to discuss the diagnosis with a physician as much as possible. A second opinion is also valuable and is worth considering. The link that can occur between a patient, his or her medical team, and other patients in a treatment can create a strong sense of support and motivation needed throughout the treatment experience. Lung cancer can develop quickly and produce severe symptoms, requiring not only medical intervention but also the support needed to get through it. The side effects can be intense, and the person might even think that the cancer is progressing even if it's getting better because the patient may feel worse. That is why open communication between the patient and his or her medical team is needed in the cancer treatment so that the medical team can help and manage the patient's needs.[1]

AVENUES FOR FINDING MOTIVATION

Hope

There should or, better, *must* be a sense of hope for the lung cancer patient. While the concept of hope is addressed extensively in chapter 20, it is important to now understand how hope is a necessary tool on the path to finding motivation. Hopes and dreams require time. What everyone hopes for can be as stressful as the efforts of lung cancer patients and caregivers to gain motivation. If a patient is told that remission is not possible, he or she can make a plan for other things he or she might want to achieve in the remaining days. These may include comfort, peace, acceptance, and even joy. Hoping can give everyone a sense of purpose and lead the way to find much-needed motivation for both the lung cancer patient and the caregiver. To build a sense of hope, the patient needs to set goals to look forward to each day. He or she should make plans and do things that are enjoyable and exciting to get his or her mind off the disease and engaged in life. The following tips from other patients who have experienced advanced-stage cancer might be helpful: [2]

- As much as possible, the patient and caregivers and family should continue to plan their days as they have always done.
- Continue with preferred activities to the extent possible.
- Find things to look forward to each day of life.
- Set dates and events to look forward to.
- Stay focused and aware of the positive things in life—time with loved ones, activities and outings, and so forth.

Inner Strength

People with cancer might find mental and physical strength that they did not know they had. Someone may have felt overwhelmed when he or she first learned that the doctors could not control the cancer and now is not coping as well as he or she did in the past. They should keep in mind that the feelings of helplessness may change. Everyone has physical and emotional reserves they did not know they had. Calling on this "inner strength" can help revive their spirit. Some lung cancer sufferers find it easier if they (1) focus their attention on the present, (2) forget about the past, and (3) think in advance for the future. They focus on incorporating the activities of intervention into their everyday daily routine. The best thing to do in that situation is to accept that it may have to be different from that point on. Others like to visualize deep into the future and plan ahead. They set personal goals, such as traveling to places they would like to visit and things to do, as if life stretches out before them. Others find motivation by focusing on the current relationships with the people they love and are close to. Inner strength manifests itself in different forms for each person, so everyone dealing with lung cancer should draw on the elements in their life that are meaningful to them.[3]

Finding Humor

Laughter can help a patient relax. A small smile or a giggle can make anyone forget, even for a small period of time, about stressful thoughts. A lung cancer patient does not *always* feel like laughing, but laughter is said to be the best "medicine." Others who have gone through the same problems have found the following ideas helpful:[4]

- Enjoy fun things children and pets do.
- Watch humorous films or television shows.
- Use a computer and view funny videos or pictures or listen to stand-up comics. If the patient does not own a computer, he or she can always use the local library or ask a friend to print out a few pages.
- Listen to comedy tapes.
- Read the comics in the newspaper or the cartoons and quotes in the magazines.
- Look for something funny and interesting in the humor section of a library or bookstore.

Ways to Cope with Lung Cancer

Many people who have lung cancer or who have been treated for cancer generate symptoms or side effects that may affect their quality of life. Everyone should try to do their regular, everyday routines and request help for those routines that may prove to be more difficult. On treatment days, planning for rest and putting off other activities will help enable well-being. Care given to help patients cope with the symptoms or side effects is called palliative care (chapter 17), comfort care, or symptom management. After a cancer diagnosis, discussing prognosis (the likely course of the disorder) can be of use to the patients and their loved ones to cope easier and to find the right type of motivation.[5]

CHALLENGES IN FINDING MOTIVATION AS A LUNG CANCER PATIENT

Lung cancer patients who may fault themselves for smoking do not have to endure the guilt that may be associated with their diagnosis. It may be difficult to put things in perspective, but what is done is done, and feelings of guilt or shame should be addressed with a therapist so that a patient can let go and focus on moving forward. Depression and "facing reality," as some call it, should be addressed with a professional, as feelings of sadness and stress may be detrimental to overall health.

If the patient went to a clinic or a hospital with some symptoms indicative of the disease or no prior symptoms at all but the cancer was found incidentally, the patient should know that there are options. For most people who have the time to review all the options and make an informed decision, they will feel better about that decision because they will know they had all the information and made the right decision based on the information they had.[6]

It can be difficult to remain optimistic when a lung cancer diagnosis is given and during treatment. Finding motivation to direct what little energy a person may have for tackling the disease and the attendant issues can be very difficult. Drawing on earlier experiences may help provide much-needed motivation. A patient who has overcome even small adversities in the past can look to the strategies he or she employed to get through those times and try to tap into those. Or a patient can seek out others who have survived their cancer and ask for additional strategies that were helpful to that person. There are some feelings, however, that everyone is experiencing. Those feelings may not come all at once, and some days will be better than others. It would probably be helpful to know that (1) others have felt the same way, (2) it won't last forever, and (3) there is a possibility of winning this battle.

Feelings will come and go, just as they always have in a person's life. It is useful to have some strategies in order to deal with the feelings. First, patients need to remember that they are not alone and that many have been in a similar situation. Some choose to reveal themselves to friends and family members. They find it helpful when they talk with others who are facing the same challenges. There is also the possibility of joining a support group so that everyone can chat whenever they prefer. Even online support groups exist if those work better for someone who doesn't feel like being face-to-face with others during their journey. If support groups are not to someone's liking, there are experts, such as psychologists, who are well trained to work with the psychological characteristics of lung cancer care.[7]

Sadness and Depression

It is normal to feel sad, and it is totally acceptable to cry or to express sadness or anger or frustration. Patients searching for motivation do not have to be upbeat all the time or pretend to be cheerful in front of other individuals. Pretending to feel fine when one actually is not does not help in the efforts to confront lung cancer. Pretending may even create barriers between a lung cancer patient and his loved ones. The idea is to refrain from "holding things in" and to do what feels natural. Depression can happen if sadness or despair seem to take over one's life. Manifesting some of the signs that are listed below is normal during a time like this, but one should keep in mind that if this state lasts longer than two weeks, a talk with a doctor is necessary. Some symptoms may appear because of physical problems, and therefore it is important to talk to a professional in the medical team about them.[8]

Grief

Everyone copes differently with loss or the threat of loss, and grief can be one of the obstacles a lung cancer patient faces on the road to finding motivation. Some feel sadness and loneliness, and others feel fear, guilt, or anger. Some find that the way they think changes, such as feeling easily confused and lost. Unfortunately, the thoughts may repeat themselves over and over again, and there might be a loss of energy. Even a generalized loss of will can appear along with a lack of specific willpower to do tasks and to see people. All these are normal reactions to grief. What a man grieves for is as varied as how he thinks or feels. There might be grief for the loss of the body as it used to be or for things the lung cancer patient used to do but cannot anymore. There can also be grief for what is left: personality, family, friends, and the future. It is understandable if the patient decides to take time for him- or herself and look inward. It is also okay to surround oneself with people to whom one is close. The goal is to let loved ones know if (1) there is anything they can do, (2) there is any way they can help, or (3) they can just sit with the patient quietly. There is no right or wrong way to grieve, and often people who are going through a major change in life need extra help. It is important to know that no one has to go through this alone. There is always a possibility to talk with a health care team, a member of a faith community, or a mental health professional. Taking all this into account would undoubtedly help the lung cancer sufferer find motivation against the disease process.[9]

Denial

It can be difficult to accept the news that the malignant cells have spread or can no longer be controlled, and it is natural to need some time to adjust and be motivated enough to accept fate. However, this can become a serious problem if it lasts longer than a few weeks. It can be an obstacle preventing one from getting the appropriate care or talking about the treatment options and choices. As time winds down, the strategy here would be to keep an open mind and listen to the qualified people's suggestions before making a decision.[10]

Anger

The feeling of "No, not me!" often changes to the question of "Why me?" or "What is next?" A lung cancer patient has lot to deal with at the moment, so it is normal to feel a bit angry. No one has to pretend that everything is fine. The sufferer might become angry with family members, neighbors, and sometimes even at him- or herself. Some people even get angry with the deity and question their faith. At first, anger can be somewhat helpful if it helps to motivate a person. An angry patient may decide to learn more about different treatment options or become more involved in the care he or she is getting, but anger does not help if it is kept inside for too long or taken out on innocent individuals. Often the people who are closest are the ones who have to deal with the outrage the most. It may help to find out the source of the anger. This is not a stress-free task, as that anger may have originated from feelings that are difficult to show, such as panic, worry, fear, or helplessness. It is easier to deal with the stress resulting from anger if the patient is open-minded in those situations and the anger can be let go. Anger is a form of energy that can be indirectly converted into motivation. It may be better to use this energy through some sort of physical activity. Simply hitting a bed with a pillow might come in handy after all.[11]

Fear and Worry

Facing the unknown can be a staggering experience for the lung cancer sufferer. At times, a patient may feel scared of losing control of his or her life. There might be fear of becoming dependent on other people or, even worse, a fear of dying. If these fears take hold, one should remember that many have felt the same way. Some people worry too much about what will happen to their loved ones in the future, and this can result in motivation loss for the whole patient and caregiver team. Many individuals have fear of being in pain or feeling sick, yet all the above concerns are normal. Sometimes patients or family members worry that talking about their fears will make the cancer worse, but it is better for the patient's health if he or she knows what to expect to a certain extent. One objective would be to learn more about the disease process and treatment options by asking all sorts of questions of the health care team. It is always best to talk to someone of trust, and if the lung cancer patient feels overwhelmed by fear, it is important to re-member that others have felt this way too.[12]

Guilt and Regret

A respiratory cancer sufferer might not have the ability to stop thinking about what he or she could have done to decelerate the rate of growth of malignant cells in his or her lungs. Thoughts about how he or she should have gone sooner to the physician or taken other precautionary measures begin to surface. It is understandable that people with offi-cially diagnosed cancer wonder if they did anything wrong that might have contributed to their clinical situation. They might (1) blame them-selves for their lifestyle choices, (2) feel guilty because treatment did not work, or (3) feel guilty because they ignored a symptom(s) and it was too late when they went to see a health care professional for assis-tance. Others worry about not following the doctor's orders the way they should have. While on the road to finding motivation, it is impor-tant to remember that the treatment failed the patient—not the other way around. No one can know why cancer happens to some and not to others. In any case, feeling guilty would certainly not make things any better for the lung cancer sufferer; instead, it can stop the patient from taking action and getting the much-needed treatment. That said, the person with lung cancer should do the following:[13]

- Try to let go of any mistakes that have been made and have caused the guilt in the first place.
- Focus on things worthy of one's time and energy.
- Forgive themselves.

Patients may want to share these feelings with their loved ones and caregivers. Some people blame themselves for upsetting the people they love. Others worry that they will be a burden on their families. They should all take comfort in the fact that many family members might consider it an honor and a privilege to take care of their loved one, while others consider it a time to share experiences and become emotionally closer to one another. Caring for someone else helps an individual take life more seriously and hence devise a way for motivat-ing the patient.

Loneliness

Ironically, a lung cancer patient may feel alone if he or she has too many people in his or her social circle, possibly because he or she is the only one in the group suffering from such a chronic illness. This scenario undeniably presents difficulties on the road to finding motivation. Lung cancer sufferers may feel that no one really understands them and that no one is really aware of what they are going through. As the cancer progresses, they may see close friends, family members, and colleagues less often and find themselves alone more than they would like. Some people may even distance themselves from the patients because they have a difficult time coping with their condition. Not only can this make the lung cancer sufferer feel really alone and abandoned, but it also hinders any possibility of finding motivation. There will be some days that will be more stressful than the others, but it is important for sufferers to know that they are not alone. They should not step aside from daily routines, and they should keep doing the things they have always done in the best way they can. If they feel the need, they should tell others around them that they do not *want* to be alone. Lung cancer sufferers should simply allow others to know that they welcome their visits. It is more than likely that the patient's loved ones are experiencing somewhat similar feelings and may also feel as if they are disconnected from the patient if they are unable to establish a connection. Talking openly and giving others a chance to be closer emotionally can work wonders, and, after all, the only thing friends and family want is to help a loved one who could use a little motivation.[14]

19

PREVENTION AND COLLECTIVE EFFORTS

Both smokers and nonsmokers are exposed to a number of risk factors that, especially in combinations such as tobacco smoking and exposure to environmental toxins, increase overall lung cancer risk. Lifestyle changes in industrialized countries related mainly to smoking, unhealthy diet, and lack of regular physical activity only make the global lung cancer situation worse. Taking measures that collectively address risk factors is one way of combatting this terrible disease; cutting down on one's own risk factors is another way to help prevent the development of lung cancer.

HOW CORPORATIONS CAN HELP

Primary Prevention

Collective efforts to prevent lung cancer are possible; as a starting point, corporations can implement measures that help contribute to lung cancer prevention strategies. The most effective but difficult-to-achieve effort is primary prevention to protect individuals from carcinogens. Primary prevention is difficult because of the numerous risk factors surrounding us at all times: industrial pollution, automobile fumes, eating habits, medicines, lifestyle, and smoking. Moreover, the environment has enormous significance for the occurrence of cancer even when lung cancer has a genetic origin, and this could be an important concern for corporations looking to participate in the efforts to rid the world of lung cancer. Corporations could make efforts to curb their use of carcinogenic materials, improve workplace conditions, provide cleaner-running vehicles, implement smoking policies designed to make smoking on the job more inconvenient, and supporting healthier living for their workers.

Reduction of Smoking

Primary prevention requires that drastic action be taken by public, private, and community organizations. First, companies can institute clean air policies that limit smoking on work grounds. Tobacco smoking is the reason for about 85 to 90 percent of all new cancer cases that lead to death.[1] Smoking within a foot or so of a building can allow secondhand smoke to move indoors, thereby affecting even those who do not choose to smoke. Secondhand smoke contains the full range of the same carcinogenic elements that have been found in the smoke inhaled by smokers but in different amounts.[2]

Dietary Habits

In accordance with the American Cancer Society's recommendations, organizations (including businesses and corporations) should work diligently to create social and physical environments that are beneficial for teaching the habits of consuming healthy foods and regularly performing physical activities. Efforts should be directed to (1) increasing access to healthy food and (2) providing safe, enjoyable, and accessible environments for physical activity and for transportation and recreation.

The working life of the individual suffering from lung cancer is tightly connected to eating and habits of physical activity, such as exercise. While a lung cancer patient who is suffering from the end stages of cell malignancy most likely will *not* be working, employees are the corporation's most precious capital, so applicable actions should be taken to improve the staff's health and subsequently reduce the risk of employees experiencing lung cancer in the future. Long working hours and overtime assignments, for example, decrease spare time for cooking and could increase fast-food consumption. Diet has been shown to have a dual effect on the appearance of lung cancer, including both protective and harmful aspects. A diet rich in antioxidant nutrients may protect against cancer.[3] There is significant evidence that individuals consuming larger quantities of fruits and vegetables face a smaller risk of suffering lung cancer—a reduction of approximately 25 percent.[4] All these points can be taken into consideration by corporations providing free lunches to their employees on a regular basis.

Physical Activity

Physical activity (and weight loss as a byproduct) represents another element of primary prevention. The role of corporations in supporting a healthy working and social environment for employees may have substantial effect on designing each individual's habits as a whole. Companies could consider offering incentives for those who get regular exercise or provide on-site fitness centers for those taking lunch breaks or those who must work overtime. Not only do such efforts help reduce illness, but they often are seen as perks to those working there or hoping to be employed by such companies.[5] Nine different clinical studies have shown that higher physical activity reduces lung cancer risk by about 30 percent.[6]

Reducing Occupational Exposure to Lung Carcinogens

Corporations involved in manufacturing or construction businesses might require contact with environmental toxins (chapter 5) in any form, thus increasing their employees' risk of lung cancer incidence. Occupational exposure to carcinogens increases lung cancer risk, with an estimated 3 to 40 percent of all lung cancer cases attributable to occupational exposures.[7] Unfortunately, full removal of these occupational substances is unrealistic considering that these toxins are present in the natural environment. Many corporations, especially those in developing countries or employing staff from lower socioeconomic classes, do not have any incentive to reduce individuals' exposure to toxic substances. Such production or construction sites represent an imminent threat not only to the employees but also to citizens residing in the neighborhood. A long-term collective strategy for reducing occupational exposure to lung cancer–associated substances should be a corporate priority.

Secondary Prevention

For corporations, the goal of secondary prevention is to avoid lung cancer appearing in advanced stages and to allow treatment of precancerous conditions for employees facing a high risk of lung cancer. Priority is given to the early detection of malignant cells. Treatment and outcome of cancers is by far more favorable when (1) the disorder is established prior to the appearance of symptoms and (2) the disease process is localized in the organ, so early cancer detection should be a top priority of corporate policy. Corporations may effectively participate in secondary prevention activities by funding investigations and trials on the effect of lung cancer screening methods on respective mortality rates. Today, numerous companies (operating mainly in the pharmaceutical business) raise funds for such investigations.

GOVERNMENT AND COLLECTIVE EFFORTS

Role of Government in Economic Losses from Lung Cancer

In addition to the devastating number of people who die from lung cancer is the side effect of economic losses, something that governments should continue to pay attention to. Such losses are methodically investigated in the United States, where tobacco smoking has caused early expenditures in the area of government-sponsored public health services, including expenses for (1) treatment of adults, (2) newborn children with medical problems, (3) decreased productivity, and (4) increased death rate. The yearly losses for 1997–2001 in the U.S. economy caused by the increased death rate due to tobacco smoking are calculated to be $92 billion, an increase of over $10 billion compared to the period 1995–1999. Medical expenses connected to tobacco smoking during 1998 were $75.5 billion, or 8 percent of all personal medical expenditures.[8]

Government Interventions

Taking the tragic consequences of tobacco smoking into consideration, it would be normal to expect a reduction in the number of smokers along with an increase in the number of people who gave up smoking. In 2003, the number of smokers in the world was reported to be 1.3 billion (over 1 billion men and around 250 million women), and over 30 million adolescents are now smoking too. The number of smokers is expected to increase to 1.7 billion by 2025. The most significant increase in tobacco smoking in the past 10 years is attributed to developing countries from Asia and Africa. When it comes to government efforts to reduce the global prevalence of lung cancer, these statistics pose a great concern.[9]

The most developed and wealthy governments do promise better outlooks. For example, the yearly consumption of cigarettes in the United States has decreased drastically. In 2004, the number of cigarettes consumed per capita decreased by about 60 percent compared to the 1960s, when consumption was very high. Even though for the period 1983–2003 the percentage of smokers among all educational levels decreased, the largest decrease was seen among college graduates.[10]

It is more than convincing that tobacco smoking and lung cancer are directly related, so governments are challenged to provide decisive measures against smoking. Quitting smoking is noticeably beneficial for the smoker. The preventive effect of quitting, however, depends on the number of years and the intensity of prior smoking. It has been noted that after 10 years of quitting smoking, the mortality risk of lung cancer is reduced from 50 to 30 percent when compared to permanent smokers.[11] The benefits of tobacco control on the population provide strong evidence that reducing exposure to cigarettes at the population level results in respective declines in the incidence of lung cancer. Fewer cases of starting to smoke and more government antismoking efforts are the real reasons behind the overall decline in the number of men dying from lung cancer since the mid-1980s. Since the 1960s, smoking among men has been gradually declining.[12]

Tobacco addiction was discovered long ago, and numerous trials and guidelines have been developed in a search for ways for people to quit permanently. Governments are not designed to be able to guide heavy smokers in their efforts to quit, but numerous investigations have found solid evidence supporting early tobacco smoking cessation as beneficial for eventual lung cancer prevention at the collective scale.

Government and Smoking Guidelines

A step to collectively addressing the grave lung cancer statistics may be the government's support of health care systems in helping nicotine-dependent patients. Nicotine-dependent smokers are exposed to carcinogenic and *genotoxic* (gene-damaging) elements that cause lung cancer, and severe dependence is often difficult to overcome. A set of guidelines for quitting smoking was developed by the government to assist nicotine-dependent patients and formal caregivers.[13] Major elements of the guidelines include the following:

- Clinicians must document the tobacco use status of every patient.
- Every smoking patient should be provided with at least one brief intervention session for effective smoking cessation.
- The long-term abstinence of tobacco is attributable to intense interventions reflecting the response of the body in relation to nicotine consumed and the overall interventional outcome.
- The approaches aimed at smoking cessation should include one or more of the following:

- Nicotine replacement (e.g., nicotine patches or gums) or other evidence-based smoking cessation pharmacotherapy
- Social support from the clinician in the form of encouragement and assistance
- Skills training or problem solving

In order to be effective, health care systems must change institutionally to identify tobacco consumers and provide interventions on a continual basis. In addition to individually focused efforts for quitting smoking, a number of strategies for tobacco control at the community, state, and national government levels have led to reducing smoking prevalence. Strategies include the following:[14]

- Reducing minors' access to tobacco products
- Disseminating effective school-based prevention curricula together with media strategies
- Adopting smoke-free laws and policies
- Using tobacco excise taxes to fund community-level interventions including mass media

- Raising the cost of tobacco products by raising taxes
- Providing proven quitting strategies through collaboration with health care organizations

Smoke-Free Workplace Legislation

Smoke-free workplace legislation has been linked to reductions of nicotine levels, as well as dust, benzene, and particulate matter, that were consistent and statistically significant. Studies have reported health indicators including respiratory systems, other symptoms, and hospital admissions as outcomes, and a consistent finding related to health reported a decreased number of admissions in hospitals for cardiac events. Evidence has been gathered in favor of the fact that smoke-free workplace legislation may also result in a reduced prevalence of active cigarette smoking. For instance, research has shown a 32 percent reduction in smoking prevalence in a country that enacted smoke-free workplace legislation, compared to a 2.8 percent reduction in neighboring countries with no smoke-free legislation in force.[15]

Although there is overwhelming public support in almost every country that has introduced a smoking ban, large groups of heavy smokers are still opposed to such legislation. People in bars, casinos, and restaurant can be separated into two groups: staff and customers. To grant customers the freedom to smoke, employees afterward become victims of constant exposure to secondhand smoke. There are ongoing arguments whether smoking bans have negative economic effects on the hospitality industry and on tourism as a whole. Studies that have been undertaken in the United States show that smoking bans have either a neutral or a favorable effect on tourist businesses. Smoke-free eating areas and rooms that have not been exposed to smoke may serve as better advertisements than any other positive characteristics of, for example, a hotel. Surveys demonstrating mainly negative economic consequences of smoke-free legislation have been funded by tobacco manufacturers and thus are not necessarily objective and of high quality. A key challenge for all governments, however, is not only to place a nationwide voting system for a smoking ban but also to issue compliance orders for restaurants, bars, casinos, and all other indoor premises covered by the provisions of legislation. In some countries, smoking bars or smoking clubs have received permission to allow smoking indoors.

Their growing number is raising questions about the effectiveness of smoking bans as well as what the general public is "paying" for these bars' and clubs' negligence. It is up to the government to decide whether to acknowledge the guidelines of medical organizations for supporting the well-being of the population or to grant the freedom to smoke to everyone regardless of the cost.[16]

Government Efforts Aimed at Children and Adolescents

Passive smoke is also a leading cause of asthma in children. Because of their exposure to tobacco or environmental smoke, children and adolescents are suffering a higher rate of asthma morbidity, including decreased lung function and asthma symptoms. Even though smoke-free legislation has become a way to reduce exposure to secondhand smoke, children are still exposed to tobacco smoke at home (chapter 17). More than one in six children suffering from asthma is reported to live with a smoking parent.[17] Despite the worldwide tendency of governments to raise the prices of cigarettes and other tobacco products, low-income families expose their children to in-home secondhand smoke more often than do non–low-income families. Additionally, adolescents suffering from asthma are consumers of tobacco smoke products, having a direct effect on the incidence and aggravation of asthma symptoms. Such results show the need for additional government efforts aimed at educating low-income families, especially adolescents, on the harmful effects of consuming tobacco smoke products. These implications are especially important for youngsters who are more vulnerable to lung problems, such as asthma, or who have already been diagnosed with a lung disorder.

Society today has easy access to all forms of information, and everyone interested in preventing lung cancer or in having a healthy life may find scientific advice on this. Generally, people with higher educational degrees live healthier lives.[18] Statistics show a reduced number of heavy smokers among college students, and academic interest in the environment may be the reason behind the statistics. Government agendas, however, may be aimed at providing broader access to education on the one hand and information regarding lung cancer prevention presented to the broader audience starting in high school on the other. A young person should not begin smoking in response to peer pressure but should be informed of the harms related to the addiction of tobacco smoking. Governments can certainly help in this effort.[19]

HOW LUNG CANCER PATIENTS CAN ASSIST EACH OTHER

Cancer Diagnosis

Hearing a cancer diagnosis is a personal experience that may be shocking and life altering. Each individual's feelings are grounded in his or her strengths, beliefs, and difficult situations that may have been faced. The acceptance of the lung cancer diagnosis, however, is not immediate; it should be a *continuous* process of adaptation. Regardless of the degree of disease, every cancer patient suffers a state of confusion and desperation. In such moments, patients may help each other since not every family member or friend can grasp the problem the way the patient can. Attention to the emotional burden of having cancer is often a part of a patient's treatment plan. The help of respiratory patient networks can make lung cancer sufferers feel less isolated and distressed and, moreover, provide them with access to the most recent information regarding available treatments.

A lung cancer support group represents a secure "space" where everyone can (1) talk about concerns stemming from their particular situations in life, (2) provide unbiased decisions, or (3) be willing to cater specifically to other patients' needs whenever possible. The beneficial effects of support groups on the confidence, feelings of stress, and interpersonal comfort of the lung cancer patient are only supplements to the direct improvement of support group members' health. The patient support group may provide information regarding treatment issues, specialist medical care, and other information pertinent to their overall struggle with the disease process.

A major aspect of collective patient–patient support is the financial assistance that lung cancer support communities grant. When the emotional shock is over, a newly diagnosed lung cancer patient has to face clinical treatment and all its complications—be it physical difficulties or financial costs that insurance may not cover.[20] For example, palliative care procedures have a beneficial effect on the overall treatment and condition of the patient. Some support communities raise funds and help their patient members cover the cost of such palliative approaches. Another example may be the financial support for transporting the patient for specialized care at a medical center in a remote location. Access to medical treatment may represent a hefty obstacle for many lung cancer patients, especially those who live far away from a qualified hospital or those of advanced age. In such cases, the proper and timely diagnosis, as well as the treatment itself, is closely related first to transportation costs and then to medical costs. The role of patient–patient groups may therefore be played by an intermediary that provides funds to lung cancer patients in need. Moreover, such support groups may shorten the time wondering which medical centers or hospitals to choose as a starting point since the major goal of these communities is to inform and provide counseling from a collective standpoint.

Virtual Patient-to-Patient Support Groups

Today, just about everyone is online. Virtual lung cancer patient communities provide a widespread availability of peer-to-peer venues where people having common interests meet online to talk about their experiences, ask questions, or provide emotional support collectively. Such virtual patient gatherings represent a solution to the "distance" problem. Using online technologies, a lung cancer patient living in Europe can easily receive the help and support from his or her peers in North America. Moreover, medical practices are shared worldwide, and the newest information on lung cancer treatment is within easy reach. It is already common for patients to get diagnosed by a doctor using online technology. Examination results, anamnesis, and medical history reports (chapter 7) are widely available in electronic form, making it easier for the medical specialist to interact and communicate about a certain case. For example, lung cancer patients can receive the opinion of a renowned medical school professor located miles and miles away in just a matter of seconds, minutes, or hours. This is extremely important for lung cancer–diagnosed individuals since (1) the emotional burden can be noteworthy and (2) a clear picture of the treatment and its risks, as well as expected longevity, is needed as soon as possible. Recent communication technologies are also cost effective since there is no need to spend much money getting diagnosed. Financial expenses, as well as emotional stress, may be too great an obstacle for a cancer patient to undertake simply to get diagnosed. In developing regions, however, access to proper medical services, information, and virtual support groups remains a luxury. It is not only problematic to get a timely discovery of a disease process such as lung cancer but also almost impossible to receive surefire medical and psychological interventions. Patient organizations continue to face the ongoing challenge of trying to collectively provide a dignified and healthy life to everyone.

In summary, people must conjoin their efforts in fighting a major cause of premature death all over the world, namely, lung cancer in all its manifestations. It is everyone's responsibility to take a long look at life and take steps to block exposure to risk factors familiar to the general public, such as tobacco smoking. Many toxins that are considered risk factors for instigating cell malignancy in the lung may not be easily avoided, yet still individuals may have have a friend, a relative, or someone else they know who has been diagnosed with lung cancer. In anticipation of further medical advances for fighting lung cancer, corporations, governments, and patient peer groups continue to show concern and to take action in a collective manner.

20

CONCLUSION

So far, the different types along with the history, causes, signs, and symptoms, of lung cancer have been analyzed. The inpatient and outpatient experiences of people who have been affected by lung cancer and those who have overcome it have also been reviewed. All in all, lung cancer poses a dangerous threat to those who are diagnosed, but with hope, patience, confidence, and support, patients can learn more about their diagnoses and make informed decisions about their own treatment and care. Once diagnosed with lung cancer, proper steps have to be taken by the patient and caregivers to undergo treatment, chemotherapy sessions, taking medication on time, following physicians' advice, and also having the right spirit throughout the ordeal.

HOPE DESPITE THE DESTRUCTIVE NATURE OF LUNG CANCER

Lung cancer can be very depressing and emotionally draining apart from the physical damage and stress taking place within the body. In turn, having a strong sense of hope can be challenging. Clinicians working with patients suffering from lung cancer can, however, intervene to give hope by enhancing quality of life from diagnosis both during the development of the disease and throughout the process of treatment. Simply put, hopeful interventions need to be developed to support both patients and caregivers.[1]

Caregivers and patients alike undergo significant stress and trauma, and it becomes necessary for both to not get "bogged down" by the negative turn of events in their lives and to ignite the spark that will give them the confidence and energy to fight the disease process. This is easier said than done, but in order not to give up and continue to keep the "fighting spirit" alive, it is necessary to keep one's willpower and always hope for a better tomorrow. Relying on friends, family, and neighbors for emotional, physical, and spiritual support and learning to ask for help when it is needed will help energize patients and keep them going when things turn difficult.

Survivors Setting Examples of Hope

There are cancer patient success stories as well as many cases of losing battles, but there are also many instances of clinical miracles. Unfortunately, lung cancer patients can give up too soon when hope is lost. Keeping the patient in cheerful surroundings and doing away with self-pity can help give some level of hope. Being patient and honest with a cancer sufferer may make decision making easier and the final days more enjoyable if a prognosis is dire. Diverting the mind from the depressing situation by doing things that the lung cancer patient enjoys can help keep a person's spirits up and may contribute to enhanced resilience. Lung cancer sufferers derive inspiration and hope from other survivors through their art, writing, poetry, and tips on life as a patient.

Trial medicines and therapies have given hope to countless patients, and those stories can provide for hope and perseverance for those still battling the disease process. Guest speeches are an excellent medium through which lung cancer survivors can tell their stories to the world. The purpose in recounting experiences of survivors or patients is twofold: it offers hope, and it acts as a "window" that brings some "fresh air" into the life of someone living with terminal lung cancer. Some survivors want to document the various thoughts and emotions that they encounter during this arduous journey. If this helps the sufferer rationalize the situation, it is a therapy in itself against becoming swallowed up by a lack of hope.

Hope after the Diagnosis

The day someone finds out that either he or she or a loved one has cancer can be one of the toughest days in one's life. For many, there is an overwhelming sense that they are alone. There are resources that help the recently diagnosed find inspiration from the people who've been there. Sometimes there is a hope that patients will find healing by speaking about it as well. It is important to show love and support to families who suffer disturbance in their lives, and it is believed that positive attitudes and friendship should be stimulated, especially at such difficult times. It is important for people to be in touch with others in the same situation, who can empathize so deeply. Hearing that a person has lung cancer can come as a shock. After learning about the diagnosis, lung cancer patients might feel numb, frightened, or angry to the point where they are unable to secure any hope. They may not believe what the doctor is saying and may feel all alone, even if their friends and family were in the same room with them. These feelings are completely normal.

The first few weeks following diagnosis are very difficult. Perhaps after hearing the word *cancer*, patients have some trouble listening to what is being said afterward or have difficulty breathing. People with cancer and those close to them will experience a wide array of emotions and feelings. These feelings can change often and without warning. At times, they may be angry, afraid, or worried, and they will not really believe that they have cancer. Nonetheless, some patients suffering from lung cancer might have a positive outlook for the future. Once they accept that they have cancer and put in place a treatment plan that they feel comfortable with, they are able to see many reasons for having hope.

Living with Hopeful Change

Millions of people around the world have cancer, and for them cancer has become a chronic, ongoing health problem, much like high blood pressure or diabetes.[2] In ways similar to that of everyone else, people who have lung cancer must get regular checkups for the rest of their lives, even after treatment ceases. Unlike other chronic health issues, however, a cancer patient probably will not need to take medicine or eat special foods once he or she has completed cancer-ending treatment, such as surgical resection, but he or she may wish to make some lifestyle choices that will enhance overall health (chapter 14). Still, once a cancer is "cured," many survivors continue to live in fear that it will return. Minor aches may make them worry and possibly even think about dying. While it is normal to ponder these thoughts, it is also important to focus on *living*. Although some people do die of lung cancer, many are treated successfully. Others will live a long time before passing away from it, so it is best that they try to make the most of each day while living with cancer and its treatment. A person will have many feelings after they learn that they have lung cancer. These feelings can alter each day, even on an hour-to-hour basis. Some of the feelings the patient may go through include denial, anger, fear, stress, anxiety, depression, sadness, guilt, and loneliness. All these feelings are normal but can inevitably stand in the way of finding hope.

A marked improvement is realized when considering the odds of living *with* versus living *past* the cancer. Some survivors go on to live for many more years in good health. A true caregiver would believe that that hope will help the body deal with cancer. Today, scientists are also considering the question of whether having a hopeful outlook and positive attitude will help people feel better in general. In cancer support groups, leaders may suggest to the patient a few ways to build a sense of hope, such as writing down hopeful feelings and talking about those feelings with others. The idea is to somehow avoid the limitations of what lung cancer sufferers prefer to do as part of their daily living routines.

Persons with lung cancer can also do things that are more meaningful to them—hence another lifestyle change in the path to achieving hope. People have hobbies, both large and small, that bring more meaning to their lives. For these individuals, it may be visiting a garden in their city or town. It could be praying in a religious place of their choice or playing golf or some other sport. At first, finding hope in the midst of change may be tough, but patients can eventually find joy in their lives. Taking note of what makes them smile and paying attention to the things they do can help when it comes to finding hope. These can be as simple as drinking coffee in the morning, sitting down somewhere next to a pet, or talking with a friend.

Some people might see their cancer making a comeback as a "wake-up call." They might realize the importance of enjoying the little things in life while having hope. Some may be interested in going to places they have never been, while others finish projects they had started but put aside a while. There are people who also mend broken relationships. Although feelings of denial, anger, fear, stress and anxiety, depression, sadness, guilt, and loneliness are all normal, so is a sense of hope. While no one is cheerful all the time, hope is a positive element of the lung cancer experience.

PATIENCE AND CONFIDENCE WHEN APPROACHING LUNG CANCER

Lung cancer can be like a frightening ride in a roller coaster. Patients have good days and some bad days. Impatient mood swings can be common among cancer patients, and caregivers need to keep that in mind. It is a known fact that cancer causes much situational stress (chapter 16); it affects family relationships, and it quickly brings forth issues in the family that might have been lying repressed or dormant for many years. That in turn can tax the patience of both the lung cancer sufferer and his or her caregiver. Some people might have short-term memory problems caused by a variety of features, such as chemotherapy, pain relievers, and sleeping patterns. It is of absolute importance to give personal space to the patient, but it is equally important to let the sufferer know that his or her loved ones care and love him or her with all their heart. At times, cancer patients may expect family members to behave in certain ways, such as by (1) coming closer together, (2) showing more love, and (3) making them feel that they are wanted by the family and not ignored. If things do not go the way in which they (the patient) had expected, it is possible that they may become even more depressed or angry or feel alienated. All these factors may diminish the patience of the individual with lung cancer.[3]

Caregivers and Caring

Caring for a family member with a disease process as serious as lung cancer can be stressful for the caregiver, but if the latter follows certain points, the course can be much less stressful. It is essential to give oneself and the patient time to adjust to the fact that lung cancer has stricken his or her life. Maintaining positivity will help the patient adjust to treatment easily and quickly. As the topic of this section suggests, patience is important when dealing with lung cancer. The caregiver has to develop a lot of patience (especially if he or she is known to lose it often), courage, and, possibly, a good sense of humor. Living with a serious disorder such as lung cancer is not easy. If certain steps are followed, it can be helpful for the patient throughout the treatment. One has to adopt a fighting spirit, which is, of course, easier said than done.

Apart from this, one has to make positive changes in lifestyle that will improve the outcomes, such as quitting smoking, regularly exercising, and eating proper and healthy food. Paying attention to how one is feeling and getting plenty of rest, good nutrition, and time for personal care are also important. By extension, these modifications will only boost the lung cancer patient's confidence.

In addition to the above, four themes related to the process of developing confidence in a caregiver can be identified. These are: increasing one's credibility, training, emotional burden, and trying to making a difference. Managing the care of patients with lung cancer can be rewarding for caregivers and nurse specialists, but it can also be emotionally challenging. Training and backing for such roles is vital and requires further in-depth research.[4]

The moment a person learns that he or she or a loved one has lung cancer, confidence can be reduced. It can also change the lives of those who are close to the patient. These changes can be difficult to handle. It is normal for the patient, family, and friends to need help coping with the feelings that a diagnosis of cancer can bring, as there may be concerns about treatments and side-effect management, hospital stays, and medical bills. The patient may also worry about caring for the family, retaining a job, or continuing daily activities. In an effort to increase confidence and patience, the individual with lung cancer who is facing such concerns can pay a visit to the following:

- Doctors, nurses, and other members of the patient's health care team can answer questions about treatment, working, or any other activities.

- Social workers, counselors, or members of the clergy can be help-ful if the patient wants to talk about his or her feelings and con-cerns. Usually, social workers can suggest resources for financial aid, transportation, home care, or emotional support.
- Support groups can also be of help. In these groups, people with lung cancer or their family members meet with other patients or their families to share what they have learned about coping with the disease and the effects of treatment. Different support groups may offer support in different forms, such as support in person, over the telephone, or on the Internet. The patient may want to talk with a member of his or her health care team about finding a support group that will boost his or her patience and confidence in the struggle against lung cancer.

The patient can be supported by family and friends in many ways, but at times the latter may want the patient to ask for what he or she needs. It can be as simple as offering the patient company, holding a hand, or giving him or her a hug. Sometimes they may provide a helping hand with meals, errands, or household chores. The patient could request them to accompany him or her on doctor's visits or treatment sessions, as people seem to feel better when they help others. There are numer-ous ways in which family, friends, other people who have cancer, spiri-tual or religious leaders, and health care providers can boost the suffer-er's confidence levels.

Alternatively, cancer support groups also matter when it comes to raising the lung cancer patient's confidence. These groups conduct meetings for people with cancer and those known to be at a risk of cancer. Depending on the patient's comfort level, they can be done in person, by phone, or on the Internet. These groups permit the patient and his or her loved ones to talk with others confronting the same issues. Many support groups host lectures and provide time for discus-sions.[5]

SEEING A DOCTOR RATHER THAN USING SELF-APPROACH

Any form of cell malignancy must be treated under a clinician's supervision only. Regularly updating doctors of the patient's progress will enable doctors to document the disease process and how the medication or therapy is working. It can be traumatic for the patient to undergo all sorts of treatment, but that is really the only way forward to getting completely relieved from the tumor. Most health care professionals are happy to explain things in language that makes sense to patients.

Patient–Doctor Communication

Talking often with the doctor is important in making informed decisions about the patient's health regimen. Wanting to be informed and asking questions give some control over the cancerous disorder and may help the patient cope. Individuals with cancer who are fully informed about their disease and treatment options usually tend to fare better and have fewer side effects than those who simply follow doctors' orders. Some people may feel overwhelmed by too much information or do not want to know as many details about their medical condition.[6]

Speaking to the doctor about the cancer sometimes may seem challenging. Some experience "information overload" during these conversations and are unable to understand what they hear, while others might feel that asking too many questions constitutes impolite behavior. It is nonetheless essential for the patient to find ways to (1) effectively communicate his or her needs to the professional caregiver, (2) ask questions to understand his or her options and learn the doctor's opinion, and (3) express his or her preferences. The lung cancer patient can also consider adopting some of the following ideas to further strengthen the likelihood of proper patient–doctor communication:

- The patient could make a note of the symptoms as a record to help remember the details he or she might want to discuss with the doctor when going for regular appointments.
- During the appointment, the patient could take notes, record important conversations, or bring along a friend or maybe a family member to keep track of the details. This would permit the pa-

tient to review the information more precisely after the appointment.

- When the patient feels there might be information overload, he or she could tell the doctor up front how much information he or she wants. This is because some patients might prefer to know each and every detail about their disease, such as statistics and the chances for recovery, while others might prefer to hear the least amount of information necessary to make good decisions about their treatment plan.

- The patient must not be afraid to "speak up" if the information received ceases to make any sense. If this is difficult for a particular patient, bringing along an advocate to assist with communicating when the patient is unable or unwilling is a good strategy. Physicians want to ensure that the lung cancer patient fully understands the information they provide.

- The patient must ensure that he or she knows the next step of care before leaving the caregiver's office.

- Occasionally, the patient might want to take home any written information to help remember what was discussed during the appointment or to share with friends and family.

Even after taking these steps, at times it is possible that the person suffering from lung cancer still has some apprehensions. In such cases, it is advisable to talk with a third person, such as another oncologist or a pulmonologist.[7]

In accordance with the doctor's instructions, it is advisable to engage in regular checkups for lung cancer. Checkups help ensure that any changes in the health of the patient are noted and treated if need be. The lung cancer sufferer may be given oxygen through a mask or nasal cannula to make breathing easier, but it is essential that the patient not smoke or let anyone else smoke in the same room while the oxygen is on.

Last, this book has been written in hopes of covering as much information about lung cancer as possible, with the additional intention of helping both patients and caregivers who have been affected by this disease process.

APPENDIX A

Lung Cancer–Related Links

www.asbestos.com/cancer/lung-cancer/prognosis.php
www.cancer.gov/cancertopics/cancerlibrary/what-is-cancer
www.cancer.ie/cancer-information/lung-cancer/symptoms-and-diagnosis
www.cancer.org/cancer/lungcancer/index
www.cancercenter.com/lung-cancer.cfm
www.cancercouncil.com.au/lung-cancer
www.cancermonthly.com/cancer_basics/lung.asp
www.cancerresearchuk.org/cancer-help
www.cdc.gov/cancer
www.emedicine.medscape.com/article/320261-overview
www.everydayhealth.com/lung-cancer/lung-cancer-diagnosis.aspx
www.guidance.nice.org.uk/CG121
www.ielcap.org/lungcancer/lcfaqs.html
www.lungcancer.about.com
www.lungcancer.org/find_information
www.lung.org/lung-disease/lung-cancer
www.lungcanceralliance.org/get-information
www.lungcancercoalition.org
www.lungcancerjournal.info
www.lungcancerprofiles.com/lung_cancer_information.aspx
www.macmillan.org.uk/cancerinformation
www.mayoclinic.org/lung-cancer
www.mdanderson.org/patient-and-cancer-information
www.medicinenet.com/lung_cancer/article.htm
www.mskcc.org/cancer-care/adult/lung
www.nationallungcancerpartnership.org
www.netdoctor.co.uk/diseases/facts/lungcancer.htm
www.nlm.nih.gov/medlineplus/lungcancer.html
www.patient.co.uk/health/lung-cancer
www.psychcentral.com/lib/2006/stress-a-cause-of-cancer
www.seer.cancer.gov
www.uspreventiveservicestaskforce.org/uspstf/uspslung.htm
www.webmd.com/lung-cancer/guide

APPENDIX B

Research and Training

American Association for Cancer Research
615 Chestnut Street, 17th Floor
Philadelphia, PA 19106
(866) 423-3965
Fax: (215) 440-9313
aacr@aacr.org
www.aacr.org

American Cancer Society
250 Williams Street NW
Atlanta, GA 30303
(800) 227-2345
www.cancer.org/research

Birmingham Comprehensive Cancer Center at University of Alabama
1720 2nd Avenue South NP 2500
Birmingham, AL 35294
(800) 822-0933
jtill@uab.edu

www.ccc.uab.edu

Brigham and Women's Hospital
75 Francis Street
Boston, MA 02115
(617) 732-5500
www.brighamandwomens.org

British Lung Foundation
73–75 Goswell Road
London EC1V 7ER
England
+44 (0)20 7688 5555
enquiries@blf.org.uk
www.blf.org.uk

Cancer Institute of New Jersey
195 Little Albany Street
New Brunswick, NJ 08903
(732) 235-2465
www.cinj.org

Cancer Treatment Centers of America
1336 Basswood Road
Schaumburg, IL 60173
(847) 342-7400
www.cancercenter.com

Center for Cancer Research, National Cancer Institute
31 Center Drive
Building 31, Room 3A11
Bethesda, MD 20892
(301) 496-4345
www.ccr.cancer.gov

City of Hope Comprehensive Cancer Center
1500 East Duarte Road
Duarte, CA 91010
(800) 826-4673
www.cityofhope.org

Dana-Farber Cancer Institute
450 Brookline Avenue
Boston, MA 02215
(866) 408-3324
dana-farbercontactus
@dfci.harvard.edu
www.dana-farber.org

Duke Cancer Institute
DUMC Box 3917
10 Bryan Searle Drive
Seeley Mudd Building, 2nd Floor
Durham, NC 27710
(888) 275-3853
www.dukecancerinstitute.org

Fox Chase Cancer Center
333 Cottman Avenue
Philadelphia, PA 19111
(888) 369-2427
www.foxchase.org

Fred Hutchinson Cancer Research Center
1100 Fairview Avenue North
PO Box 19024
Seattle, WA 98109
(206) 667-5000
externalrel@fhcrc.org
www.fhcrc.org

H. Lee Moffitt Cancer Center and Research Institute
12902 Magnolia Drive
Tampa, FL 33612
(800) 456-3434
www.moffitt.org

Huntsman Cancer Institute, University of Utah
2000 Circle of Hope
Salt Lake City, UT 84112
(877) 585-0303
www.huntsmancancer.org

Intercultural Cancer Council, Baylor College of Medicine
One Baylor Plaza MS 620
Houston, TX 77030
(713) 798-4614
Fax: (713) 798-3990
icc@uh.edu
www.iccnetwork.org

International Early Lung Cancer
Action Program
925 W. Baseline Road, Suite 105,
#G4
Tempe, AZ 85283
(480) 560-5516
coordinator@ielcap.org
www.ielcap.org

Irish Cancer Society
4345 Northumberland Road
Dublin 4, Ireland
+353 (01) 2310-500
Fax: +353 (01) 2310-555
research@irishcancer.ie
www.cancer.ie

James Graham Brown Cancer
Center
529 South Jackson Street
Louisville, KY 40202
(866) 530-5516
info@ulh.org
www.browncancercenter.org

Lung Cancer Research Foundation
845 Third Avenue, 6th Floor
New York, NY 10022
(646) 290-5154
Fax: (888) 638-8563
info@lungfund.org
www.lungcancerresearchfoundati
on.org

LUNGevity Foundation
218 South Wabash Avenue, Suite
540

Chicago, IL 60604
(312) 464-0716
Fax: (312) 464-0737
info@lungevity.org
lungevity.org

Manchester Cancer Research Cen
tre, University of Manchester
Wilmslow Road
Manchester M20 4BX
England
+44 0161 446 3156
Fax: +44 0161 446 3109
mcrc@manchester.ac.uk
www.mcrc.manchester.ac.uk

Massachusetts General Hospital
Cancer Center
55 Fruit Street
Boston, MA 02114
(877) 789-6100
mghcancercenter@partners.org
www.massgeneral.orgcancer

MD Anderson Cancer Center,
University of Texas
1515 Holcombe Boulevard
Houston, TX 77030
(713) 792-2121
www.mdanderson.org

Memorial Sloan-Kettering Cancer
Center
1275 York Avenue
New York, NY 10065
(800) 525-2225
publicaffairs@mskcc.org
www.mskcc.org

Moores Cancer Center, University of California, San Diego
3855 Health Sciences Drive
La Jolla, CA 92093
(858) 657-7000
www.cancer.ucsd.edu

Modern Cancer Hospital Guangzhou
42 Lianquan Road
Tianhe District
Guangzhou
People's Republic of China
+86 020 22221111 ext. 3333
Fax: +86 020 22830688
service@asiancancer.com
www.asiancancer.com

National Cancer Institute
6116 Executive Boulevard, Suite 300
Bethesda, MD 20892
(800) 422-6237
www.cancer.gov

National Lung Cancer Partnership
1 Point Place, Suite 200
Madison, WI 53719
(608) 833-7905
Fax: (608) 833-7906
info@nationallungcancerpartnership.org
www.nationallungcancerpartnership.org

Ohio State University Comprehensive Cancer Center, James Cancer Hospital and Solove Research Institute
300 West 10th Avenue
Columbus, OH 43210
(800) 293-5066
www.cancer.osu.edu

Providence Portland Medical Center
4805 Northeast Glisan Street
Portland, OR 97213
(800) 833-8899

Robert H. Lurie Comprehensive Cancer Center of Northwestern University
676 North St. Clair, Suite 1200
Chicago, IL 60611
(312) 695-1301
Fax: (312) 695-1352
www.cancer.northwestern.edu

Roswell Park Cancer Institute
Elm and Carlton Streets
Buffalo, NY 14263
(877) 275-7724
www.roswellpark.org

Sidney Kimmel Comprehensive Cancer Center at Johns Hopkins Medicine
Harry and Jeanette Weinberg Building, Suite 1100
401 North Broadway
Baltimore, MD 21287
(410) 955-5222

kpr@jhmi.edu
www.hopkinskimmelcancercenter
.org

Simmons Cancer Center, University of Texas Southwestern Medical Center
Seay Biomedical Building
2201 Inwood Road
2nd Floor, Suite 106
Dallas, TX 75390
(214) 645-4673
www.utswmedicine.org

Siteman Cancer Center at Barnes, Jewish Hospital and Washington University School of Medicine
660 South Euclid Avenue
Box 8100
St. Louis, MO 63110
(800) 600-3606
Fax: (314) 414-0204
www.siteman.wustl.edu

St. Jude Children's Research Hospital
262 Danny Thomas Place
Memphis, TN 38105
(901) 595-3300
www.stjude.org

Stanford Cancer Institute
Lorry Lokey Building, SIM 1
265 Campus Drive, Suite G2103
Stanford, CA 94305
(877) 668-7535
Fax: (650) 736-0607
www.cancer.stanford.edu

Swedish Cancer Institute
1221 Madison Street
Seattle, WA 98104
(855) 922-6237
www.swedish.org

Terry Fox Research Institute
675 West 10th Avenue
14th Floor
Vancouver, BC
Canada V5Z1L3
(604) 675-8222
Fax: (604) 675-8118
info@tfri.ca
www.tfri.ca

UCLA Lung Cancer Program, University of California, Los Angeles
Division of Cardiac and Thoracic Surgery
Ronald Reagan UCLA Medical Center
Room 64-128 CHS
10833 Le Conte Avenue
Los Angeles, CA 90095
(310) 825-8061
Fax: (310) 794-7335
lungcancerprogram@mednet.ucla.edu
www.lungcancer.ucla.edu

Union for International Cancer Control
62 Route de Frontenex
1207 Geneva
Switzerland

+41 22 809 1811
Fax: +41 22 809 1810
info@uicc.org
www.uicc.org

University of California Davis
Comprehensive Cancer Center
2279 45th Street
Sacramento, CA 95817
(916) 734-5935
can-
cer.center@ucdmc.ucdavis.edu
www.ucdmc.ucdavis.educancer

University of California San Diego
Moores Cancer Center
3855 Health Sciences Drive
La Jolla, CA 92093
(858) 657-7000
www.cancer.ucsd.edu

University of California San Francisco Helen Diller Family Comprehensive Cancer Center
Box 0875, UCSF
San Francisco, CA 94143
(800) 689-8273
communications@cc.ucsf.edu
cancer.ucsf.edu

University of Colorado Cancer
Center
Cancer Research Administration
Office
13001 East 17th Place
Campus Box F434
Aurora, CO 80045
(303) 724-3155

Fax: (303) 724-3162
www.coloradocancercenter.org

University of Michigan Comprehensive Cancer Center
1500 East Medical Center Drive
Floor B1, Room 363
Ann Arbor, MI 48109
(800) 865-1125
www.mcancer.org

University of Pittsburgh Cancer
Institute
5150 Centre Avenue
Pittsburgh, PA 15232
(412) 647-2811
Fax: (412) 623-7768
contactUPCI@upmc.edu
www.upci.upmc.edu

University of Tennessee Health
Science Center, West Clinic
100 North Humphreys Boulevard
Memphis, TN 38120
(901) 683-0055
www.westclinic.com

University of Texas MD Anderson
Cancer Center
1515 Holcombe Boulevard
Houston, TX 77030
(877) 632-6789
www.mdanderson.org

UNMC Eppley Cancer Center
985950 Nebraska Medical Center
Omaha, NE 68198
(800) 999-5465

Fax: (402) 559-4970   691 Preston Building
www.unmc.educancercenter   Nashville, TN 37232
                                             (800) 811-8480
Vanderbilt-Ingram Cancer Center   www.vicc.org

APPENDIX C

Lung Cancer–Related Organizations

American Academy of Allergy Asthma & Immunology
555 East Wells Street
Suite 1100
Milwaukee, WI 53202
(414) 272-6071
www.aaaai.org

American Association for Respiratory Care
9425 North MacArthur Boulevard, Suite 100
Irving, TX 75063
(972) 243-2272
Fax: (972) 484-2720
info@arc.org
www.aarc.org

American College of Chest Physicians
3300 Dundee Road
Northbrook, IL 60062

(847) 498-1400
Fax: (847) 498-5460
www.chestnet.org

American Cancer Society
250 Williams Street NW
Atlanta, GA 30303
(800) 227-2345
www.cancer.org

American Lung Association
1301 Pennsylvania Avenue NW, Suite 800
Washington, DC 20004
(212) 315-8700
Fax: (202) 452-1805
www.lung.org

American Thoracic Society
25 Broadway, 18th Floor
New York, NY 10004
(212) 315-8600

Fax: (212) 315-6498
atsinfo@thoracic.org
www.thoracic.org

Bettie R. May Foundation for
Small Cell Lung Cancer PO Box
2515
Southfield, MI 48076
(248) 496-9145
info@brmay.org
www.brmay.org

Bonnie J. Addario Lung Cancer
Foundation
1100 Industrial Road, Suite 1
San Carlos, CA 94070
(650) 598-2857
info@lungcancerfoundation.org
www.lungcancerfoundation.org

Cancer Care
275 Seventh Avenue, 22nd Floor
New York, NY 10001
(212) 712-8400
Fax: (212) 712-8495
info@cancercare.org
www.cancercare.org

Cancer Research Institute
National Headquarters
One Exchange Plaza
55 Broadway, Suite 1802
New York, NY 10006
(212) 688-7515
Fax: (212) 832-9376
www.cancerresearch.org

Gianni Ferrarotti Lung Cancer
Foundation
17345 Kinloch
Redford Township, MI 48240
(313) 532-0983
info@gianniscause.com
www.gianniscause.org

Lung Cancer Alliance
888 16th Street NW, Suite 150
Washington, DC 20006
(202) 463-2080
info@lungcanceralliance.org
www.lungcanceralliance.org

Lung Cancer Circle of Hope
7 Carnation Drive, Suite A
Lakewood, NJ 08701
(732) 363-4426
Fax: (732) 370-9180
www.lungcancercircleofhope.org

LUNGevity Foundation
218 S. Wabash Avenue, Suite 540
Chicago, IL 60604
(312) 464-0716
Fax: (312) 464-0737
www.events.lungevity.org

National Heart, Lung, and Blood
Institute
P.O. Box 30105
Bethesda, MD 20824
(301) 592-8573
Fax: (240) 629-3246
nhlbiinfo@nhlbi.nih.gov
www.nhlbi.nih.gov

Thomas G. Labrecque Foundation
1414 Prince Street Suite 400
Alexandria, VA 22314

(703) 299-9610
Fax: (703) 997-8907
www.tglclassic.com

APPENDIX D

Nationally Recognized Lung Cancer Clinics

Abramson Cancer Center, University of Pennsylvania
3400 Spruce Street
Philadelphia, PA 19104
(800) 789-7366
www.penncancer.org

Albert Einstein Cancer Center, Yeshiva University
1300 Morris Park Avenue
Bronx, NY 10461
(718) 430-2302
www.einstein.yu.edu

Alvin J. Siteman Cancer Center, Washington University School of Medicine and Barnes-Jewish Hospital
660 South Euclid Avenue
Campus Box 8109
St. Louis, MO 63110
(800) 600-3606

www.siteman.wustl.edu

Arizona Cancer Center, University of Arizona
1515 North Campbell Avenue
Tucson, AZ 85724
(800) 524-5928
www.azcc.arizona.edu

Assarian Cancer Center
47601 Grand River
Novi, MI 48374
(866) 246-4673
www.stjohnprovidence.org

Barbara Ann Karmanos Cancer Institute, Wayne State University School of Medicine
4100 John R Street
Detroit, MI 48201
(800) 527-6266
www.karmanos.org

Cancer Institute of New Jersey
Robert Wood Johnson Medical
School
195 Little Albany Street
New Brunswick, NJ 08903
(732) 235-8515
www.cinj.org

Cancer Therapy and Research
Center, University of Texas
Health Science Center
7979 Wurzbach Road
Urschel Tower, Room U627
San Antonio, TX 78229
(800) 340-2872
www.ctrc.net

Case Comprehensive Cancer
Center
Case Western Reserve University
11100 Euclid Avenue
Cleveland, OH 44106
(216) 844-8797
www.cancercase.edu

Chao Family Comprehensive
Cancer Center, University of California, Irvine
101 The City Drive
Building 56, Route 81, Room 209
Orange, CA 92868
(877) 824-3627
www.cancer.uci.edu

City of Hope Comprehensive
Cancer Center
1500 East Duarte Road

Duarte, CA 91010
(800) 826-4673
www.cityofhope.org

Coborn Cancer Center
1900 CentraCare Circle, Suite
1600
St. Cloud, MN 56303
(877) 229-4907
Fax: (320) 229-5160
coborncancercen-
ter@centracare.com
www.centracare.com

Cold Spring Harbor Laboratory
Cancer Center
1 Bungtown Road
Cold Spring Harbor, NY 11724
(516) 367-8800
www.cshl.edu

Comprehensive Cancer Center of
Wake Forest University
Medical Center Boulevard
Winston-Salem, NC 27157
(336) 716-9253
www.wfubmc.edu

Dan L. Duncan Cancer Center,
Baylor College of Medicine
One Baylor Place
Houston, TX 77030
(713) 798-1354
www.bcm.edu

Dana-Farber/Harvard Cancer
Center
450 Brookline Avenue

Boston, MA 02215
(617) 632-3000
www.dfhcc.harvard.edu

David H. Koch Institute for Integrative Cancer Research at MIT
77 Massachusetts Avenue, 76-158
Cambridge, MA 02139
(617) 253-6403
www.ki.mit.edu

Duke Cancer Institute, Duke University Medical Center
Box 2714
2424 Erwin Road
Durham, NC 27710
(888) 275-3853
www.dukecancerinstitute.org

Eppley Cancer Center, University of Nebraska Medical Center
985950 Nebraska Medical Center
Omaha, NE 68198
(800) 922-0000
www.unmc.edu

Fox Chase Cancer Center
333 Cottman Avenue
Philadelphia, PA 19111
(888) 369-2427
www.fccc.edu

Fred Hutchinson/University of Washington Cancer Consortium
PO Box 19024
Seattle, WA 98109
(206) 288-7222
www.fhcrc.org

Georgetown Lombardi Comprehensive Cancer Center, Georgetown University
3970 Reservoir Road NW
Washington, DC 20007
(202) 444-4000
www.lombardi.georgetown.edu

H. Lee Moffitt Cancer Center and Research Institute
12902 Magnolia Drive
MCC-CEO
Tampa, FL 33612
(888) 860-2778
www.moffitt.org

Harold C. Simmons Cancer Center, University of Texas Southwestern Medical Center
2201 Inwood Road
Dallas, TX 75390
(866) 460-4673
www.simmonscancercenter.org

Herbert Irving Comprehensive Cancer Center, Columbia University
1130 St. Nicholas Avenue, Room 508
New York, NY 10032
(877) 697-9355
www.hiccc.columbia.edu

Holden Comprehensive Cancer Center
University of Iowa
200 Hawkins Drive

5970Z JPP
Iowa City, IA 52242
(800) 237-1225
www.uihealthcare.org

Hollings Cancer Center, Medical University of South Carolina
86 Jonathan Lucas Street
Charleston, SC 29425
(800) 424-6872
www.hcc.musc.edu

Huntsman Cancer Institute, University of Utah
2000 Circle of Hope
Salt Lake City, UT 84112
(877) 585-0303
www.huntsmancancer.org

Indeterminate Lung Nodule Clinic, University of Maryland
22 South Greene Street
Baltimore, MD 21201
(800) 888-8823
www.umgcc.org

Jackson Laboratory Cancer Center
600 Main Street
Bar Harbor, ME 04609
(207) 288-6051
www.jax.org

Jonsson Comprehensive Cancer Center, University of California at Los Angeles
10833 Le Conte Avenue
Los Angeles, CA 90095

(888) 662-8252
www.cancer.ucla.edu

Kimmel Cancer Center, Thomas Jefferson University
233 South 10th Street
Philadelphia, PA 19107
(888) 955-1212
www.kcc.tju.edu

Knight Cancer Institute, Oregon Health and Science University
3181 SW Sam Jackson Park Road
Portland, OR 97239
(503) 494-8311
www.ohsu.edu

Lung Cancer Center, Cleveland Clinic
9500 Euclid Avenue
Cleveland, OH 44195
(800) 801-2273
www.my.clevelandclinic.org

Masonic Cancer Center, University of Minnesota
420 Delaware Street SE
Minneapolis, MN 55455
(612) 672-7422
www.cancer.umn.edu

Massey Cancer Center, Virginia Commonwealth University
PO Box 980037
401 College Street
Richmond, VA 23298
(804) 828-5116
www.massey.vcu.edu

Mayo Clinic
13400 E. Shea Boulevard
Scottsdale, AZ 85259
(480) 301-8000
Fax: (480) 301-9310
www.mayoclinic.org

Memorial Sloan-Kettering Cancer
Center
1275 York Avenue
New York, NY 10065
(212) 639-2000
www.mskcc.org

New York University Cancer Institute, New York University Lan-
gone Medical Center
550 First Avenue
1201 Smilow Building
New York, NY 10016
(888) 769-8633
www.cancer.med.nyu.edu

Norris Cotton Cancer Center,
Dartmouth-Hitchcock Medical
Center
One Medical Center Drive
Lebanon, NH 03756
(800) 639-6918
www.cancer.dartmouth.edu

Ohio State University Comprehensive Cancer Center
300 West 10th Avenue, Suite 159
Columbus, OH 43210
(800) 293-5066
www.cancer.osu.edu

Providence Cancer Center
22301 Foster Winter Drive
Southfield, MI 48075
(800) 341-0801
www.stjohnprovidence.org

Providence Hospital
16001 West 9 Mile Road
Southfield, MI 48075
(248) 849-3000
www.stjohnprovidence.org

Purdue University Center for
Cancer Research
Hansen Life Sciences Research
Building
201 South University Street
West Lafayette, IN 47907
(765) 494-9129
www.cancerresearch.purdue.edu

Robert H. Lurie Comprehensive
Cancer Center, Northwestern
University
303 East Superior Street
Chicago, IL 60611
(866) 587-4322
www.cancer.northwestern.edu

Roswell Park Cancer Institute
Elm and Carlton Streets
Buffalo, NY 14263
(800) 767-9355
www.roswellpark.org

St. Jude Children's Research Hospital

262 Danny Thomas Place
Memphis, TN 38105
(866) 278-5833
www.stjude.org

Salk Institute Cancer Center
10010 North Torrey Pines Road
La Jolla, CA 92037
(858) 453-4100
www.salk.edu

Sanford-Burnham Medical Research Institute
10901 North Torrey Pines Road
La Jolla, CA 92037
(858) 646-3100
www.sanfordburnham.org

Sidney Kimmel Comprehensive Cancer Center, Johns Hopkins University
401 North Broadway
Baltimore, MD 21231
(410) 955-8964
www.hopkinsmedicine.org

Stanford Cancer Institute, Stanford University
Lorry Lokey Stem Cell Building
265 Campus Drive, Suite G2103
Stanford, CA 94305
(877) 668-7535
www.cancer.stanford.edu

Temple Lung Center, Temple University Hospital
3401 North Broad Street
Philadelphia, PA 19140

(215) 707-2000
www.tuh.templehealth.org

University of Alabama at Birmingham
1802 Sixth Avenue South
Birmingham, AL 35294
(800) 822-0933
www3.ccc.uab.edu

University of California Davis Comprehensive Cancer Center
4501 X Street, Suite 3003
Sacramento, CA 95817
(916) 734-5959
www.ucdmc.ucdavis.edu/cancer

University of California San Diego Moores Cancer Center
3855 Health Sciences Drive
La Jolla, CA 92093
(866) 773-2703
www.cancer.ucsd.edu

University of California San Francisco Helen Diller Family Comprehensive Cancer Center
1450 3rd Street, Box 0128
San Francisco, CA 94115
(415) 353-8489
www.cancer.ucsf.edu

University of Chicago Comprehensive Cancer Center
5841 South Maryland Avenue
Chicago, IL 60637
(773) 702-6808
www.cancer.uchicago.edu

University of Colorado Center, University of Colorado Hospital
13001 East 17th Place
Aurora, CO 80045
(877) 422-3648
www.uch.edu

University of Hawaii Cancer Center
677 Ala Moana Boulevard, Suite 901
Honolulu, HI 96813
(808) 586-3010
www.uhcancercenter.org

University of Kansas Cancer Center
3901 Rainbow Boulevard
Kansas City, KS 66160
(800) 332-6048
www.kucancercenter.org

University of Maryland Marlene and Stewart Greenebaum Cancer Center
22 South Greene Street
Baltimore, MD 21201
(800) 888-8823
www.umgcc.org

University of Michigan Comprehensive Cancer Center
1500 East Medical Center Drive
Ann Arbor, MI 48109
(800) 865-1125
www.mcancer.org

University of New Mexico Cancer Center
1201 Camino de Salud NE
Albuquerque, NM 87131
(800) 432-6806
www.cancer.unm.edu

University of North Carolina Lineberger Comprehensive Cancer Center
450 West Drive, CB 7295
Chapel Hill, NC 27599
(866) 869-1856
www.unclineberger.org

University of Pittsburgh Cancer Institute
5150 Centre Avenue
Pittsburgh, PA 15232
(412) 647-2811
www.upci.upmc.edu

University of Southern California Norris Comprehensive Cancer Center
1441 Eastlake Avenue
Los Angeles, CA 90089
(800) 872-2273
www.uscnorriscancer.usc.edu

University of Texas MD Anderson Cancer Center
1515 Holcombe Boulevard, Unit 91
Houston, TX 77030
(877) 632-6789
www.mdanderson.org

University of Virginia Cancer
Center
6171 West Complex
Charlottesville, VA 22908
(800) 223-9173
www.healthysystem.virginia.edu

University of Wisconsin Carbone
Cancer Center
1111 Highland Avenue, Room
7057
Madison, WI 53705
(800) 622-8922
www.uwhealth.org

Vanderbilt-Ingram Cancer Center
691 Preston Research Building
Nashville, TN 37232
(877) 936-8422
www.vicc.org

Van Eslander Cancer Center
19229 Mack Ave.
Grosse Pointe Woods, MI 48236

(866) 246-4673
www.stjohnprovidence.org/Va-
nElslander

Winship Cancer Institute, Emory
University
1365C Clifton Road
Atlanta, GA 30322
(888) 946-7447
www.winshipcancer.emory.edu

Wistar Institute Cancer Center
3601 Spruce Street
Philadelphia, PA 19104
(215) 898-3700
www.wistar.org

Yale Cancer Center, Yale University School of Medicine
333 Cedar Street
New Haven, CT 06510
(866) 925-3226
www.yalecancercenter.org

APPENDIX E

For Further Reading

Argiris, Athanassios, and Jame Abraham. *Lung Cancer (Emerging Cancer Therapeutics V3 I1)*. New York: Demos Medical Publishing, 2012.

Azzoli, Christopher G. *Dx/Rx: Lung Cancer*. 2nd ed. Burlington, MA: Jones & Bartlett Learning, 2012.

Bernal, Samuel D., and Paul J. Hesketh. *Lung Cancer Differentiation: Implications for Diagnosis and Treatment*. Boca Raton, FL: CRC Press, 1992.

Cagle, Philip T., and Timothy Allen. *Advances in Surgical Pathology: Lung Cancer*. Philadelphia: Lippincott Williams & Wilkins, 2010.

Cooper, David N. *The Molecular Genetics of Lung Cancer*. New York: Springer, 2004.

Langwith, Jacqueline. *Lung Cancer (Perspectives on Diseases and Disorders)*. Farmington Hills, MI: Greenhaven Press, 2011.

Falk, Stephen, and Chris Williams. *Lung Cancer (The Facts)*. New York: Oxford University Press, 2010.

Fossella, Frank V., Joe B. Putnam Jr., Ritsuko Komaki, J. D. Cox, W. Ki Hong, and J. A. Roth. *Lung Cancer*. New York: Springer, 2002.

Giaccone, Giuseppe. *Systemic Treatment of Non-Small Cell Lung Cancer*. New York: Oxford University Press, 2012.

Gridelli, Cesare, and Riccardo A. Audisio. *Management of Lung Cancers in Older People*. New York: Springer, 2013.

Harper, Peter, Nasser Hanna, David Gandara, Corinne Faivre-Finn, Alejandro Corvalan, Benjamin Besse, D. Ross Cambridge, Neil Bayman, and Fred Hirsch. *Lung Cancer: State of the Art*. London: Remedica Medical Education and Publishing, 2011.

Henschke, Claudia I., and Peggy McCarthy. *Lung Cancer: Myths, Facts, Choices—and Hope*. New York: Norton, 2003.

Jeremic, Branislav. *Advances in Radiation Oncology in Lung Cancer (Medical Radiology/Radiation Oncology)*. New York: Springer, 2011.

Kernstine, Kemp H., Karen L. Reckamp, and Charles R. Thomas Jr. *Lung Cancer: A Multidisciplinary Approach to Diagnosis and Management*. New York: Demos Medical Publishing, 2010.

Keshamouni, Venkateshwa, Douglas Arenberg, and Gregory Kalemkerian. *Lung Cancer Metastasis: Novel Biological Mechanisms and Impact on Clinical Practice*. New York: Springer, 2009.

Lyss, Alan P., Humberto Fagundes, and Patricia Corrigan. *Chemotherapy and Radiation for Dummies*. Hoboken, NJ: Wiley, 2005.

Macbeth, Fergus, Robert Milroy, William Steward, and Rod Burnet. *Lung Cancer*. Boca Raton, FL: CRC Press, 1996.

Mazzone, Peter. *The Cleveland Clinic Guide to Lung Cancer*. New York: Kaplan Publishing, 2009.

Pandya, Kishan J., Julie R. Brahmer, and Manuel Hidalgo. *Lung Cancer: Translational and Emerging Therapies*. Boca Raton, FL: CRC Press, 2007.

Parles, Karen, Joan H. Schiller, and Amy Cipau. *100 Questions and Answers about Lung Cancer*. Burlington, MA: Jones & Bartlett Publishers, 2011.

Pass, Harvey I., David P. Carbone, David H. Johnson, John D. Minna, Giorgio V. Scagliotti, and Andrew T. Turrisi. *Principles and Practice of Lung Cancer: The Official Reference Text of the International Association for the Study of Lung Cancer (IASLC)*. Philadelphia: Lippincott Williams & Wilkins, 2010.

Scott, Walter J. *Lung Cancer: A Guide to Diagnosis and Treatment*. 2nd ed. Omaha, NE: Addicus Books, 2012.

Scarantino, Charles W., R. H. Choplin, C. S. Faulkner II, C. J. Kovacs, S. G. Mann, T. O'Connor, S. K. Plume, F. Richards II, and C. W. Scarantino. *Lung Cancer: Diagnostic Procedures and Therapeutic Management with Special Reference to Radiotherapy*. New York: Springer, 2012.

Torres, Varetta N. *Lung Cancer in Women*. New York: Nova Science Publishers, 2008.

Van Schil, P. *Lung Metastases and Isolated Lung Perfusion*. New York: Nova Science Publishers, 2013.

Williams, Chris. *Lung Cancer: The Facts*. New York: Oxford University Press, 1995.

GLOSSARY

A

acinar. Refers to any cluster of cells that resembles a multiple-lobed berry.

acinar adenocarcinoma. A histological subtype of gland-forming cancer whose characteristic is the formation of acini and tubules in the cuboidal- and columnar-shaped malignant cells.

actinic keratosis. A premalignant condition of thick, scaly, or crusty patches of skin.

acute leukemia. A group of rapidly progressing leukemia.

adenine (A). A purine derivative with a range of functions in biochemistry comprising a chemical component of DNA and RNA.

adenocarcinoma. Malignant tumor originating in glandular epithelium.

adenocarcinoma with mixed subtypes. Most common histologic subtype of lung cancer. Cancer cells may be a mixture of acinar, papillary, bronchioalveolar, or solid adenocarcinoma with mucin.

adenocarcinoma in situ (AIS). Precancerous cells found on different organs, usually the cervix. They typically affect glandular cells and are a precursor for adenocarcinoma.

adenomatous hyperplasia. An overgrowth of the tissue, usually of the lung or endometrium. This condition is known to be a precursor to cancer.

adenosine triphosphate (ATP). A purine nucleoside consisting of adenine and ribose that is a constituent of RNA. Also a cardiac depressant and vasodilator.

adenosquamous carcinomas. A different category of bronchogenic carcinoma, with areas of glandular, squamous, and large cell differentiation.

adenylate cyclase. An enzyme that breaks down and changes ATP to cyclic AMP.

adrenalectomy. The process of surgically removing one or both of the adrenal glands.

aerobics. Any activity that requires more oxygen and increases the respiratory and heart rate.

alkylating agent. Any cytotoxic drug containing alkyl groups, such as chlorambucil, that acts by damaging DNA. They are widely used in treating cancer by chemotherapy.

alpha-tocopherol. Also known as vitamin E.

amifostine. A chemoprotectant used to counter kidney toxicity in cisplatin chemotherapy.

aminopterin. A folic acid antagonist and inhibitor of dihydrofolate reductase. A potent cell-damaging agent formerly used to manage leukemia.

amrubicin. An ananthracycline used in the treatment of lung cancer.

anamnesis. Pertains to either a patient case history, particularly using the patient's recollections, or the body's immunologic memory.

anemia. Reduction below normal of the number of red blood cells, quantity of hemoglobin, or the volume of packed red cells in the blood; a symptom of various diseases and disorders, such as cancer.

angiosarcomas. The vascular endothelial cells have malignant neoplasms. The term may be used generally or may indicate a subtype, such as hemangiosarcoma.

anhedonia. The inability to experience gratification in normally satisfying acts.

anthracotic. A condition characterized by anthracosis, which is a kind of pneumoconiosis, typically asymptomatic, due to evidence of anthracite coal dust in the lungs.

anticoagulative. An agent that inhibits coagulation, especially of blood. Most common anticoagulative is heparin.

antiemetic. Any medication that prevents vomiting.

antigen. Any substance that can stimulate the making of antibodies and merge with them.

antihistamines. Certain compounds or medicines that counteract or inhibit the effect of histamine in the body, usually used in the treatment of allergic disorders.

antimetabolite. A substance that has a structural resemblance to one needed for normal bodily functions and whose effect interferes with the use of the essential metabolite.

apoptosis. A normal, genetically made process that results in the death of cells and triggered by the presence or absence of stimuli, as DNA damage.

argon. A colorless, inert gaseous element that constitutes about 1 percent of the earth's atmosphere, used in lightbulbs and in lasers for medical procedures.

arterial thrombosis. A blood clot that forms in an artery. It can obstruct the flow of blood to major organs.

aseptic. The state of being infection free of a septic substance. Another word for sterile.

asymptomatic. Not showing any symptom or any evidence of disease or illness.

atelectasis. Partial or complete collapse of the lung.

autoantibodies. An antibody that is produced by the body that fights any of its own tissues, cells, or cell components.

B

B72.3. A monoclonal antibody utilized in the treatment of cancers, usually of a gynecologic nature.

basal cell carcinomas. An epithelial tumor of the skin that rarely spreads but has the possibility of invading and damaging local tissues. It more often than not appears as one or several small pearly nodules with central pits on the skin of older adults who frequently get exposed to the sun.

basal cells. A keratinocyte found in the stratum basale of the epidermis.

basaloid. Bears a resemblance to that which is basal but not necessarily a basal derivation.

basaloid carcinoma. An uncommon transitional cancer of the anal canal containing areas that look like basal cell carcinoma of the skin. Basaloid carcinoma is very invasive.

B-catenin. Beta-catenin, a protein that is made by the *CTNNB1* gene.

benzodiazepine. A group of psychoactive drugs whose main chemical structure is the union of a benzene ring and a diazepine ring. It increases the effect of the neurotransmitter gamma-aminobutyric acid (GABA), which results in sedative, hypnotic, antianxiety, anticonvulsant, amnesic action and muscle relaxation. Benzodiazepines are helpful in managing anxiety, muscle spasms, insomnia, agitation, seizures, and alcohol withdrawal.

beta-integrin. A protein that is coded by the ITGB3 gene and is related to the occurrence of endemetriosis.

bevacizumab (Avastin). An angiogenesis inhibitor, a drug that slows the development of new blood vessels. It is used in managing a variety of cancers, including colorectal, kidney, lung, breast, and ovarian.

bile. Dark green to yellowish fluid made by the liver that is responsible for breaking down ingested fats for digestion in the small intestine.

bomb calorimeter. A device used in measuring the heat of combustion of a particular reaction.

bone resorption. The process of breaking down bone and releasing minerals by osteoclasts, resulting in a transfer of calcium from bone to the blood.

BP-1-102. An anticancer drug that inhibits a certain protein responsible for the growth of specific types of cancer.

breath analysis. A noninvasive test done using a machine to detect organic compounds present in the exhaled breath. Lung cancer and upper respiratory infection biomarkers are detected too.

bronchi. Plural form of bronchus. A passage in the respiratory tract that conducts air into the lungs.

bronchioalveolar carcinoma (BAC). An uncommon form of lung cancer that occurs in the cells near the small air sacs in the outer regions of the lungs. The incidence rate is higher in nonsmokers, women, and Asians than other forms of lung cancer.

bronchioles. A small branch of a bronchus.

bronchodilator. A substance that dilates constricted bronchial tubes to aid breathing. It is usually taken for the relief of asthma.

bronchoscopy. A test done by means of inserting an instrument into the airways, usually through the nose or mouth, to examine the inside of the airways.

C

cachexia. Also called wasting syndrome. It is characterized by loss of weight, muscle atrophy, fatigue, weakness, and noticeable loss of appetite in someone who is not trying to lose weight.

canalicular. Pertaining to the canaliculus, which is a small canal or duct in the body, such as the fine channels in compact bone.

cancellous bone. Also called trabecular or spongy bone. It is one of the two types of osseous tissue that form bones.

cancer. Known medically as a malignant neoplasm, it is an extensive group of different diseases, all of which involve unregulated cell growth.

cancer-related emergency. Any emergency that arises from the complications of cancer, such as cardiac tamponade, airway obstruction, or deep-vein thrombosis.

capecitabine. An orally administered anticancer medication used in the treatment of metastatic breast and colorectal cancers.

carboplatin. An anticancer drug used against some kinds of cancer, usually ovarian carcinoma, lung, head, and neck cancers.

carcinoembryonic antigen. A glycoprotein involved in cell adhesion. It is used as a tumor marker to detect the reappearance of malignant tissue or cells after surgical resection or to confine the spread of cancer.

carcinoma in situ. A premature form of carcinoma defined by the nonexistence of invasion of surrounding tissues.

carcinomata. A medical term that refers to a persistent malignant tumor made of transformed epithelial cells.

carcinosarcoma. A malignant tumor that is a mixture of carcinoma and sarcoma.

cardiac tamponade. Also known as pericardial tamponade. An acute type of pericardial effusion characterized by the accumulation of fluid in the pericardium, which encloses the heart.

cardiorespiratory. Pertaining to the heart and lungs.

catecholamine. Hormones released by the brain to stimulate the flight-or-fight response.

cauterization. The process of burning part of a body to remove or close off a part of it that destroys some tissue in order to lessen damage, take away an undesired growth, or reduce other possible medically detrimental risks, such as infections.

cavitation. Formation of small pockets of gas in liquids or tissue in the body.

centrosome. A part of the cell that serves as the major microtubule organizing center of the cell as well as a controller of cell-cycle progression.

cerebrospinal fluid. A clear bodily fluid that takes up the subarachnoid space and the ventricular system around and inside the central nervous system.

cetuximab (Erbitux). An epidermal growth factor receptor inhibitor used to treat metastatic colorectal cancer and head and neck cancer.

chemotherapy. The treatment of cancer with one or more cell-damaging antineoplastic drugs as part of a standardized regimen.

chest radiography. Commonly called a chest X-ray, a projection radiograph of the chest used to discover conditions affecting the chest and nearby structures.

chondrocyte. The only cells found in healthy cartilage.

chondrosarcoma. A cancer composed of cells derived from transformed cells that produce cartilage.

chromatography tandem mass spectrometry. A test to detect specific categories of drugs and their metabolites.

chronic bronchitis. A chronic inflammation of the bronchi in the lungs.

chronic leukemia. Slowly progressing leukemia.

chronic obstructive pulmonary diseases (COPD). A group of progressive lung diseases that make it hard to breathe. The disease gets worse over time.

cilliated cells. Cells covered in tiny hair-like projections known as cilia.

cilliated columnar epithelial cells. Rectangular-shaped cells that have hair-like protrusions called cilia.

cisplatinum. A platinum-containing white powder (chemical formula $PtCl_2 H_6 N_2$) used to treat ovarian carcinoma and other cancers.

clara cells. Dome-shaped cells with short microvilli found in the bronchioles.

claustrophobia. Fear of small spaces.

clear cell carcinoma. An uncommon kind of tumor characterized by clear cells.

clinico-pathological. Of or relating to the combined study of disease symptoms and pathology.

colony-stimulating factors. Secreted glycoproteins that attach to receptor proteins on the surfaces of hemopoietic stem cells, activating intracellular signaling pathways that can cause the cells to proliferate and differentiate into a kind of blood cell.

corticosteroids. A group of chemicals that includes steroid hormones made in the adrenal cortex; the analogues of these hormones are synthesized in laboratories. Corticosteroids are used in a wide range of physiological processes, including stress response, immune response, and regulation of inflammation, carbohydrate metabolism, protein catabolism, blood electrolyte levels, and behavior.

crizotinib (Xalkori). An anticancer drug acting as an anaplastic lymphoma kinase and c-ros oncogene 1 inhibitor used in the treatment of some types of non–small cell lung carcinoma.

cryoprobe. A tool used in cryosurgery that has a cold tip for applying intense cold to diseased tissue to remove or destroy it.

cryotherapy. Treatment by means of applications of cold or freezing.

cyclophosphamide. A nitrogen mustard alkylating agent that is used to manage different kinds of cancer and autoimmune disorders. Also known as cytophosphane.

cytologic. Pertaining to cytology, which is the branch of biology that deals with the development, structure, and uses of cells.

cytoplasmic ribonucleoprotein. A nucleoprotein that has RNA contained in the gel-like substance inside the cell membrane.

cytoprotective agent. Any medication or substance that works by protecting the cytoplasm of the cell.

cytosine (C). One of the four major bases found in DNA and RNA with adenine, guanine, and thymine. It is found in DNA, as part of RNA, or as a part of a nucleotide.

cytosol. Also known as intracellular fluid. It is the liquid found inside the cells.

D

deep-vein thrombosis (DVT). Formation of a blood clot or thrombus in a deep vein, usually in the leg or pelvic veins.

dexamethasone. A synthetic glucocorticoid that acts as an anti-inflammatory and immuno-suppressant drug.

differentiation. In relation to biology, the process that a less specialized cell undergoes to become a more specialized cell type.

digital clubbing. A deformity of the nail bed of the fingers as a complication of a variety of diseases, mostly of the heart and lungs. It signifies a lack of a considerable amount of oxygen.

disease. An abnormal condition that affects the body. It could refer to the deviation of the body's state from healthy.

docetaxel. A proven chemotherapy medication that acts by interfering with cell division. It is used chiefly for the treatment of breast, ovarian, and non–small cell lung cancer.

doxorubicin. An anticancer drug that acts by intercalating DNA, with the gravest adverse effect being life-threatening heart damage. It is used in the treatment of different cancers, such as hematological malignancies, carcinomas, and soft-tissue sarcomas.

dysgraphia. The inability to write. A transcription disability associated with impaired hand-writing, orthographic coding, and finger sequencing.

dysnomia. A condition that affects memory. It is characterized by a difficulty with recalling words or names.

dysphagia. Difficulty in swallowing.

dyspnea. Difficulty in breathing.

E

E-cadherin. A protein that is encoded by the *CDH1* gene. Also known as CAM 120/80 or epithelial cadherin or uvomorulin.

edema. Abnormal accumulation of fluid beneath the skin.

emboli. Plural for embolus, which is a medical term for either a blood clot, a fat globule, or a gas bubble in the bloodstream that could cause a blockage far from the actual site of the embolism.

endobronchial ultrasound-guided transbronchial needle aspiration (EBUS TBNA). A procedure done with the use of a tube and a bronchoscope that are inserted into the patient's airway and into the lungs, but instead of extracting a tissue sample right away, an ultrasound probe is used to locate any abnormal areas. The located abnormal region is where a small grasping needle takes a sample of the tissue for diagnosis.

endoscope. An instrument used to examine the interior of a hollow organ or cavity of the body.

endothelial growth factor (VEGF). A signal protein made by cells that fuels vasculogene-sis and angiogenesis. It is part of the system that, when blood circulation is not enough, reestablishes the oxygen supply to tissues.

endurance shuttle walk test. A regulated field exam to test the endurance capacity in patients with chronic lung disease.

epidermal growth factor receptor (EGFR) tyrosine kinase inhibitor drugs. A type of anticancer medication that acts by targeting EGFR, which, if it mutates, could lead to cancer.

erlotinib (Tarceva). An anticancer drug used to treat non–small cell lung cancer and other types of cancer. A reversible tyrosine kinase inhibitor that targets the epidermal growth factor receptor (EGFR).

erythropoietin. A hormone that is responsible for the production of red blood cells.

esophagus. A hollow muscular tube where food passes from the throat to the stomach.

etoposide. An anticancer drug that acts by forming a ternary complex with DNA and the topoisomerase II enzyme, which aids in DNA unwinding and prevents religation of the DNA strands. This results in the destruction of the DNA strand. Cancer cells depend on topoisomerase II more than healthy cells since they divide fast. This causes errors in DNA synthesis and results in apoptosis of the cancer cell.

excitotoxicity. The pathological process by which nerve cells are injured and destroyed by the overstimulation of neurotransmitters such as glutamate and similar substances.

extragonadal germ cell tumor. Occurs when cells that are supposed to form sperm in the testicles or eggs in the ovaries go to other parts of the body. They may form extragonadal germ cell tumors. These tumors may begin to grow anywhere in the body but often begin to grow in organs such as the pineal gland in the brain, in the mediastinum, or in the abdomen.

ezrin-radixin-moesin. A group of actin-binding proteins encoded by human genes that link the actin cytoskeleton and plasma membrane proteins and act as signal transducers.

F

femur. Also known as the thighbone.

fiber-optic bronchoscope. The procedure involves inserting a thin tube-like fiber-optic instrument through the nose or mouth and down into the lungs. The tube is able to carry pictures back to a video screen or camera. It is used to diagnose certain lung conditions.

fibrosarcomas. A type of cancerous tumor that is from fibrous tissues of the bone and invades long or flat bones, such as the femur, tibia, and mandible. It also involves the periosteum and overlying muscle. It is usually found in males aged 30 to 40.

fight-or-flight response. The body's natural way of reacting to a perceived harmful event, attack, or threat to survival.

filamin A. A cytoplasmic protein that is made by the *FLNA* gene that is responsible for binding actin filaments into orthogonal networks in cortical cytoplasm and participates in the anchoring of membrane proteins for the actin cytoskeleton. This in turn modulates cell shape and migrates cells.

filamin B. A cytoplasmic protein that is made by the *FLNB* gene that is responsible for regulating intracellular communication and signaling by cross-linking the protein actin to allow direct communication between the cell membrane and cytoskeletal network to control proper skeletal development.

fine-needle aspiration biopsy. A diagnostic test done to examine superficial lumps or masses.

fistula. An abnormal connection between two epithelium-lined organs or vessels that normally do not link. It is generally a disease condition, but a fistula may be surgically created for therapeutic reasons, such as to allow easier withdrawal of blood for hemodialysis.

fluorescence differential gel electrophoresis. A kind of test used to separate mixed population of DNA or proteins.

folate antimetabolite. An anticancer medication that acts by impairing the function of folic acids.

fusiform. Refers to having the characteristic of looking like a spindle that is wide in the middle and tapers at both ends.

G

gas chromatography-mass spectrometry (GG-MS). A method that merges the attributes of gas-liquid chromatography and mass spectrometry to identify various substances within a test sample.

gastroesophageal. Pertaining to the stomach and esophagus.

gastrointestinal stromal tumors (GIST). Most common mesenchymal tumors of the gastrointestinal tract. They are characterized by mutations in the KIT gene or PDGFRA gene and may or may not stain positively for KIT.

gefitinib (Iressa). An anti-cancer drug that acts by inhibiting EGFR. It interrupts signaling through the epidermal growth factor receptor (EGFR) in target cells.

glutamate. An important compound or neurotransmitter in cellular metabolism and in the disposal of waste nitrogen.

goblet cells. simple columnar epithelial cells that function to secrete mucin, which dissolves in water to form mucus. They use both apocrine and merocrine methods for secretion.

Golgi apparatus. A part of the cell found in most eukaryotic cells. It is responsible in the packaging of proteins inside the cell before they are sent to their destination. It plays a vital role in the processing of proteins for secretion.

granulosa cells. Type of cells responsible for the production of sex hormones as well as various growth factors thought to interact with the female gamete, or egg, during its development.

guanine (G). One of the four main nucleobases found in DNA and RNA, the others being adenine, cytosine, and thymine. In DNA, guanine is paired with cytosine.

H

hallucinogenic. Any substance that causes hallucinations. They cause subjective changes in perception, thought, emotion, and consciousness.

hematemesis. The vomiting of blood.

hematopoiesis. Formation of blood cellular components.

hemoptysis. Expectoration or coughing up of blood-tinged sputum.

homeostasis. The ability of the body to regulate its internal environment and maintain a stable, relatively constant condition of properties.

Horner's syndrome. A combination of the drooping of eyelids and constriction of the pupil, sometimes accompanied by decreased sweating of the face on the same side; redness of the conjunctiva of the eye. Outward displacement of the eye, or enophthalmos, is also a common symptom. It is indicative of a problem with the sympathetic nervous system.

humerus. The long bone of the upper arm.

hyaline cartilages. A kind of cartilage seen on many joint surfaces. It has no nerves or blood vessels and has an uncomplicated structure.

hypercalcaemia. Excessive amounts of calcium in the blood.

I

immunoglobulin. Also known as an antibody. A large Y-shaped protein made by beta cells that is utilized by the immune system to recognize and counteract the effects of foreign objects, such as bacteria and viruses.

immunohistochemically. Pertains to having the traits of immunohistochemistry, which is the process of detecting antigens in cells of a tissue section by making use of the principle of antibodies binding specifically to antigens in biological tissues.

incremental shuttle walk test. A test done by stimulating a cardiopulmonary exercise using a field walking test. A test of cardiopulmonary endurance.

insomnia. Difficulty falling or staying asleep.

interstitial. Space or gap between structures.

intracranial pressure. Pressure inside the skull, brain tissue, and cerebrospinal fluid.

irinotecan. An anticancer drug that acts by preventing DNA from unwinding.

J

jaundice. A yellowish pigmentation of the skin and other mucous membranes caused by excess amounts of bilirubin in the blood. It is often seen in patients with liver disease.

K

karkinos. Latin for "crab." Another term for cancer.

L

Lambert-Eaton myasthenic syndrome (LEMS). A rare autoimmune disorder that is described as muscle weakness of the limbs. It can be associated with cancer, and the direct treatment of the cancer may relieve its symptoms.

large cell neuroendocrine carcinoma (LCNEC) of the lung. The tumor cells lack light-microscopic characteristics that would identify them as a small cell carcinoma, squamous cell carcinoma, adenocarcinoma, or other, more specific histologic types of lung cancer. The anaplastic cells appear larger with no salt-and-pepper chromatin. They are also derived from neuroendocrine cells.

large cell anaplastic carcinoma. The kind of carcinoma where cells appear to be larger. There is a reverse formation of differentiation in cells, and the nuclei are darkly stained.

large cell carcinoma having the rhabdoid phenotype. A very rare form of cancer; it is a type of large cell carcinoma that appears to have tangled intermediate filaments that displace the cell nucleus outward toward the cell membrane.

large cell undifferentiated carcinoma (LCUC). Named for the cells that constitute it; the cells are large with huge nuclei, and the equivalent tumors are large with areas of necrotic or dead tissue.

larynx. Also known as the voice box. It is responsible in the production of sound and in the protection of the trachea against food aspiration.

laser-induced interstitial thermotherapy. Involves the destruction of interstitial tissue for curative or palliative purposes through the induction of increased temperature by means of laser light energy transmission.

Leydig cells. Found adjacent to the seminiferous tubules, they make testosterone or male hormone in the presence of luteinizing hormone.

liposarcomas. Cancerous tumors arising in fat cells in deep soft tissue.

lung adenocarcinoma. *See* adenocarcinoma.

lymphadenopathy. Disease of the lymph nodes characterized by swelling of lymph nodes due to infection, autoimmune diseases, or malignancy.

lymphoepitheloma-like carcinoma (LELC). A subtype of squamous cell carcinoma. A kind of malignant tumor that arises from uncontrolled mitosis of transformed cells originating in epithelial tissue.

M

macromolecule. A very large molecule normally created by polymerization of minor subunits. In biochemistry, the term is applied to nucleic acids, proteins, and carbohydrates and also to nonpolymeric molecules with a large molecular mass, such as lipids and macrocycles.

magnetic resonance imaging (MRI). A medical imaging technique utilized in radiology to look at internal structures of the body in detail.

mediastinoscopy. A surgical procedure that enables visualization of the contents of the mediastinum to obtain a tissue sample for biopsy. Mediastinoscopy is utilized to examine the lymph nodes to determine the stage of lung cancer or for diagnosing other conditions affecting structures in the mediastinum, such as sarcoidosis or lymphoma.

mediastinum. The group of structures in the thorax. It contains the heart and its great vessels, the esophagus, the trachea, phrenic and cardiac nerves, the thoracic duct, the thymus, and the lymph nodes.

medical sonography. Medical ultrasound. An imaging technique used for visualizing subcutaneous body structures for pathology or diagnostic purposes.

megestrol. An anticancer drug that is derived from progesterone. It is used in the treatment of advanced carcinoma of the breast and endometrium.

meiosis. An extraordinary type of cell division needed for sexual reproduction in eukaryotes.

mesenchyme. A kind of undifferentiated loose connective tissue that is made mostly from mesoderm, although some is derived from other germ layers. It is able to extend into the tissues of the lymphatic and circulatory systems and in connective tissues throughout the body as well.

metastasis. Spread of cancer cells from one organ to another.

methotrexate. Also known as amethopterin. An antimetabolite and antifolate drug. It is utilized in the management of cancer, autoimmune diseases, and ectopic pregnancy and for the induction of medical abortions.

mitochondrial DNA. DNA found in organelles called mitochondria, the structures within eukaryotic cells that change the chemical energy from food into a form that cells can use.

mitosis. Cell division in unicellular organisms. This process will create more identical cells.

Mohs surgery. A kind of chemosurgery done to treat common types of skin cancer. During the duration of the surgery, after each removal of tissue and while the patient waits, the pathologist checks the tissue specimen for cancer cells, and the results inform the surgeon where to remove tissue next. The surgeon performing the procedure is also the pathologist reading the specimen slides.

molecular targeted therapy. Type of treatment or medication that blocks the growth of cancer cells by directly stopping the specific targeted molecules essential for cancer cell and tumor formation.

mucin staining. Staining or dyeing of mucin for microscopic contrast with the purpose of medical diagnosis.

multiple sclerosis. An inflammatory disease characterized by the destruction of myelin sheaths around axons of the brain and spinal cord resulting in the loss of myelin and scarring. It often results in physical and mental difficulties.

muscle-sparing incision. Creating limited or small incisions to reduce the effect of surgery on the muscles at the surgical site.

myc. A regulator gene that codes for a transcription factor.

N

necrosis. Death of cells in living tissue.

needle phobia. Fear of needles.

non–small cell lung cancer (NSCLC). Any type of epithelial lung cancer other than small cell lung carcinoma. They are unresponsive to chemotherapeutic agents and can be treated by surgery.

nucleotide. Biological molecules that form the building blocks of DNA and RNA and serve to carry packets of energy within the cell.

O

oncogenes. A gene that has the potential to cause cancer in tumor cells.

oncology. The branch of medicine that deals with tumors and cancer, including the study of their development, diagnosis, treatment, and prevention.

oncoproteins. The resultant protein in the mutation or increased expression of a normal gene to an oncogene.

oophorectomy. Surgical removal of one or both ovaries.

Oregon Death with Dignity Act. Legalizes physician-assisted dying, commonly referred to as physician-assisted suicide, with certain restrictions.

organoid. Resembling an organ.

osteogenesis. Bone tissue formation.

osteolytic lesions. Characteristic areas of damage due to myeloma, a type of cancer of plasma cells.

otolaryngologic. Pertaining to ENT (ear, nose, and throat).

P

paclitaxel. An anticancer medication that acts by inhibiting mitosis.

palliative. Treatment that focuses on relieving and preventing the suffering of patients.

palm healing. A type of Japanese alternative medicine that is believed to transfer universal energy in the form of qi through the palms. Qi is believed to help in self-healing and equilibrium.

Pancoast tumors. Also known as pulmonary sulcus tumor or superior sulcus tumor. Tumor of the pulmonary apex, which is the top end of either the right or the left lung.

paraneoplastic syndromes. A disease that is the result of the presence of cancer in the body but is not due to the presence of cancer cells.

parasternal. Vertical line on the front of the thorax.

parenchymal. Pertaining to the parenchyma, the tissue characteristic of an organ.

pathogenesis. The mechanism that causes a disease.

pathologic. Characteristic of a disease.

pathologist. One who studies and diagnoses diseases.

pemetrexed (Alimta). An anticancer drug that is used to treat pleural mesothelioma and non–small cell lung cancer. It acts by inhibiting the formation of precursor purine and pyrimidine nucleotides. Pemetrexed prevents the creation of DNA and RNA, which are needed for the growth and survival of both normal cells and cancer cells.

perfusion. Process of the circulation of blood to capillaries in tissues.

peritoneal mesothelioma. Kind of cancer that attacks the lining of the abdomen.

phagocytes. Cells that protect the body by ingesting harmful foreign materials, such as bacteria or dying cells.

pharmacology. The study of medications and their compositions, structure, mechanisms of action, indications, reactions, and effects.

phospholipid. A type of lipids that is a major component of all cell membranes as it makes lipid bilayers.

physician-assisted suicide. When one or more doctors help another person commit suicide directly or intentionally and voluntarily cause his or her own death. This may be done by providing one with drugs or equipment to end one's own life but may extend to other actions.

plasma membrane. The semipermeable wall that separates the inside of the cell from the outside environment.

pleura. The serous membrane that covers the lungs and adjoining structures.

pleural effusion. Excess fluid that accumulates between the visceral and parietal pleura.

pleural mesothelioma. A rare form of cancer that develops from cells of the protective lining that covers the pleura.

pleurodesis. A procedure done to prevent recurrence of pneumothorax or recurrent pleural effusion.

pleuroperitoneal shunt. A catheter implanted to transfer pleural fluid into the peritoneal cavity. It requires manual pumping.

pneumocytes. Lung cells. They are responsible in the exchange of gas, secretion of pulmonary surfactant, and self-regeneration.

pneumonectomy. Surgical removal of a lung.

pneumothorax. Abnormal accumulation of air or gas in the pleural space that separates the lung from the chest wall.

polymerase. An enzyme that is solely responsible in the synthesis of polymers of nucleic acids.

porfimer. A miscellaneous anticancer medication that is used to treat esophageal and endo-brachial non–small cell lung cancer.

positron emission tomography (PET). A nuclear medical imaging procedure that creates a three-dimensional image of functional processes in the body. It detects pairs of gamma rays emitted indirectly by a positron-emitting radionuclide or tracer that is introduced into the body on a biologically active molecule.

posterolateral thoracotomy. Chest surgery technique in which an incision is made in the fold below the breast, below the tip of the scapula. The incision is continued downward along the course of the ribs and upward as far as the spine of the scapula. It requires the division of the trapezius, rhomboideus, latissimus dorsi, and serratus anterior muscles.

posttraumatic stress disorder (PTSD). Anxiety disorder due to an intensely traumatic event, characterized by mentally reexperiencing the trauma, avoidance of trauma-associated stimuli, numbing of emotional responsiveness, and hyperalertness and difficulty in sleeping, remembering, or concentrating.

prednisone. An immunosuppressing medication used to treat various inflammatory diseases, such as moderate allergic reactions and some types of cancer.

preganglionic fibers. Fibers arising from the central nervous system to the ganglion.

prophylactic cranial irradiation (PCI). Type of radiotherapy to the brain used to decrease the risks of the spread of cancer cells to different organs.

provisional diagnosis. The initial diagnosis, even when all test results have not been received and/or analyzed yet.

pseudoglandular. Resembling that of a gland but not glandular in nature.

pulmonary acini. Acini of the respiratory system. *See also* acini.

pulmonary embolus. Blockage of an artery of the lung by fat, tumor, tissue, or a clot originating from a vein.

pulmonary nodules. Mass formation in the lung.

pulmonary sulcus tumors. *See* Pancoast tumors.

Q

quercetin. A flavonol, a plant-derived flavonoid found in fruits, vegetables, leaves, and grains. It is used as an ingredient in supplements, beverages, or foods.

R

radical mastectomy. The surgical removal of the breast, underlying chest muscle, and lymph nodes of the axilla as a treatment for breast cancer.

replicative senescence. A restriction in the number of times that cells can divide. A basic feature of somatic cells except for most tumor cells and possibly some stem cells.

ribonucleic acid (RNA). An ever-present classification of large biological molecules that serve important roles in the coding, decoding, regulation, and expression of genes.

ribonucleotide reductase. An enzyme that catalyzes the formation of deoxyribonucleotides from ribonucleotides.

ribosome. A large and complex molecular machine, found within all living cells, that serves as the main site of biological protein synthesis.

rough endoplasmic reticulum (rough ER). A membranous network of cisterns studded with protein-manufacturing ribosomes. It is responsible in the creation of lysosomal enzymes; secreted proteins, either secreted constitutively with no tag or secreted in a regulatory manner involving clathrin and paired basic amino acids in the signal peptide; integral membrane proteins; and initial glycosylation.

S

salvage therapy. Also known as rescue therapy. A kind of treatment provided when an ailment does not respond to standard treatment.

sarcomatoid carcinoma. A comparatively rare form of cancer whose malignant cells have histological, cytological, or molecular properties of epithelial tumors and mesenchymal tumors.

scalene muscles. A group of three pairs of muscles in the lateral neck. They are composed of the scalenus anterior, scalenus medius, and scalenus posterior muscles.

secretory component. A component of immunoglobulin A (IgA) that is made of a portion of the polymeric immunoglobulin receptor.

segmentectomy. Surgical removal of a part of an organ or a gland.

single-detector computed tomography scanner. A type of computed tomographic (CT) study using a single detector row CT scanner to produce detailed images of a body part for diagnosis.

small cell lung cancer (SCLC). A disease in which the cells of the lung tissues grow uncontrollably and form tumors.

spinal cord compression. Occurs when the spinal cord is compressed by bone fragments from a vertebral fracture, a tumor, an abscess, a ruptured intervertebral disc, or another lesion. It is identified as a medical emergency independent of its cause and requires fast diagnosis and treatment to prevent long-term disability due to irreversible spinal cord injury.

sputum cytology. A sputum test to determine the presence of a pulmonary system malignancy.

squamous cell carcinoma. A cancer of a kind of epithelial cell, the squamous cell, which is the main component of the epidermis of the skin. They can also be found in the lining of the digestive tract, lungs, and other areas of the body.

Stat3. Short for signal transducer and activator of transcription 3. A transcription factor that is encoded by the *STAT3* gene.

stereotactic body radiation treatment (SBRT). Also known as stereotactic ablative radiotherapy (SABR), a kind of radiation therapy in which a small number of very high doses of radiation are delivered to small, well-defined tumors. The purpose is to deliver a radiation dose that is high enough to eliminate the cancer while minimizing contact to surrounding healthy organs.

stereotactic body radiosurgery. Treatment that delivers high doses of radiation at the same time that it saves nearby tissues and organs. In spite of its name, it is a nonsurgical radiation therapy that can be used as an alternative to invasive surgery.

suicidal ideation. Medical term for thoughts about or an atypical preoccupation with suicide.

superior sulcus tumors. *See* Pancoast tumor.

superior vena cava obstruction. Outcome of the direct obstruction of the superior vena cava by malignancies such as compression of the vessel wall by right upper lobe tumors or thymoma and/or mediastinal lymphadenopathy. Also known as superior vena cava syndrome.

superior vena cava syndrome. *See* superior vena cava obstruction.

surfactant. The compounds that lower the surface tension. They coat the walls of the alveoli in the lungs, allowing it to expand properly.

symptomatic. Showing symptoms or subjective details indicative of a disease or illness.

syndrome of inappropriate antidiuretic hormone secretion (SIADH). Characterized by excessive release of antidiuretic hormone from the posterior pituitary gland or another source. The result is hyponatremia and sometimes fluid overload.

T

telomerase. An enzyme found in the telomeres of specific chromosomes that is active in cell division and may play a part in the proliferation of cancer cells.

thoracentesis. Also known as a pleural tap. An invasive procedure to remove fluid or air from the pleural space for diagnostic or therapeutic purposes.

thoracic outlet syndrome. A syndrome involving compression at the superior thoracic outlet in which excess pressure is placed on a neurovascular bundle passing between the anterior scalene and middle scalene muscles.

thrombophlebitis. A vein inflammation due to a blood clot or thrombus.

thymine (T). One of the four nucleobases in the nucleic acid of DNA.

Thyroid transcription factor I (TTF-1). Also known as NK2 homeobox 1 NKX2-1. A protein that in humans is encoded by the *NKX2-1* gene.

thyroxine. Also known as T4, one of the three hormones produced by the thyroid gland. It is responsible for the regulation of metabolism.

topotecan. An anticancer agent that is a topoisomerase inhibitor. A water-soluble derivative of camptothecin. It is used in form of the hydrochloride to treat ovarian cancer, lung cancer, and other forms of cancer.

trachea. The windpipe. It is the cartilaginous and membranous tube descending from the larynx into the bronchi.

transbronchial biopsy. A procedure in which a thin, lighted tube is inserted through the nose or mouth to collect several pieces of lung tissue.

transitional cell carcinomas. Kind of cancer that classically arises in the urinary system: the kidney, urinary bladder, and accessory organs.

transthoracic needle aspiration. A procedure in which a thin, lighted tube is inserted through the thorax to collect several pieces of lung tissue.

tropomyosins. Two-stranded alpha-helical coiled proteins found in muscle. They are responsible for regulating the function of actin filaments in both muscle and nonmuscle cells.

tuberculosis. An infectious disease caused by a variety of strains of mycobacteria, usually *Mycobacterium tuberculosis*. It usually attacks the lungs but can also involve other parts of the body.

tubulin. One of the many members of a small family of globular proteins. The most common members of the tubulin family are α-tubulin and β-tubulin, the proteins that make up microtubules.

tumor-suppressor genes. Also known as an anti-oncogene. They protect the cell from cancer.

tyrosine kinase. An enzyme that can transfer a phosphate group from ATP to a protein in a cell. They can mutate and cause unregulated growth, causing cancer.

V

vesicular chromatin. A protein in which large amounts of euchromatin are present.

video-assisted thoracoscopic surgery (VATS). A kind of thoracic or chest surgery performed using a small video camera that is introduced into the patient's chest via a scope. The surgeon is able to see the instruments that are being used along with the anatomy on which the surgeon is operating.

vinca alkaloid. A set of antimitotic and antimicrotubule agents that were originally derived from the periwinkle plant *Catharanthus roseus*.

vincristine. An anticancer medication that acts by inhibiting mitosis.

vinorelbine. An anticancer medication that acts by inhibiting mitosis. It is used to treat some types of cancer, such as breast cancer and non–small cell lung cancer.

W

wedge resection. A surgical procedure to remove a triangle-shaped slice of tissue. It is used to remove a tumor or other types of tissue that need to be removed and typically includes a small amount of normal tissue around it.

white-coat hypertension. Also known as white-coat syndrome. Patients exhibit elevated blood pressure in a clinical setting or when seeing a doctor but not in other settings. It is believed to be due to the anxiety that some people experience during a clinic visit.

white-coat syndrome. *See* white-coat hypertension.

X

xeroderma. A condition that involves the skin and that can be treated with moisturizers. People with this condition experience scaling, itching, and cracking of the skin.

NOTES

PREFACE

1. "What is lung cancer," www.lungcancer.org, accessed March 28, 2013.

2. Peter Crosta, "What is lung cancer," , www.medicalnewstoday.com, accessed August 14, 2012.

3. "Five most common cancers in each racial/ethnic group," www.seer.cancer.gov, accessed March 29, 2013.

4. American Cancer Society, "Cancer facts and figures," www.cancer.org, accessed April 28, 2013.

5. "The report on carcinogens, eleventh edition," National Toxicology Program, Department of Health and Health Services, www.ntp.niehs.nih.gov, accessed April 8, 2013.

6. C. G. Humble, D. R. Pathak, and J. M. Samet, "Personal and family history of respiratory disease and lung cancer risk," *American Review of Respiratory Disease* 134, no. 3 (1986): 466–70.

7. M. Inoue, M. Iwasaki, N. Nagai, J. Nitadori, T. Otani, S. Sasazuki, and S. Tsugane, "Association between lung cancer incidence and family history of lung cancer: Data from a large-scale population-based cohort study, the JPHC study," *Chest* 130, no. 4 (2006): 968–75.

8. "Radon in the home," www.cdc.gov, accessed April 2, 2013.

9. P. Boffetta, W. Ye, H. O. Adami, L. A. Mucci, and O. Nyrén, "Risk of cancers of the lung, head and neck in patients hospitalized for alcoholism in Sweden," *British Journal of Cancer* 85, no. 5 (2001): 678–82.

10. "What are clinical trials?," www.nhlbi.nih.gov, accessed April 8, 2013.

11. "How do clinical trials protect participants?," www.nhlbi.nih.gov, accessed March 3, 2013.

12.   Lynne Eldridge, "Cancer support groups," http://lungcancer.about.com, accessed May 21, 2013.

13.   "Nutrition for the person with cancer during treatment," www.cancer.org, accessed March 29, 2012.

14.   "Nutrition for the person with cancer during treatment," www.cancer.org, accessed March 29, 2012.

15.   L. Ovesen, J. Hannibal, and M. Sørensen, "Taste thresholds in patients with small-cell lung cancer," *Journal of Cancer Research and Clinical Oncology* 117, no. 1 (1991): 70–72.

16.   Lynne Eldridge, "Lung cancer smoker's guilt" http://lungcancer.about.com, accessed May 14, 2013; "Asbestos exposure and cancer risk," www.cancer.gov, accessed April 8, 2013.

17.   Zoe T. Raleigh, "A biopsychosocial perspective on the experience of lung cancer," *Journal of Psychosocial Oncology* 28, no. 1 (2010): 116–25.

18.   Lynne Eldridge, "12 tips for supporting a loved one with cancer," http://lungcancer.about.com, accessed March 3, 2013.

19.   Lynne Eldridge, "Tips for caregivers of cancer patients," http://lungcancer.about.com, accessed April 5, 2013.

20.   Melissa Conrad Stöppler, "Lung cancer," www.medicinenet.com, accessed March 29, 2013.

21.   S. P. Riaz, M. Lüchtenborg, R. H. Jack, V. H. Coupland, K. M. Linklater, M. D. Peake, and H. Møller, "Variation in surgical resection for lung cancer in relation to survival: Population-based study in England 2004–2006," *European Journal of Cancer* 48, no. 1 (2012): 54–60.

22.   T. Treasure and M. Utley, "Survival after resection for primary lung cancer," *Thorax, An International Journal of Respiratory Medicine* 61, no. 8 (2006): 710–15.

23.   Department of Health, "Improving outcomes: A strategy for cancer, January 2011," https://www.gov.uk, accessed March 29, 2013.

I. INTRODUCTION TO THE LUNG CELL

1.   Alison C. MacKinnon, Jens Kopatz, and Tariq Sethi, "The molecular and cellular biology of lung cancer: Identifying novel therapeutic strategies," *Oxford Journals—British Medical Bulletin* 95, no. 1 (2010): 47–61.

2.   A. Matakidou, T. Eisen, and R. S. Houlston, "Systematic review of the relationship between family history and lung cancer risk," *British Journal of Cancer* 93, no. 7 (2005): 825–33.

3.   MacKinnon et al., "The molecular and cellular biology of lung cancer."

4. Arnold Berk, Harvey Lodish, Lawrence Zipursky, Paul Matsudaira, David Baltimore, and James Darnel, "The dynamic cell," *Molecular Cell Biology*, 4th ed. (New York: W. H. Freeman, 2000).

5. "Monad," Biology Online, www.biology-online.org/dictionary/Monad, accessed May 1, 2013.

6. "A basic introduction to the science underlying NCBI resources—What is a cell," www.ncbi.nlm.nih.gov, accessed May 2, 2013.

7. SEER Training Modules, "Anatomy and physiology module," U.S. National Institutes of Health, National Cancer Institute, http://training.seer.cancer.gov, accessed March 26, 2013.

8. "Epithelial tissues," www.bcb.uwc.ac.za/sci_ed/grade10/mammal/epithelial.htm, accessed May 1, 2013.

9. Louise Tremblay, "3 major cell types," last updated August 18, 2013, accessed March 13, 2013, www.livestrong.com.

10. Ian Murnaghan, "Learn about DNA structure," last updated February 21, 2013, www.exploredna.co.uk/learn-about-dna-structure.html, accessed March 23, 2013.

11. "What is DNA?," published May 6, 2013, http://ghr.nlm.nih.gov/handbook/basics/dna, accessed June 2, 2013.

12. "DNA-RNA-protein introduction," www.nobelprize.org/educational/medicine/dna, accessed May 8, 2013.

13. "What is DNA?"

14. "DNA-RNA-protein introduction," www.nobelprize.org/educational/medicine/dna, accessed May 8, 2013.

15. "What is DNA?"

16. "DNA-RNA-protein introduction."

17. "What is RNA?"

18. Francis Crick, "Central dogma of molecular biology," *Nature* 227, no. 5258 (1970): 561–63.

19. "Cells and DNA," published April 29, 2013, http://ghr.nlm.nih.gov/handbook/basics, accessed May 10, 2013.

20. "Cytoskeleton," www.cellsalive.com/cells/cytoskel.htm, accessed March 12, 2013.

21. "What is a cell?," National Center for Biotechnology Information, last modified March 30, 2004, www.ncbi.nlm.nih.gov, accessed March 17, 2013.

22. "Cells and DNA."

23. "Cells and DNA."

24. "Cells and DNA."

25. "Cells and DNA."

26. "Cells and DNA."

27. "Lung Disease and Respiratory Health Center: Lung treatments," last reviewed August 1, 2009, www.webmd.com/lung/picture-of-the-lungs?page=3, accessed March 3, 2013.

28. "Respiratory, trachea, bronchioles and bronchi," www.histology.leeds.ac.uk/respiratory/conducting.php, accessed May 12, 2013.

29. Bhakti Satalkar, "Trachea function," posted July 23, 2010, www.buzzle.com/articles/trachea-function.html, accessed March 22, 2013.

30. Satalkar, "Trachea function."

31. Satalkar, "Trachea function."

32. "Ciliated columnar epithelium," Davidson College Biology Department, www.bio.davidson.edu, accessed May 13, 2013.

33. Bruce Alberts, Alexander Johnson, Julian Lewis, Martin Raff, Keith Roberts, and Peter Walter, "Desmosomes connect intermediate filaments from cell to cell," in *Molecular Biology of the Cell*, 4th ed. (New York: Garland Science, 2002).

34. "Major zones and divisions of the respiratory system," www.getbodysmart.com/ap/respiratorysystem/zonesdivisions/tutorial.html, accessed May 12, 2013.

35. B. Alberts, D. Bray, J. Lewis, M. Raff, and J. Watson, "Cilia and centrioles," in *Molecular Biology of the Cell*, 3rd ed. (New York: Garland Science, 1994).

36. Jun Atsuta, Sherry A. Sterbinsky, Jim Plitt, Lisa M. Schwiebert, Bruce S. Bochner, and Robert P. Schleimer, "Phenotyping and cytokine regulation of the BEAS-2B human bronchial epithelial cell: Demonstration of inducible expression of the adhesion molecules VCAM-1 and ICAM-1," *American Journal of Respiratory Cell and Molecular Biology* 17, no. 5 (1997): 571–82.

37. Atsuta et al., "Phenotyping and cytokine regulation of the BEAS-2B human bronchial epithelial cell."

38. "Anatomy review: Respiratory structures," Winona State University Biology, www.winona.edu, accessed May 12, 2013.

39. Susan D. Reynolds and Alvin M. Malkinson, "Clara cell: Progenitor for the bronchiolar epithelium," *International Journal of Biochemistry and Cell Biology* 42, no. 1 (2011): 1–4.

40. "Pulmonary alveolus," www.sciencedaily.com/articles/p/pulmonary_alveolus.htm, accessed May 12, 2013.

41. M. Ochs, J. R. Nyengaard, A. Jung, L. Knudsen, M. Voigt, T. Wahlers, J. Richter, and H. J. Gundersen, "The number of alveoli in the human lung," *American Journal of Respiratory and Critical Care Medicine* 169, no. 1 (2004): 120–24.

42.   James F. Thompson, "Exam 3 review: Chapter 22: Alveoli," Austin Peay State University Biology, http://apbrwww5.apsu.edu/thompsonj, accessed May 15, 2013.

43.   M. Johnson, Jonathan H. Widdicombe, Lennel Allen, Pascal Barbry, and Leland G. Dobbs, "Alveolar epithelial type I cells contain transport proteins and transport sodium, supporting an active role for type I cells in regulation of lung liquid homeostasis," *Proceedings of the National Academy of Sciences of the United States of America* 99, no. 4 (2002): 1966–971.

44.   Kenneth S. Saladin, *Anatomy and Physiology: The Unity of Form and Function* (New York: McGraw -ill, 2007).

45.   Carlyn Main, "The difference between male and female skeletons," http://human-skeleton-model-review.toptenreviews.com/the-difference-between-male-and-female-skeletons.html, accessed May 2, 2013.

46.   Michael W. King, "Introduction," The Medical Biochemistry Page, last modified February 10, 2013, http://themedicalbiochemistrypage.org/steroid-hormones.php, accessed March 7, 2013.

47.   Miller-Keane and Marie T. O'Toole, *Miller-Keane Encyclopedia and Dictionary of Medicine, Nursing, and Allied Health*, 7th ed. (New York: Saunders/Elsevier, 2007).

48.   "Definition of adrenal cortex," last reviewed June 14, 2012, www.medterms.com, accessed May 4, 2013.

49.   Peter A. Torjesen and Liv Sandnes, "Serum testosterone in women as measured by an automated immunoassay and a RIA," *Clinical Chemistry* 50, no. 3 (2004): 678–79.

50.   Dick F. Swaab and Alicia Gracia-Falgueras, "Sexual differentiation of the human brain in relation to gender identity and sexual orientation," *Functional Neurology* 24, no. 1 (2009): 17–28.

51.   Swaab and Gracia-Falgueras, "Sexual differentiation of the human brain in relation to gender identity and sexual orientation."

52.   Rex A. Hess, David B. Unick, Ki-Ho Lee, Janice Bahr, Julia A. Taylor, Kenneth S. Korach, and Dennis Lubahn, "A role for oestrogens in the male reproductive system," *Nature* 390, no. 6659 (1997): 509–12.

53.   "Somatic cells," www.biology-online.org/dictionary/Somatic_cells, accessed May 14, 2013.

54.   Main, "The difference between male and female skeletons."

55.   Main, "The difference between male and female skeletons."

56.   Nicholas Wade, "Male chromosome may evolve fastest," *New York Times*, published online January 13, 2010, www.nytimes.com, accessed March 12, 2013.

57.   Renee Twombly, "Estrogen's dual nature? Studies highlight effects on breast cancer," *Journal of the National Cancer Institute* 103, no. 12 (2011): 920–21.

58.   A. Morgentaler and C. Schulman, "Testosterone and prostate safety," *Frontiers of Hormone Research* 37 (2009): 197–203.

59.   Andrew Sullivan, "The he hormone," *New York Times Magazine*, April 2, 2000, www.photius.com/feminocracy/testosterone.html, accessed May 14, 2013.

60.   Swaab and Gracia-Falgueras, "Sexual differentiation of the human brain in relation to gender identity and sexual orientation."

61.   J. M. Berg, J. L. Tymoczko, and L. Stryer, "Section 27.6 mutations involve changes in the base sequence of DNA," in *Biochemistry*, 5th ed. (New York: W. H. Freeman, 2002).

62.   "Better health channel," Amherst College, last reviewed November 2005, www3.amherst.edu/~dmirwin/Reports/BetterHealth.htm, accessed May 11, 2013.

63.   "Mitochondrial DNA," reviewed October 2012, http://ghr.nlm.nih.gov/chromosome/MT, accessed May 5, 2013.

64.   Bruce Alberts, Alexander Johnson, Julian Lewis, Martin Raff, Keith Roberts, and Peter Walter, "Most cancers derive from a single abnormal cell," in *Molecular Biology of the Cell*.

65.   "Lung cancer (small cell)," www.cancer.org/cancer/lungcancer-small-cell/detailedguide/small-cell-lung-cancer-what-is-small-cell-lung-cancer, accessed May 5, 2013.

2. LUNG CELL HEALTH VERSUS LUNG CELL DISORDER

1.   M. S. Wold, "Replication protein A: A heterotrimeric, single-stranded DNA-binding protein required for eukaryotic DNA metabolism," *Annual Review of Biochemistry* 66 (1997): 61–92.

2.   "How cells multiply," updated September 2009, www.cancerresearchuk.org, accessed February 27, 2013.

3.   G. M. Cooper, "The eukaryotic cell cycle," in *The Cell: A Molecular Approach*, 2nd ed. (Sunderland, MA: Sinauer Associates, 2000).

4.   "Cell energy and cell functions," http://www.nature.com/scitable/topic-page/cell-energy-and-cell-functions-14024533, accessed May 11, 2013.

5.   Emilie Blond, Christine Maitrepierre, Sylvie Normand, Monique Sothier, Hubert Roth, Joelle Goudable, and Martine Laville, "A new indirect calorimeter is accurate and reliable for measuring basal energy expenditure, thermic effect of food and substrate oxidation in obese and healthy subjects,"

European e-Journal of Clinical Nutrition and Metabolism 6, no. 1 (2011): e7–e15.

6. "Cellular oxidation vs. burning of sugar" www.accessexcellence.org/RC/VL/GG/ecb/cellular_oxidation_burning_sugar.php, accessed May 12, 2013.

7. Bruce Alberts, Alexander Johnson, Julian Lewis, Martin Raff, Keith Roberts, and Peter Walter, "The universal features of cells on earth," in *Molecular Biology of the Cell*, 4th ed. (New York: Garland Science, 2002).

8. Alberts et al., "The universal features of cells on earth."

9. Bruce Alberts, Alexander Johnson, Julian Lewis, Martin Raff, Keith Roberts, and Peter Walter, "The lipid bilayer," in *Molecular Biology of the Cell*.

10. Geoffrey M. Cooper, "Chromosomes and chromatin," in *The Cell*; Leigh Eisenman and Jill Hunter, "The cell," Dartmouth College Biology, www.dartmouth.edu/~cbbc/courses/bio4/bio4-lectures/theCell.html, accessed April 28, 2013.

11. Kirstie Saltsman, "Cellular reproduction: Multiplication by division: Inside the cell," National Institute of General Medical Services, last modified April 22, 2011, http://publications.nigms.nih.gov/insidethecell/chapter4.html, accessed April 7, 2013.

12. Kirstie Saltsman, "The last chapter: Cell aging and death," National Institute of General Medical Services, last modified April 22, 2011, http://publications.nigms.nih.gov/insidethecell/chapter5.html, accessed March 6, 2013.

13. Genetic Science Learning Center, "The inside story of cell communication," August 6, 2012, http://learn.genetics.utah.edu/content/begin/cells/inside-story, accessed March 23, 2013.

14. F. Calvo and E. Sahai, "Cell communication networks in cancer invasion," *Current Opinion in Cell Biology* 23, no. 5 (2011): 621–29.

15. Genetic Science Learning Center, "When cell communication goes wrong," August 6, 2012, http://learn.genetics.utah.edu/content/begin/cells/bad-com, accessed March 23, 2013.

16. Sami I. Said, "Glutamate receptor activation in the pathogenesis of acute lung injury," in *Cell Signalling in Vascular Inflammation*, ed. J. Bhattacharya (New York: Humana Press, 2005), 47–50.

17. M. Trojano and D. Paolicelli, "The differential diagnosis of multiple sclerosis: Classification and clinical features of relapsing and progressive neurological syndromes," *Neurological Sciences* 22, suppl. 2 (2001): S98–102.

18. R. J. Shaw and L. C. Cantley, "Ras, PI(3)K and mTOR signalling controls tumour cell growth," *Nature* 441, no. 7092 (2006): 424–30.

19. David Shier, Jackie Butler, and Ricki Lewis, *Hole's Essentials of Human Anatomy and Physiology*, 10th ed. (New York: McGraw-Hill, 2009).

20. K. T. Chang, C. M. Tsai, Y. C. Chiou , C. H. Chiu, K. S. Jeng, and C. Y. Huang, "IL-6 induces neuroendocrine dedifferentiation and cell proliferation in non-small cell lung cancer cells," *American Journal of Physiology—Lung Cellular and Molecular Physiology* 289, no. 3 (2005): L446–53.

21. K. Matsuyama, Y. Chiba, M. Sasaki, H. Tanaka, R. Muraoka, and N. Tanigawa, "Tumor angiogenesis as a prognostic marker in operable non-small cell lung cancer," *Annals of Thoracic Surgery* 65, no. 5 (1998): 1405–9.

22. "How a cancer spreads," Cancer Research UK, last updated November 11, 2011, www.cancerresearchuk.org, accessed March 18, 2013.

23. M. Bacac and I. Stamenkovic, "Metastatic cancer cell," *Annual Review of Pathology: Mechanisms of Disease* 3 (2008): 221–47.

24. H. Gerhardt and H. Semb, "Pericytes: Gatekeepers in tumor cell metastasis," *Journal of Molecular Medicine* 86, no. 2 (2008): 135–44.

25. L. Kopfstein and G. Christofori, "Metastasis: Cell-autonomous mechanisms versus contributions by the tumor microenvironment," *Cellular and Molecular Life Sciences* 63, no. 4 (2006): 449–68.

26. D. S. Tan, R. Agarwal, and S. B. Kaye, "Mechanisms of transcoelomic metastasis in ovarian cancer," *Lancet Oncology* 7, no. 11 (2006): 925–34.

27. M. Rath, *Cellular Health Series—Cancer* (Santa Clara, CA: MR Publishing, 2001), 13.

28. John E. Hall, *Guyton & Hall Medical Physiology*, 12th ed. (Philadelphia: Elsevier Saunders, 2011).

29. T. Sadler, *Langman's Medical Embryology*, 9th ed. (Baltimore: Lippincott Williams & Wilkins, 2003).

30. Jean-Claude Yernault, "Lung aging," Encyclopaedia of Aging, 2002, www.encyclopedia.com, accessed March 25, 2013.

31. Yernault, "Lung aging."

32. R. Effros, "Anatomy, development, and physiology of the lungs," May 2006, www.nature.com/gimo/contents/pt1/full/gimo73.html#f3, accessed March 19, 2013.

3. REAL MEANING AND ANATOMY OF LUNG CANCER

1. Freddie Bray, H. R. Shin, F. Bray, D. Forman, C. Mathers, and D. M. Parkin, "Estimates of worldwide burden of cancer in 2008: GLOBOCAN 2008," *International Journal of Cancer* 127, no. 12 (2010): 2893–917.

2. Anne S. Tsao, "Lung carcinoma: Tumors of the lungs," in *Merck Manual Professional Edition* (Whitehouse Station, NJ: Merck, Sharp and Dohme Corp., 2011).

3. "Cancer nomenclature," Radlink PET and Cardiac Imaging Centre, www.molecularimaging.com.sg/cancer_nomenclature.asp, accessed April 25, 2013.

4. "Cancer overview," Stanford University, www.cancer.stanford.edu/information/cancerOverview.html, accessed February 17, 2013.

5. "Cancer classification," National Cancer Institute, http://training.seer.cancer.gov/disease/categories/classification.html, accessed April 25, 2013.

6. Ramaswamy Govindan and Janakiraman Subramanian, "Lung cancer in never-smokers: A review," *Journal of Clinical Oncology* 25, no. 5 (2007): 561.

7. "Lung adenocarcinoma," College of American Pathologists, www.cap.org, accessed May 2, 2013.

8. "Cancer classification."

9. Sharon Lane, "Rare cancer: Types," www.rare-cancer.org/types-of-cancer.php, accessed May 3, 2013.

10. Kevin G. Billingsley, M. E. Burt, E. Jara, R. J. Ginsberg, J. M. Woodruff, D. H. Leung, and M. F. Brennan, "Pulmonary metastases from soft tissue sarcoma: Analysis of patterns of disease and postmetastasis survival," *Annals of Surgery* 229, no. 5 (1999): 602.

11. "Cancer classification."

12. H. I. Libshitz, J. Zornoza, and J. W. McLarty, "Lung cancer in chronic leukemia and lymphoma," *Radiology* 127, no. 2 (1978): 297.

13. "Cancer classification."

14. F. Coster, R. Somers, B. G. Taal, P. van Heerde, B. Coster, T. Dozeman, S. J. Huisman, and A. A. Hart, "Increased risk of lung cancer, non-Hodgkin's lymphoma, and leukemia following Hodgkin's disease," *Journal of Clinical Oncology* 7, no. 8 (1989): 1046.

15. "Cancer nomenclature."

16. J. Pont, N. Pridun, N. Vesely, H. R. Kienzer, E. Pont, and F. J. Spital, "Extragonadal malignant germ cell tumor of the lung," *Journal of Thoracic and Cardiovascular Surgery* 107 (1994): 311.

17. Peter Crosta, "What is cancer? What causes cancer?," last modified March 21, 2013, www.medicalnewstoday.com/info/cancer-oncology, accessed April 21, 2013.

18. Carlo M. Croce, "Oncogenes and cancer," *New England Journal of Medicine* 358 (2008): 502–11.

19. R. S. Mitchell, V. Kumar, A. K. Abbas, and N. Fausto, "Neoplasms of the thyroid," in *Robbins Basic Pathology* (Philadelphia: Saunders, 2007).

20. Arnold J. Levine, "Tumor suppressor genes." *Sci & Med* 2, no. 1 (1995): 28–37.

21. Crosta, "What is cancer?"

22. Catherine Paddock, "New clue to how cancer cells spread," www.medicalnewstoday.com/articles/251306.php, accessed April 27, 2013.

23. Tina St. John, "Lung cancer staging and diagnosis," in *With Every Breath: A Lung Cancer Guidebook* (Vancouver, WA: Lung Cancer Caring Ambassadors Program, 2009), 33.

24. Tina St. John, "The lungs and respiratory system," in *With Every Breath: A Lung Cancer Guidebook* (Vancouver, WA: Lung Cancer Caring Ambassadors Program, 2009), 7.

25. I. Koko, N. Mullai, J. Samuel, and L. P. Hussein," *Journal of Clinical Oncology* 22, no. 14S (2004): 7306.

26. St. John, "Lung cancer staging and diagnosis," 39.

27. Anne S. Tsao, "Lung carcinoma: Tumors of the lungs," in *Merck Manual Professional Edition*.

28. "Symptoms of lung cancer," www.lungcancer.co/symptoms, accessed April 29, 2013.

29. "Fact sheet: Symptoms of lung cancer," http://oreilly.com/onconurse/factsheets/symptoms_lung.pdf, accessed April 30, 2013.

30. St. John, "Lung cancer staging and diagnosis," 38.

31. Lucian Sulica, "Voice disorders," www.voicemedicine.com/unilateral.htm, accessed May 3, 2013.

32. "Lung cancer symptoms," Cancer Research UK, www.cancerresearchuk.org, accessed April 29, 2013.

33. "Symptoms of lung cancer."

34. Anne S. Tsao, "Lung carcinoma."

35. "Symptoms of lung cancer."

36. St. John, "Lung cancer staging and diagnosis," 38.

37. J. E. Raber-Durlacher, M. T. Brennan, I. M. Verdonck-de Leeuw, R. J. Gibson, J. G. Eilers, T. Waltimo, C. P. Bots, M. Michelet, T. P. Sollecito, T. S. Rouleau, A. Sewnaik, R. J. Bensadoun, M. C. Fliedner, S. Silverman Jr., and F. K. Spijkervet, "Swallowing dysfunction in cancer patients," *Supportive Care in Cancer* 20, no. 3 (2012): 433.

38. St. John, "The lungs and respiratory system," 7.

39. St. John, "Lung cancer staging and diagnosis," 38.

40. "Causes of breathlessness."

41. C. Chiles, P. K. Woodard, F. R. Gutierrez, and K. M. Link, "Metastatic involvement of the heart and pericardium: CT and MR imaging," *RadioGraphics* 21 (2001): 439.

42. "Fact sheet."

43. H. L. Devalia and G. T. Layer, "Current concepts in gynaecomastia," *Surgeon* 7, no. 2 (2009): 114.

44. "Fact sheet."

45. St. John, "Lung cancer staging and diagnosis," 38.

46. "Fact sheet."

47. C. Villas, A. Collía, J. D. Aquerreta, J. Aristu, W. Torre, P. Díaz De Rada, and S. Gocci, "Cervicobrachialgia and pancoast tumor: Value of standard anteroposterior cervical radiographs in early diagnosis," *Orthopedics* 27, no. 10 (2004): 1092–94.

48. "Thoracic outlet syndrome," American Academy of Orthopaedic Surgeons, http://orthoinfo.aaos.org, accessed May 3, 2013.

49. "Metastatic lung cancer," www.bonetumor.org/metastatic-tumors/metastatic-lung-cancer, accessed April 30, 2013.

50. "Fact sheet."

51. K. Yokoi, R. Tsuchiya, T. Mori, K. Nagai, T. Furukawa, S. Fujimura, K. Nakagawa, and Y. Ichinose, "Results of surgical treatment of lung cancer involving the diaphragm," *Journal of Thoracic and Cardiovascular Surgery* 120, no. 4 (2004): 799.

52. St. John, "Lung cancer staging and diagnosis," 42.

53. St. John, "Lung cancer staging and diagnosis," 40.

54. "Symptoms of lung cancer"; J. I. Martin Parra, Gomez A. Naranjo, and J. C. Sanjuan Rodriguez, "Obstructive jaundice as a presentation form of bronchogenic small cell carcinoma," *Revista Espanola De Enfermedades Digestivas* 88, no. 4 (1996): 299.

55. David C. Dugdale, "Liver metastasis," www.nlm.nih.gov/medlineplus/ency/article/000277.htm, accessed May 3, 2013.

56. St. John, "Lung cancer staging and diagnosis," 42.

57. "Fact sheet."

58. St. John, "The lungs and respiratory system," 8–9.

59. J. Cai, G. Liang, Z. Cai, T. Yang, S. Li, and J. Yang, "Isolated renal metastasis from squamous cell lung cancer," *Multidisciplinary Respiratory Medicine* 8, no. 1 (2013): 2.

60. "Symptoms of lung cancer."

61. H. Sugiura, K. Yamada, T. Sugiura, T. Hida, and T. Mitsudomi, "Predictors of survival in patients with bone metastasis of lung cancer," *Clinical Orthopaedics and Related Research* 466, no. 3 (2008): 729.

62. "Metastatic lung cancer."

63. "Understanding bone metastasis," Yale Medical Group, www.yalemedicalgroup.org, accessed May 3, 2013.

64. Sugiura et al., "Predictors of survival in patients with bone metastasis of lung cancer," 729.

65. Laurie Gutmann and Michael Mareska, "Lambert-Eaton myasthenic syndrome," *Seminars in Neurology* 24, no. 2 (2004): 149; J. R. Jiang, J. Y. Shih, H. C. Wang, R. M. Wu, C. J. Yu, and P. C. Yang, "Small-cell lung cancer

presenting with Lambert-Eaton myasthenic syndrome and respiratory failure," *Journal of the Formosan Medical Association* 101, no. 12 (2002): 871–74.

66. "Fact sheet."

67. Muhammad W. Saif, Imran A. P. Siddiqui, and Muhammad A. Soheil, "Management of ascites due to gastrointestinal malignancy," *Annals of Saudi Medicine* 29, no. 5 (2009): 369–77.

68. Huntsman Cancer Institute, "Edema," in *Cancer Chemotherapy Manual* (St. Louis, MO: Facts and Comparisons, 2001).

69. Mortimer B. Lipsett, "Effects of cancers of the endocrine and central nervous system on nutritional status," *Cancer Research* 37 (1977): 2373.

70. D. Vaudry, B. J. Gonzalez, M. Basille, L. Yon, A. Fournier, and H. Vaudry, "Pituitary adenylate cyclase-activating polypeptide and its receptors: From structure to functions," *Pharmacological Reviews* 52, no. 2 (2000): 269.

71. "Lung cancer non-small cell overview," American Cancer Society, www.cancer.org, accessed April 30, 2013.

72. Vaudry et al., "Pituitary adenylate cyclase-activating polypeptide and its receptors," 269.

73. "Lung cancer non-small cell overview."

74. "Fact sheet."

75. "What is perforated bowel?," www.minahealth.com/what_is_perforated_bowel.htm, accessed May 3, 2013.

76. J. S. Woo, K. R. Joo, Y. S. Woo, J. Y. Jang, Y. W. Chang, J. Lee II, and R. Chang, "Pancreatitis from metastatic small cell lung cancer successful treatment with endoscopic intrapancreatic stenting," *Korean Journal of Internal Medicine* 21, no. 4 (2006): 256.

77. T. Maeno, H. Satoh, H. Ishikawa, Y. T. Yamashita, T. Naito, M. Fujiwara, H. Kamma, M. Ohtsuka, and S. Hasegawa, "Patterns of pancreatic metastasis from lung cancer," *Anticancer Research* 18, no. 4B (1998): 2881.

78. "Fact sheet."

79. Richard W. Hyde, Benjamin Interiano, and Donald Stuard, "Acute respiratory distress syndrome in pancreatitis," *Annals of Internal Medicine* 77, no. 6 (1972): 923.

80. "Fact sheet."

81. St. John, "Lung cancer staging and diagnosis," 41.

82. Huntsman Cancer Institute, "Edema," www.hci.utah.edu/patientdocs/hci/drug_side_effects/edema.html, accessed April 25, 2013.

83. "Edema," University of Maryland Medical Center, www.umm.edu/altmed/articles/edema-000055.htm, accessed April 30, 2013.

4. HISTORY OF LUNG CANCER

1. "Oncology," Dictionary.com, http://dictionary.reference.com/browse/oncology, accessed March 28, 2013.

2. S. I. Hajdu, "A note from history: Landmarks in history of cancer, part 1," *Cancer* 117, no. 5 (2011): 1097–102.

3. "Science diction: The origin of the word 'cancer,'" National Public Radio, www.npr.org/templates/story/story.php?storyId=130754101, accessed April 24, 2013.

4. "The history of cancer," American Cancer Society, last modified June 8, 2012, www.cancer.org, accessed May 8, 2013.

5. Hajdu, "A note from history,"

6. "The history of cancer."

7. Marilyn Yalom, *A History of the Breast* (New York: Ballantine Books, 1998).

8. S. Farber, L. K. Diamond, R. D. Mercer, R. F. Sylvester Jr., and J. A. Wolff, "Temporary remissions in acute leukemia in children produced by folic acid antagonist, 4-aminopteroyl-glutamic acid (aminopterin)," *New England Journal of Medicine* 238, no. 23 (1948): 787–93

9. P. Hunter, "The fourth front against cancer: The first clinical trials to test engineered viruses that attack tumour cells have yielded promising results for future cancer therapies," *EMBO Reports* 12, no. 8 (2011): 769–71.

10. "Cancer causes: Theories throughout history," American Cancer Society, www.cancer.org, accessed May 24, 2013.

11. "The history of cancer."

12. D. Wagener, *The History of Oncology* (New York: Springer, 2009), 19.

13. "Cancer causes."

14. Lynne Eldridge, "Famous people with lung cancer," http://lungcancer.about.com, accessed February 23, 2013; "10 celebrities who fought lung cancer," CBS News, www.cbsnews.com, accessed March 14, 2013.

15. B. E. Johnson, J. Grayson, R. W. Makuch, R. I. Linnoila, M. J. Anderson, M. H. Cohen, E. Glatstein, J. D. Minna, and D. C. Ihde, "Ten-year survival of patients with small-cell lung cancer treated with combination chemotherapy with or without irradiation," *Journal of Clinical Oncology* 8, no. 3 (1990): 396–401.

16. "SEER stat fact sheets: Lung and bronchus," http://seer.cancer.gov/statfacts/html/lungb.html, accessed April 23, 2013.

17. Johnson et al., "Ten-year survival of patients with small-cell lung cancer treated with combination chemotherapy with or without irradiation."

5. CAUSES AND RISK FACTORS OF LUNG CANCER

1.   H. Hein, P. Suadicani, and F. and Gyntelberg, "Lung cancer risk and social class: The Copenhagen Male Study," *Danish Medical Bulletin* 39, no. 2 (1992): 173–76.

2.   Peter Crosta, "What is cancer? What causes cancer?," last modified March 21, 2013, www.medicalnewstoday.com/info/cancer-oncology, accessed March 23, 2013.

3.   Anne S. Tsao, "Lung carcinoma: Tumors of the lungs," in *Merck Manual Professional Edition* (Whitehouse Station, NJ: Merck, Sharp and Dohme Corp., 2011).

4.   "Risk factors," Centers for Disease Control and Prevention, www.cdc.gov/cancer/lung/basic_info/risk_factors.htm, accessed July 20, 2013; E. Schairer and E. Schöniger, "Lungenkrebs und Tabakverbrauch [Lung cancer and tobacco consumption]," *Zeitschrift für Krebsforschung* 1, no. 4 (1943): 69.

5.   "Risk factors"; Schairer and Schöniger, "Lungenkrebs und Tabakverbrauch."

6.   M. R. Alderson, P. N. Lee, and R. Wang, "Risks of lung cancer, chronic bronchitis, ischaemic heart disease, and stroke in relation to type of cigarette smoked," *Journal of Epidemiol Community Health* 39, no. 4 (1985): 286–93.

7.   Schairer and Schöniger, "Lungenkrebs und Tabakverbrauch."

8.   Jeffrey E. Harris, "Social and economic causes of cancer," Massachusetts Institute of Technology, http://archive.org/stream/socialeconomicca00harr/socialeconomicca00harr_djvu.txt, accessed April 10, 2013.

9.   Harris, "Social and economic causes of cancer."

10.   M. Pavia, A. Bianco, C. Pileggi, and I. F. Angelillo, "Meta-analysis of residential exposure to radon gas and lung cancer," *Bulletin of the World Health Organization* 81, no. 10 (2003): 732–38.

11.   Harris, "Social and economic causes of cancer."

12.   Harris, "Social and economic causes of cancer."

13.   I. Szadkowska-Stanczyk and N. Szeszenia-Dabrowska , "Lung cancer due to occupational exposures—A review of epidemiological evidences," *Medycyna Pracy* 51 (2001): 27–34 .

14.   M. Ocke, H. Bueno-de-Mesquita, E. J. Feskens, W. A. van Staveren, and D. Kromhout, "Repeated measurements of vegetables, fruits, beta-carotene, and vitamins C and E in relation to lung cancer: The Zutphen Study," *American Journal of Epidemiology* 145, no. 4 (1997): 65.

15.   Harris, "Social and economic causes of cancer."

16. C. Lu, A. Onn, and A. A. Vaporciyan, "Cancer of the lung," in *Holland-Frei Cancer Medicine* (Beijing: People's Medical Publishing House, 2010), chap. 78.

17. T. R. Devereux, J. A. Taylor, and J. C. Barrett, "Molecular mechanisms of lung cancer: Interaction of environmental and genetic factors," *Chest* 1996: 14S–19S. doi:10.1378/chest.109.3_Supplement.14S.

18. Harris, "Social and economic causes of cancer."

19. Shannon M. Stare and James J. Jozefowicz, "The effects of environmental factors on cancer prevalence rates and specific cancer mortality rates in a sample of OECD developed countries," *International Journal of Applied Economics* 5, no. 2 (2008): 92–115.

20. K. B. Moysich, R. J. Menezes, A. Ronsani, H. Swede, M. E. Reid, K. M. Cummings, K. L. Falkner, G. M. Loewen, and G. Bepler, "Regular aspirin use and lung cancer risk," *BMC (BioMed Central) Cancer* 2 (2002): 31.

21. Ocke et al., "Repeated measurements of vegetables, fruits, beta-carotene, and vitamins C and E in relation to lung cancer."

22. A. Kubik, P. Zatloukal, L. Tomasek, J. Dolezal, L. Syllabova, J. Kara, P. Kopecky, and I. Plesko, "A case-control study of lifestyle and lung cancer associations by histological types," *Neoplasma* 55, no. 3 (2008): 192–99; K. E. Powell and S. N. Blair, "The public health burdens of sedentary living habits: Theoretical but realistic estimates," *Medicine and Science in Sports and Exercise* 26, no. 7 (1994): 851–56.

23. M. C. Alavanja, M. Dosemeci, C. Samanic, J. Lubin, C. F. Lynch, C. Knott, J. Barker, J. A. Hoppin, D. P. Sandler, J. Coble, K. Thomas, and A. Blair, "Pesticides and lung cancer risk in the agricultural health study cohort," *American Journal of Epidemiology* 160, no. 9 (2004): 876–85.

24. Harris, "Social and economic causes of cancer."

25. V. Bagnardi, G. Randi, J. Lubin, D. Consonni, T. K. Lam, A. F. Subar, A. M. Goldstein, S. Wacholder, A. W. Bergen, M. A. Tucker, A. Decarli, N. E. Caporaso, P. A. Bertazzi, and M. T. Landi, "Alcohol consumption and lung cancer risk in the Environment and Genetics in Lung Cancer Etiology (EAGLE) study," *American Journal of Epidemiology* 171, no. 1 (2010): 36–44.

26. Stare and Jozefowicz, "The effects of environmental factors on cancer prevalence rates and specific cancer mortality rates in a sample of OECD developed countries."

27. Stare and Jozefowicz, "The effects of environmental factors on cancer prevalence rates and specific cancer mortality rates in a sample of OECD developed countries."

28. M. R. Alderson, P. N. Lee, and R. Wang, "Risks of lung cancer, chronic bronchitis, ischaemic heart disease, and stroke in relation to type of cigarette smoked," *Journal of Epidemiological Community Health* 39, no. 4 (1985):

286–93.; A. J. Littman, M. D. Thornquist, E. White, L. A. Jackson, G. E. Goodman, and T. L. Vaughan, "Prior lung disease and risk of lung cancer in a large prospective study," *Cancer Causes Control* 15, no. 8 (2004): 819–27.

29. Stare and Jozefowicz, "The effects of environmental factors on cancer prevalence rates and specific cancer mortality rates in a sample of OECD developed countries."

30. Stare and Jozefowicz, "The effects of environmental factors on cancer prevalence rates and specific cancer mortality rates in a sample of OECD developed countries."

31. Stare and Jozefowicz, "The effects of environmental factors on cancer prevalence rates and specific cancer mortality rates in a sample of OECD developed countries."

32. Stare and Jozefowicz, "The effects of environmental factors on cancer prevalence rates and specific cancer mortality rates in a sample of OECD developed countries."

33. Stare and Jozefowicz, "The effects of environmental factors on cancer prevalence rates and specific cancer mortality rates in a sample of OECD developed countries."

34. Stare and Jozefowicz, "The effects of environmental factors on cancer prevalence rates and specific cancer mortality rates in a sample of OECD developed countries."

35. Stare and Jozefowicz, "The effects of environmental factors on cancer prevalence rates and specific cancer mortality rates in a sample of OECD developed countries."

6. PATHOLOGY OF LUNG CANCER

1. H. Celis and R. H. Fagard, "White-coat hypertension: A clinical review," *European Journal of Internal Medicine* 15, no. 6 (2004): 348–57.

2. M. Lloyd-Williams, "Depression—The hidden symptom in advanced cancer," *Journal of the Royal Society of Medicine* 96, no. 12 (2003): 577–81.

3. N. Murray and A. T. Turrisi, "A review of first-line treatment for small-cell lung cancer," *Journal of Thoracic Oncology* 2006: 270–78.

4. T. Miyaoka, M. Nagahama, K. Tsuchie, M. Hayashida, A. Nishida, T. Inagaki, and J. Horiguchi, "Charles Bonnet syndrome: Successful treatment of visual hallucinations due to vision loss with Yi-gan san," *Progress in Neuro-Psychopharmacology and Biological Psychiatry* 33, no. 2 (2009): 382–83.

5. L. H. Iyer, "Exposure to nonsteroidal anti-inflammatory drugs and weight loss and hospitalization in non-small cell lung cancer patients," *Texas Medical Center Dissertations*, paper AAI1518776 (January 1, 2012); D. J. Sher,

B. T. Gielda, M. J. Liptay, W. H. Warren, M. Batus, M. J. Fidler, S. Garg, and P. Bonomi, "Prognostic significance of weight gain during definitive chemo-radiotherapy for locally advanced non–small-cell lung cancer," *Clinical Lung Cancer* 14, no. 4 (2013): 370–75.

6. M. Merad-Taoufik, S. Antoun, and P. Ruffié, "Fever and infectious complications in patient with lung cancer [in French]," *Revue de Pneumologie Clinique* 64, no. 2 (2008): 99–103.

7. C. Visovsky and S. M. Schneider, "Cancer-related fatigue," *Online Journal of Issues in Nursing* 8, no. 3 (2003): 8.

8. E. B. Reitschuler-Cross and B. Arnold, "ACP Journal Club: Parenteral hydration did not improve dehydration or quality of life in advanced cancer," *Annals of Internal Medicine* 158, no. 6 (2013): JC10.

9. R. Krenke, J. Klimiuk, P. Korczynski, W. Kupis, M. Szolkowska, and R. Chazan, "Hemoptysis and spontaneous hemothorax in a patient with multifocal nodular lung lesions," *Chest* 140, no. 1 (2011): 245–51; G. L. Colice, "Detecting lung cancer as a cause of hemoptysis in patients with a normal chest radiograph: Bronchoscopy vs CT," *Chest* 111, no. 4 (1997): 877–84.

10. P. Katsinelos, G. Paroutoglou, A. Beltsis, I. Pilpilidis, B. Papaziogas, K. Mimidis, and P. Tsolkas, "Hematemesis as a presenting symptom of lung cancer with synchronous metastases to the esophagus and stomach: A case report," *Romanian Journal of Gastroenterology* 13, no. 3 (2004): 251–53.

11. A. Winter, J. MacAdams, and S. Chevalier, "Normal protein anabolic response to hyperaminoacidemia in insulin-resistant patients with lung cancer cachexia," *Clinical Nutrition* 31, no. 5 (2012):765–73; Y. Shimizu, N. Nagaya, T. Isobe, M. Imazu, H. Okumura, H. Hosoda, M. Kojima, K. Kangawa, and N. Kohno, "Increased plasma ghrelin level in lung cancer cachexia," *Clinical Cancer Research* 9, no. 2 (2003): 774–78; H. R. Levine, E. Tingle, B. Carter, and D. Dockery, "Synovial metastasis from lung cancer," *Proceedings (Baylor University Medical Center)* 26, no. 1 (2013): 25–27; F. Cantini, L. Niccoli, C. Nannini, D. Chindamo, M. Bertoni, E. Cassarà, and C. Salvarani, "Isolated knee monoarthritis heralding resectable non-small-cell lung cancer: A paraneoplastic syndrome not previously described," *Annals of the Rheumatic Diseases* 66, no. 12 (2007): 1672–674.

12. H. M. Bae, S. H. Lee, T. M. Kim, D. W. Kim, S. C. Yang, H. G. Wu, Y. W. Kim, and D. S. Heo, "Prognostic factors for non-small cell lung cancer with bone metastasis at the time of diagnosis," *Lung Cancer* 77, no. 3 (2012): 572–77; H. Sugiura, K. Yamada, T. Sugiura, T. Hida, and T. Mitsudomi, "Predictors of survival in patients with bone metastasis of lung cancer," *Clinical Orthopaedics and Related Research* 466, no. 3 (2008): 729–36; N. Katakami, "Lung cancer with bone metastasis [in Japanese]," *Gan To Kagaku Ryoho* 33, no. 8 (2006): 1049–53.

13. J. Tajti, K. Sas, D. Szok, E. Vörös, and L. Vécsei, "Clusterlike headache as a first sign of brain metastases of lung cancer," *Headache* 36, no. 4 (1996): 259–60; E. Sarlani, A. H. Schwartz, J. D. Greenspan, and E. G. Grace, "Facial pain as first manifestation of lung cancer: A case of lung cancer-related cluster headache and a review of the literature," *Journal of Orofacial Pain* 17, no. 3 (2003): 262–67.

14. N. Tatsumi, S. Fumiyuki, H. Eisaku, H. Akihiro, F. Yasushi, and F. Satoshi, "A study of TS-1 in patients with recurrent head and neck cancer—Regard as lung metastasis," *Head and Neck Cancer* 30, no. 1 (2004): 111–.15; I. Yoichi, K. Akira, F. Madoka, and T. Mamoru, "Case of lung cancer which appeared after the first treatment for head and neck cancer: The efficacy of chest x-ray examination in search of lung metastasis," *Journal of the Japan Broncho-Esophagological Society* 53, no. 3 (2002): 264–70.

15. A. J. Hoffman, B. A. Given, A. von Eye, A. G. Gift, and C. W. Given, "Relationships among pain, fatigue, insomnia, and gender in persons with lung cancer," *Oncology Nursing Forum* 34, no. 4 (2007): 785–92; S. L. Kozachik and K. Bandeen-Roche, "Predictors of patterns of pain, fatigue, and insomnia during the first year after a cancer diagnosis in the elderly," *Cancer Nursing* 31, no. 5 (2008): 334–44.

16. Hoffman et al., "Relationships among pain, fatigue, insomnia, and gender in persons with lung cancer"; Kozachik and Bandeen-Roche, "Predictors of patterns of pain, fatigue, and insomnia during the first year after a cancer diagnosis in the elderly."

17. R. Amin, "Dysphagia in lung cancer," *Journal of the Royal Society of Medicine* 95, no. 1 (2002): 55–56; D. R. Camidge, "The causes of dysphagia in carcinoma of the lung," *Journal of the Royal Society of Medicine* 94, no. 11 (2001): 567–72.

18. I. Henoch, B. Bergman, and E. Danielson, "Dyspnea experience and management strategies in patients with lung cancer," *Psychooncology* 17, no. 7 (2008): 709–15; D. Xue and A. P. Abernethy, "Management of dyspnea in advanced lung cancer: recent data and emerging concepts," *Current Opinion in Supportive and Palliative Care* 4, no. 2 (2010): 85–91; C. F. Lee, P. N. Carding, and M. Fletcher, "The nature and severity of voice disorders in lung cancer patients," *Logopedics Phoniatrics Vocology* 33, no. 2 (2008): 93–103.

7. LUNG CANCER SCREENING AND DIAGNOSTICS

1. D. Samson, "Evidence for management of small cell lung cancer," *Chest* 132 (2007): 314S–323S.

2. J. E. Dowell, "Small cell lung cancer: are we making progress?," *American Journal of the Medical Sciences* 339 (2010): 68–76.

3. A. A. Ponomareva, E. I. Rykova , N. V. Cherdyntseva, E. L. Choĭnzonov, P. P. Laktionov, and V. V. Vlasov, "Molecular-genetic markers in lung cancer diagnostics [in Russian]," *Molecular Biology (Mosk)* 45, no. 2 (2011): 203–17; N. Lindeman, "Molecular diagnostics of lung cancers at the Brigham and Women's Hospital and Dana-Farber Cancer Institute: Technology in rapid evolution," *Archives of Pathology and Laboratory Medicine* 136, no. 10 (2012): 1198–200.

4. "Introduction to cancer detection and diagnosis," Winship Cancer Institute, October 24, 2011, www.cancerquest.org/cancer-detection-diagnosis.html, accessed March 16, 2013.

5. "Lung cancer—Small cell," National Center for Biotechnology Information, August 24, 2011, www.ncbi.nlm.nih.gov, accessed March 16, 2013.

6. "Lung cancer—Small cell."

7. World Health Organization, "Early detection of cancer," www.who.int/cancer/detection/en, accessed March 16, 2013.

8. Georg Klemperer, *The Elements of Clinical Diagnosis* (London: Macmillan, 1904), chap. 1.

9. Scottish Intercollegiate Guidelines Network, *Management of Patients with Lung Cancer* (Edinburgh: Scottish Intercollegiate Guidelines Network, 2005), 3.

10. Scottish Intercollegiate Guidelines Network, *Management of Patients with Lung Cancer*, 3.

11. "What is screening?," National Cancer Institute, November 2, 2011, www.cancer.gov, accessed March 23, 2013.

12. "What is screening?"

13. Edmund S. Cibas and Barbara S. Ducatman, *Cytology: Diagnostic Principles and Clinical Correlate* (Philadelphia: Elsevier Health Sciences, 2009), 67.

14. Cibas and Ducatman, *Cytology*, 67.

15. Cibas and Ducatman, *Cytology*, 67.

16. "What is a macrophage?," AZoNetwork, www.news-medical.net/health/What-is-a-Macrophage.aspx, accessed March 23, 2013.

17. Cibas and Ducatman, *Cytology*, 67.

18. Cibas and Ducatman, *Cytology*, 67.

19. David Zieve and David R. Eltz, "Venipuncture," September 31, 2011, www.nlm.nih.gov/medlineplus, accessed March 22, 2013.

20. "Blood test accurately detects early stages of lung, breast cancer in humans," Science Daily, September 26, 2012, www.sciencedaily.com, accessed March 23, 2013.

21. "Blood test accurately detects early stages of lung, breast cancer in humans."

22. "Blood test accurately detects early stages of lung, breast cancer in humans."

23. "Blood test accurately detects early stages of lung, breast cancer in humans."

24. Kemp H. Kernstine, *Lung Cancer: A Multidisciplinary Approach to Diagnosis and Management* (New York: Demos Medical Publishing, 2011), 61–62.

25. Kernstine, *Lung Cancer*.

26. "Lung cancer: Detection and diagnosis," Winship Cancer Institute, October 24, 2011, www.cancerquest.org/cancer-detection-diagnosis.html, accessed March 16, 2013.

27. Peter Hertrich, *Practical Radiography* (Hoboken, NJ: Wiley, 2005), 34.

28. Alfred P. Fishman, Jack A. Elias, Jay A. Fishman, Michael A. Grippi, Larry R. Kaiser, and Robert M. Senior, *Fishman's Manual of Pulmonary Diseases and Disorders* (New York: McGraw-Hill, 2002), 486.

29. Healthwise Staff, "Computed tomography (CT) scan of the body," WebMD, June 13, 2011, http://www.webmd.com, accessed May 16, 2013.

30. Healthwise Staff, "Computed tomography (CT) scan of the body"

31. Kernstine, *Lung Cancer*, 55.

32. Kernstine, *Lung Cancer*, 55.

33. Kernstine, *Lung Cancer*, 55.

34. National Cancer Institute, "Lung cancer trial results show mortality benefit with low-dose CT," April 11, 2010, www.cancer.gov, accessed March 24, 2013.

35. National Cancer Institute, "Lung cancer trial results show mortality benefit with low-dose CT."

36. National Cancer Institute, "Lung cancer trial results show mortality benefit with low-dose CT."

37. "MRI scan," Cancer Research UK, www.cancerresearchuk.org, accessed March 21, 2013.

38. "MRI scan."

39. "MRI scan."

40. "MRI scan."

41. "MRI scan."

42. "What is ultrasound?," AZoNetwork, www.news-medical.net/health/What-is-an-Ultrasound.aspx, accessed March 22, 2013.

43. "What is ultrasound?"

44. "What is ultrasound?"

45. Tim Kenny, "Endobronchial ultrasound-guided transbronchial needle aspiration," July 27, 2010, www.patient.co.uk, accessed March 22, 2013.

46. Tim Kenny, "Endobronchial ultrasound-guided transbronchial needle aspiration."

47. Suzanne C. Smeltzer, *Brunner and Suddarth Textbook of Medical Surgical Nursing* (Philadelphia: Lippincott Williams and Wilkins, 2010), 575.

48. Johns Hopkins Hospital, "Lung biopsy," John Hopkins Medicine, www.hopkinsmedicine.org, accessed March 16, 2013.

49. "How reliable is the diagnosis of lung cancer using small biopsy specimens?," Department of Pathology, Western General Hospital, Edinburgh, 1993, www.ncbi.nlm.nih.gov, accessed March 16, 2013.

50. "How reliable is the diagnosis of lung cancer using small biopsy specimens?"

51. "How reliable is the diagnosis of lung cancer using small biopsy specimens?"

52. Johns Hopkins Hospital, "Lung biopsy."

53. Johns Hopkins Hospital, "Lung biopsy."

54. Johns Hopkins Hospital, "Lung biopsy."

55. Johns Hopkins Hospital, "Lung biopsy."

56. Johns Hopkins Hospital, "Lung biopsy."

57. Johns Hopkins Hospital, "Lung biopsy."

58. Johns Hopkins Hospital, "Lung biopsy."

59. Johns Hopkins Hospital, "Lung biopsy."

60. Johns Hopkins Hospital, "Lung biopsy."

61. R. S. Fontana, "The Mayo Lung Project: A perspective," *Cancer* 89 (2000): 2352–55; L. L. Humphrey, S. Teutsch, and M. Johnson, "Lung cancer screening with sputum cytologic examination, chest radiography, and computed tomography: an update for the U.S.," *Annals of Internal Medicine* 140, no. 9 (2004): 740–53.

62. C. I. Henschke, D. I. McCauley, D. F. Yankelevitz, D. P. Naidich, G. McGuinness, O. S. Miettinen, D. M. Libby, M. W. Pasmantier, J. Koizumi, N. K. Altorki, and J. P. Smith, "Early Lung Cancer Action Project: Overall design and findings from baseline screening," *Lancet* 354 (1999): 99–105; C. I. Henschke, D. P. Naidich, D. F. Yankelevitz, G. McGuinness, D. I. McCauley, J. P. Smith, D. Libby, M. Pasmantier, M. Vazquez, J. Koizumi, D. Flieder, N. Altorki, and O. S. Miettinen, "Early Lung Cancer Action Project: Initial findings on repeated screenings," *Cancer* 92 (2001): 153–59; M. Kaneko, M. Kusumoto, and T. Kobayashi, "CT screening for lung cancer in Japan," *Cancer* 89 (2000): 2485–88; J. L. Mulshine, "Screening for lung cancer: In pursuit of the pre-metastatic disease," *Nature Reviews Cancer* 3 (2003): 65–73.

63. A. Jemal, R. C. Tiwari, T. Murray, A. Ghafoor, A. Samuels, E. Ward, E. J. Feuer, and M. J. Thun, "Cancer statistics, 2004," *CA: A Cancer Journal for Clinicians* 54 (2004): 8–29 ; Henschke et al., "Early Lung Cancer Action Project"; T. Sobue, N. Moriyama, M. Kaneko, M. Kusumoto, T. Kobayashi, R. Tsuchiya, R. Kakinuma, H. Ohmatsu, K. Naqai,H. Nishiyama, E. Matsui, and K. Equchi, "Screening for lung cancer with low-dose helical computed tomography: Anti-lung cancer association project," *Journal of Clinical Oncology* 20 (2002): 911–20; T. Nawa, T. Nakagawa, S. Kusano, Y. Kawasaki, Y. Sugawara, and H. Nakata, "Lung cancer screening using low-dose spiral CT: Results of baseline and 1-year follow-up studies," *Chest* 122 (2002): 15–20; S. J. Swensen, J. R. Jett, T. E. Hartman, D. E. Midthun, J. A. Sloan, A. M. Sykes, G. L. Aughenbaugh, and M. A. Clemans, "Lung cancer screening with CT: Mayo Clinic experience," *Radiology* 226 (2003): 756–61; U. Pastorino, M. Bellomi, and C. Landoni, "Early lung-cancer detection with spiral CT and positron emission tomography in heavy smokers: 2-year results," *Lancet* 362 (2003): 593–97.

64. S. J. Swensen, J. R. Jett, D. E. Midthun, and T. E. Hartman, "Computer tomographic screening for lung cancer: Home run or foul ball?," *Mayo Clinic Proceedings* 78 (2003): 1187–88.

65. Pastorino et al., "Early lung-cancer detection with spiral CT and positron emission tomography in heavy smokers."

66. D. L. Sackett and J. E. Wennberg, "Choosing the best research design for each question," *British Medical Journal* 315 (1997): 1636; J. Concato, N. Shah, and R. I. Horwitz, "Randomized, controlled trials, observational studies, and the hierarchy of research designs," *New England Journal of Medicine* 342 (2000): 1887–92.

67. C. I. Henschke, D. F. Yankelevitz, J. P. Smith, D. Libby, M. Pasmantier, D. McCauley, G. McGuinness, D. P. Naidich, A. Farooqi, M. Vasquez, and O. S. Miettinen, "CT screening for lung cancer: Assessing a regimen's diagnostic performance," *Clinical Imaging* 28 (2004): 317–21; W. J. Kostis, A. P. Reeves, D. F. Yankelevitz, and C. I. Henschke, "Three-dimensional segmentation and growth-rate estimation of small pulmonary nodules in helical CT images," *Institute of Electrical and Electronics Engineers Transaction on Medical Imaging* 22 (2003): 1259–74.

68. R. A. Smith, V. Cokkinides, and H. J. Eyre, "American Cancer Society guidelines for the early detection of cancer 2004," *CA: A Cancer Journal for Clinicians* 54 (2004): 41–52.

8. OUTPATIENT AND INPATIENT EXPERIENCES

1.   "About internal medicine," American College of Physicians, www.acponline.org, accessed May 2, 2013.

2.   "Pulmonology," American College of Physicians, accessed May 2, 2013, www.acponline.org/patients_families/about_internal_medicine/subspecialties/pulmonology, accessed May 2, 2013.

3.   Gregory Cosby, reviewer, "Lung cancer doctors," July 29, 2010, www.healthline.com/health/doctors-for-lung-cancer, accessed May 2, 2013.

4.   Michéle Aubin, Rénald Bergeron, Lise Fillion, Eveline Hudon, Francois Lehmann, Yvan Ledue, Diane Morin, Daniel Reinharz, René Verreault, and Lucie Vézina, "Family physician involvement in cancer care follow-up: The experience of a cohort of patients with lung cancer," *Annals of Family Medicine* 8, no. 6 (2010): 526–32.

5.   "Medical oncology," American College of Physicians, www.acponline.org/patients_families/about_internal_medicine/subspecialties/oncology, accessed May 2, 2013.

6.   "Types of oncologists," May 2011, www.cancer.net/all-about-cancer/newly-diagnosed/find-oncologist/types-oncologists, accessed May 14, 2013.

7.   Laureano Molins, Juan J. Fibla, Jose M. Mier, and Ana Sierra, "Outpatient thoracic surgery," *Thoracic Surgery Clinics* 18, no. 3 (2008): 321–27.

8.   "Lung cancer surgery terms," Society of Thoracic Surgeons, www.sts.org/patient-information/other-resources/lung-cancer-surgery-terms#23, accessed May 14, 2013.

9.   "Stereotactic body radiosurgery lung cancer surgery alternative," Cancer Treatment Group, www.cancertreatmentgroup.com, accessed May 15, 2013.

10.   Lyenne Eldridge, "Complementary/alternative treatments for lung cancer," updated October 31, 2012, www.lungcancer.about.com/od, accessed May 15, 2013.

11.   "Questions to ask," www.lungcancer.org, accessed May 13, 2013.

12.   "After surgery for lung cancer," Cancer Research UK, www.cancerresearchuk.org, accessed May 15, 2013.

13.   Lyenne Eldridge, "Choosing a lung cancer treatment center," updated October 11, 2012, www.lungcancer.about.com, accessed May 13, 2013.

14.   Peter B. Bach, Colin B. Begg, Laura C. Cramer, Robert J. Downey, Sarah E. Gelfand, and Deborah Schrag, "The influence of hospital volume on survival after resection for lung cancer," *New England Journal of Medicine* 345, no. 3 (2001): 181–88.

9. SQUAMOUS CELL CARCINOMAS AND BRONCHIOALVEOLAR CARCINOMAS

1. Anne S. Tsao, "Lung carcinoma: Tumors of the lungs," in *Merck Manual, Professional Edition* (Whitehouse Station, NJ: Merck, Sharp and Dohme Corp., 2011).

2. Tsao, "Lung carcinoma."

3. "Non-small cell lung cancer treatment @PDQ," National Cancer Institute, www.cancer.gov/cancertopics/pdq/treatment/non-small-cell-lung/Patient/page2, accessed May 3, 2013.

4. N. Isohata, Y. Naritaka, T. Shimakawa, S. Asaka, T. Katsube, S. Konno, M. Murayama, S. Shiozawa, K. Yoshimatsu, M. Aiba, H. Ide, and K. Ogawa, "Occult lung cancer incidentally found during surgery for esophageal and gastric cancer," *Anticancer Research* 28 (2008): 1841.

5. Tsao, "Lung carcinoma."

6. Tina St. John, "Lung cancer overview," in *With Every Breath: A Lung Cancer Guidebook* (Vancouver, WA: Lung Cancer Caring Ambassadors Program, 2009), 28–29.

7. "Cancer classification," National Cancer Institute, http://training.seer.cancer.gov/disease/categories/classification.html, accessed April 25, 2013.

8. "Squamous cell lung carcinoma," College of American Pathologists, www.cap.org, accessed May 3, 2013.

9. Sharon Lane, "Rare cancer: Types," www.rare-cancer.org/types-of-cancer.php, accessed May 3, 2013.

10. Suzanne Robin, "Characteristics of squamous cell carcinoma," updated March 23, 2010, www.livestrong.com, accessed May 3, 2013.

11. Robin, "Characteristics of squamous cell carcinoma."

12. G. L. Bayle, *Recherches Sur la Phthisie Pulmonaire* (Paris: Gabon, 1810).

13. "Lung cancer incidence statistics," Cancer Research UK, www.cancerresearchuk.org, accessed April 23, 2013; Y. C. Chen, D. C. Christiani, H. J. Su, Y. M. Hsueh, T. J. Smith, L. M. Ryan, S. C. Chao, J. Y. Lee, and Y. L. Guo, "Early-life or lifetime sun exposure, sun reaction, and the risk of squamous cell carcinoma in an Asian population," *Cancer Causes and Control* 21, no. 5 (2010): 771–76.

14. Chen et al., "Early-life or lifetime sun exposure, sun reaction, and the risk of squamous cell carcinoma in an Asian population."

15. C. F. Mountain, "Revisions in the international system for staging lung cancer," *Chest* 111, no. 6 (1997): 1710–717.

16. D. R. Aberle, A. M. Adams, C. D. Berg, W. C. Black, J. D. Clapp, R. M. Fagerstrom, I. F. Gareen, C. Gatsonis, P. M. Marcus, and J. D. Sicks, "Re-

duced lung-cancer mortality with low-dose computed tomographic screening," *New England Journal of Medicine* 365, no. 5 (2011): 395–409.

17. M. Noguchi, A. Morikawa, M. Kawasaki, Y. Matsuno, T. Yamada, S. Hirohashi, H. Kondo, and Y. Shimosato, "Small adenocarcinoma of the lung: Histologic characteristics and prognosis," *Cancer* 75, no. 12 (1995): 2844–52.

18. K. E. Finberg, L. V. Sequist, V. A. Joshi, A. Muzikansky, J. M. Miller, M. Han, J. Beheshti, L. R. Chirieac, E. J. Mark, and A. J. Iafrate, "Mucinous differentiation correlates with absence of EGFR mutation and presence of KRAS mutation in lung adenocarcinomas with bronchioloalveolar features," *Journal of Molecular Diagnostics* 9, no. 3 (2007): 320–26.

19. O. S. Breathnach, D. J. Kwiatkowski, D. M. Finkelstein, J. Godleski, D. J. Sugarbaker, B. E. Johnson, and S. Mentzer, "Bronchioloalveolar carcinoma of the lung: Recurrences and survival in patients with stage I disease," *Journal of Thoracic and Cardiovascular Surgery* 121, no. 1 (2001): 42–47; Finberg et al., "Mucinous differentiation correlates with absence of EGFR mutation and presence of KRAS mutation in lung adenocarcinomas with bronchioloalveolar features."

20. L. Zhong, M. S. Goldberg, Y. T. Gao, and F. Jin, "Lung cancer and indoor air pollution arising from Chinese-style cooking among nonsmoking women living in Shanghai, China," *Epidemiology* 10, no. 5 (1999): 488–94; X. R. Wang, Y. L. Chiu, H. Qiu, J. S. Au, and I. T. Yu, "The roles of smoking and cooking emissions in lung cancer risk among Chinese women in Hong Kong," *Annals of Oncology* 20, no. 4 (2009): 746–51.

21. J. E. Barkley and M. R. Green, "Bronchioloalveolar carcinoma," *Journal of Clinical Oncology* 14, no. 8 (1996): 2377–86; K. H. Albertine, R. M. Steiner, D. M. Radack, D. M. Golding, D. Peterson, H. E. Cohn, and J. L. Farber, "Analysis of cell type and radiographic presentation as predictors of the clinical course of patients with bronchioalveolar cell carcinoma," *Chest* 113, no. 4 (1998): 997–1006.

22. G. A. Otterson, M. A. Villalona-Calero, S. Sharma, M. G. Kris, A. Imondi, M. Gerber, D. A. White, M. J. Ratain, J. H. Schiller, A. Sandler, M. Kraut, S. Mani, and J. R. Murren, "Phase I study of inhaled doxorubicin for patients with metastatic tumors to the lungs," *Clinical Cancer Research* 13, no. 4 (2007): 1246–52; H. L. West, J. J. Crowley, R. B. Vance, W. A. Franklin, R. B. Livingston, S. R. Dakhil, J. K. Giguere, S. E. Rivkin, M. Kraut, K. Chansky, and D. R. Gandara, "Advanced bronchioloalveolar carcinoma: A phase II trial of paclitaxel by 96-hour infusion (SWOG 9714): A Southwest Oncology Group study," *Annals of Oncology* 16, no. 7 (2005): 1076–80.

23. International Agency for Research on Cancer, *Pathology and Genetics of Tumors of the Lung, Pleura, Thymus and Heart (IARC WHO Classification of Tumors)* (New York: World Health Organization, 2004).

24.   International Agency for Research on Cancer, *Pathology and Genetics of Tumors of the Lung, Pleura, Thymus and Heart (IARC WHO Classification of Tumors)*.

25.   International Agency for Research on Cancer, *Pathology and Genetics of Tumors of the Lung, Pleura, Thymus and Heart (IARC WHO Classification of Tumors)*.

10. UNDIFFERENTIATED CARCINOMAS AND ADENOCARCINOMAS OF THE LUNG

1.   Alfred E. Chang, Daniel F. Hayes, Harvey I. Pass, Richard M. Stone, Patricia A. Ganz, Timothy J. Kinsella, Joan H. Schiller, and Victor J. Strecher, *Oncology: An Evidence-Based Approach* (New York: Springer, 2006), 558.

2.   "What is non-small cell lung cancer?," American Cancer Society, last updated January 17, 2013, www.cancer.org, accessed March 19, 2013.

3.   Chang et al., *Oncology*, 558.

4.   Lynne Eldridge, "Large cell carcinoma of the lungs," last updated September 12, 2012, http://lungcancer.about.com, accessed March 19, 2013.

5.   Eldridge, "Large cell carcinoma of the lungs."

6.   Dani S. Zander, Helmut H. Popper, Jaishree Jagirdar, Abida K. Haque, Philip T. Cagle, and Roberto Barrios, *Molecular Pathology of Lung Diseases* (New York: Springer, 2008).

7.   René Hagea, Kees Seldenrijkb, Peter de Bruinb, Henry van Swieten, and Jules van den Boscha, "Pulmonary large-cell neuroendocrine carcinoma (LCNEC)," *European Journal Cardio-Thoracic Surgery* 23 (2003): 457–60.

8.   Zander et al., *Molecular Pathology of Lung Diseases*.

9.   Zander et al., *Molecular Pathology of Lung Diseases*.

10.   Zander et al., *Molecular Pathology of Lung Diseases*.

11.   Zander et al., *Molecular Pathology of Lung Diseases*.

12.   Zander et al., *Molecular Pathology of Lung Diseases*.

13.   Eldridge, "Large cell carcinoma of the lungs."

14.   Jun-ichi Nitadori, Genichiro Ishii, Koji Tsuta, Tomoyuki Yokose, Yukinori Murata, Tetsuro Kodama, Kanji Nagai, Harubumi Kato, and Atsushi Ochiai, "Immunohistochemical differential diagnosis between large cell neuroendocrine carcinoma and small cell carcinoma by tissue microarray analysis with a large antibody panel," *American Journal of Clinical Pathology* 125 (2006): 682–92.

15.   Nitadori et al. "Immunohistochemical differential diagnosis between large cell neuroendocrine carcinoma and small cell carcinoma by tissue microarray analysis with a large antibody panel."

16. Nitadori et al., "Immunohistochemical differential diagnosis between large cell neuroendocrine carcinoma and small cell carcinoma by tissue microarray analysis with a large antibody panel."

17. Zander et al., *Molecular Pathology of Lung Diseases.*
18. Zander et al., *Molecular Pathology of Lung Diseases.*
19. "What is non-small cell lung cancer?"
20. "Lung adenocarcinoma," College of American Pathologists, last updated April 13, 2011, www.cap.org, accessed March 21, 2013.
21. Zander et al., *Molecular Pathology of Lung Diseases.*
22. Zander et al., *Molecular Pathology of Lung Diseases.*
23. Zander et al., *Molecular Pathology of Lung Diseases.*
24. "Lung adenocarcinoma."
25. Eldridge, "Large cell carcinoma of the lungs."
26. Giuseppe Pelosi, "The new taxonomy of lung adenocarcinoma stemming from a multidisciplinary integrated approach: Novel pathology concepts and perspectives," *Journal of Thoracic Oncology* 6 (2011): 241–43.
27. "Lung adenocarcinoma."
28. "Lung adenocarcinoma."
29. Zander et al., *Molecular Pathology of Lung Diseases.*
30. Zander et al., *Molecular Pathology of Lung Diseases.*
31. Bryan L. Betz, Catherine A. Dixon, Helmut C. Weigelin, Stewart M. Knoepp, and Michael H. Roh, "The use of stained, cytologic direct smears for ALK gene rearrangement analysis of lung adenocarcinoma," *Cancer Cytopathology* 121 (2013): 10.
32. Zander et al., *Molecular Pathology of Lung Diseases.*
33. Zander et al., *Molecular Pathology of Lung Diseases.*
34. Zander et al., *Molecular Pathology of Lung Diseases.*

11. OAT CELL CARCINOMAS AND COMBINED SMALL CELL CARCINOMAS

1. D. S. Ettinger, L. Goldman, and D. Ausiello, *Lung Cancer and Other Pulmonary Neoplasms* (Philadelphia: Cecil Medicine, 2011), chap. 197.
2. Ettinger et al., *Lung Cancer and Other Pulmonary Neoplasms.*
3. W. A. Fry, H. R. Menck, and D. P. Winchester, *The National Cancer Data Base Report on Lung Cancer* (Chicago: American College of Surgeons, 1996), 1947–55.
4. L. M. Krug, M. G. Kris, K. Rosenzweig, W. D. Travis, V. T. DeVita Jr., S. Hellman, and A. A. Rosenberg, "Cancer of the lung," in *Cancer: Principles*

and Practice of Oncology, 8th ed. (Philadelphia: Lippincott Williams & Wilkins, 2008), 66.

5. Krug et al., "Cancer of the lung," 66.

6. D. F. Shore and M. Paneth, "Survival after resection of small cell carcinoma of the bronchus," *Thorax* 35, no. 11 (1980): 819–22; J. Deslauriers, "Current surgical treatment of nonsmall cell lung cancer 2001," *European Respiratory Journal* 35 (Suppl. 2002): 61s–70s; V. Levison, "Pre-operative radiotherapy and surgery in the treatment of oat cell carcinoma of the bronchus," *Clinical Radiology* 31, no. 3 (1980): 345–48.

7. Shore and Paneth, "Survival after resection of small cell carcinoma of the bronchus"; Deslauriers, "Current surgical treatment of nonsmall cell lung cancer 2001"; Levison, "Pre-operative radiotherapy and surgery in the treatment of oat cell carcinoma of the bronchus."

8. N. Ismaili, "A rare bladder cancer—Small cell carcinoma: Review and update," *Orphanet Journal of Rare Diseases* 6 (2011): 75.

9. C. F. Mountain, "Clinical biology of small cell carcinoma: Relationship to surgical therapy," *Seminars in Oncology* 5, no. 3 (1978): 272–79.

10. Apar Kishor Ganti, Anne Kessinger, and Weining Zhen, "Limited-stage small cell lung cancer: Therapeutic options," *Oncology* 21, no. 3 (2007): 303–12.

11. Anne S. Tsao, "Lung carcinoma: Tumors of the lungs," Merck Manual Professional Edition, www.merckmanuals.com, accessed April 25, 2013.

12. William D. Travis, Elisabeth Brambilla, and H. Konrad Muller-Hermelink, *Pathology and Genetics of Tumors of the Lung, Pleura, Thymus and Heart: World Health Organization Classification of Tumors* (Lyon: IARC Press, 2004), 242.

13. J. E. Dowell, "Small cell lung cancer: Are we making progress?," *American Journal of the Medical Sciences* 339 (2010): 68–76.

14. R. Stupp, C. Monnerat, A. T. Turrisi, M. C. Perry, and S. Leyvraz, "Small cell lung cancer: State of the art and future perspectives," *Lung Cancer* 45 (2004): 105–17.

15. Stupp et al., "Small cell lung cancer."

16. Shore and Paneth, "Survival after resection of small cell carcinoma of the bronchus"; Deslauriers, "Current surgical treatment of nonsmall cell lung cancer 2001"; Levison, "Pre-operative radiotherapy and surgery in the treatment of oat cell carcinoma of the bronchus."

17. C. W. Deal and J. R. Belcher, "A comparison between the influence of oat cell and undifferentiated bronchial carcinoma on the prognosis after resection," *British Journal of Diseases of the Chest* 57 (1963): 182–86.

18. American Cancer Society, *Cancer Facts and Figures 2009* (Atlanta: American Cancer Society, 2009).

19. G. R. Simon and A. Turrisi, "Management of small cell lung cancer: ACCP evidence-based clinical practice guidelines (2nd edition)," *Chest* 132 (2007): 324S–339S.

20. P. A. Jänne, B. Freidlin, and S. Saxman, "Twenty-five years of clinical research for patients with limited-stage small cell lung carcinoma in North America," *Cancer* 95 (2002): 1528–38.

12. OTHER MANIFESTATIONS OF LUNG CANCER

1. "Lung disease," American Lung Association, www.lung.org/lung-disease, accessed March 14, 2013.

2. "Cancer facts and figures 2009," American Cancer Society, ww2.cancer.org/downloads/STT/500809web.pdf, accessed June 8, 2013.

3. Carol Mattson Porth and Glenn Matfin, *Essentials of Pathophysiology* (Philadelphia: Lippincott Williams and Wilkins, 2010), 665–68.

4. Suzanne C. Smeltzer, *Brunner and Suddarth Textbook of Medical Surgical Nursing* (Philadelphia: Lippincott Williams and Wilkins, 2010), 574.

5. M. Salsali and E. E. Cliffton, "Superior vena caval obstruction in carcinoma of lung," *New York State Journal of Medicine* 69, no. 22 (1969): 2875–80.

6. Salsali and Cliffton, "Superior vena caval obstruction in carcinoma of lung."

7. M. Noda, T. Seike, K. Fujita, Y. Yamakawa, M. Kido, and H. Iguchi, "Role of immune cells in brain metastasis of lung cancer cells and neuron tumor cell interaction," *Russian Journal of Physiology* 95, no. 12 (2009): 1386–96.

8. R. Perez-Soler, P. McLaughlin, W. S. Velasquez , F. B. Hagemeister, J. Zornoza, J. T. Manning, L. M. Fuller, and F. Cabanillas, "Clinical features and results of management of superior vena cava syndrome secondary to lymphoma," *Journal of Clinical Oncology* 2, no. 4 (1984): 260–66.

9. D. C. Dugdale, K. J. Ritter, and D. E. Wilhyde, "Lung abscess causing Horner's syndrome," *Western Journal of Medicine* 153, no. 2 (1990): 196–97.

10. D. L. Reede, E. Garcon, W. R. Smoker, and R. Kardon, "Horner's syndrome: Clinical and radiographic evaluation," *Neuroimaging Clinics of North America* 18, no. 2 (2008): 369–85.

11. Haralabos Parissis and Vincent Young, "Treatment of pancoast tumors from the surgeons prospective: Re-appraisal of the anterior-manubrial sternal approach," *Journal of Cardiothoracic Surgery* 5 (2010): 102; Christopher Bardorf, "Horner syndrome," Medscape Reference, http://emedicine.medscape.com, accessed June 14, 2013.

12. Dugdale et al., "Lung abscess causing Horner's syndrome."

13. Allan Bruckheim, "How a drooping eye can be linked to lung cancer," *Chicago Tribune*, March 18, 1991, 5; Reede et al., "Horner's syndrome: clinical and radiographic evaluation."

14. U.S. Cancer Statistics Working Group, *United States Cancer Statistics: 1999–2009 Incidence and Mortality Web-Based Report* (Atlanta: U.S. Department of Health and Human Services Centers for Disease Control and Prevention and National Cancer Institute, 2013).

15. Dong Peng, Deng Kaihong, and Xiao Jiahe, "Study of relation between MRI findings of supratentorial metastasis of lung cancer and blood distribution," *West China Medical Journal* 18, no. 1 (2003): 6–8; Gao Xulan, Wu Shan, and Zhong Yujie, "The interstitial blood vessels of lung cancer and metastasis," *Chinese Journal of Clinical and Experimental Pathology* 3 (1994).

16. Suzanne C. Smeltzer, *Brunner and Suddarth's Textbook of Medical Surgical Nursing*, 2009–11.

17. H. Al-Husaini, P. Wheatley-Price, M. Clemons, and F. Shepherd, "Prevention and management of bone metastases in lung cancer: A review," *Journal of Thoracic Oncology* 4, no. 2 (2009): 251–59.

18. Al-Husaini et al., "Prevention and management of bone metastases in lung cancer."

19. Al-Husaini et al., "Prevention and management of bone metastases in lung cancer."

20. Smeltzer, *Brunner and Suddarth's Textbook of Medical Surgical Nursing*, 1831–40.

21. A. L. Quan, G. M. Videtic, and J. H. Suh, "Brain metastases in small cell lung cancer," CancerNetwork: *Home Journal of Oncology* 18, no. 8 (2004): 1; Boone Goodgame and Ramswamy Govindan, "Lung cancer-related brain metastases: Further considerations," CancerNetwork: *Home Journal of Oncology* 22, no. 2 (2008): 1.

22. Goodgame and Govindan, "Lung cancer-related brain metastases"; M. Noda, T. Seike, K. Fujita, Y. Yamakawa, M. Kido, and H. Iguchi, "Role of immune cells in brain metastasis of lung cancer cells and neuron tumor cell interaction," *Neuroscience and Behavioral Physiology* 41, no. 3 (2011): 243–51; J. A. Shields, N. Perez, C. L. Shields, S. Foxman, and B. Foxman, "Simultaneous choroidal and brain metastasis as initial manifestations of lung cancer," *Ophthalmic Surgery and Lasers* 33, no. 4 (2002): 323–25.

23. Goodgame and Govindan, "Lung cancer related brain metastases"; Noda et al., "Role of immune cells in brain metastasis of lung cancer cells and neuron tumor cell interaction"; Shields et al., "Simultaneous choroidal and brain metastasis as initial manifestations of lung cancer."

24. Smeltzer, *Brunner and Suddarth's Textbook of Medical Surgical Nursing*, 1275–79.

25. Charisios Karanikiotis, Apostolos Tentes, Sotirios Marakidis, and Konstantinos Vafiadis, "Large bilateral adrenal metastases in non-small cell lung cancer," *World Journal of Oncology* 2 (2004): 37.

26. Jeffrey Goh, "Imaging in adrenal metastases," Medscape Reference, http://emedicine.medscape.com, accessed June 19, 2013; Richard Holy, Marc Piroth, Michael Pinkawa, and Michael J. Eble, "Stereotactic body radiation therapy (SBRT) for treatment of adrenal gland metastases from non-small cell lung cancer," *Strahlentherapie und Onkologie* 187, no. 4 (2011): 245–51; D. Uden, E. Ullmann, and M. Reijnen, "Adrenalectomy for isolated adrenal metastasis after gamma knife surgery for an intracerebral metastasis of non-small-cell lung carcinoma," *Journal of Cancer Research and Therapeutics* 7, no. 1 (2011): 75–77.

27. K. Kagohashi, H. Satoh, I. Hiroaki, Hiroichi, M. Ohtsuka, and K. Sekizawa, "Liver metastasis at the time of initial diagnosis of lung cancer," *Medical Oncology* 20, no. 1 (2003): 25-28.

28. Kagohashi et al., "Liver metastasis at the time of initial diagnosis of lung cancer."

13. INITIAL APPROACHES TO LUNG CANCER

1. "Lung cancer—Small cell," National Center for Biotechnology Information, August 24, 2011, www.ncbi.nlm.nih.gov, accessed May 16, 2013.

2. Alfred P. Fishman, Jack A. Elias, Jay A. Fishman, Michael A. Grippi, Larry R. Kaiser, and Robert M. Senior, *Fishman's Manual of Pulmonary Diseases and Disorders* (New York: McGraw-Hill, 2002), 486.

3. "Lung cancer—Small cell."

4. "Lung cancer—Small cell."

5. Amanda Chan, "The 10 deadliest cancers and why there's no cure," My Health News Daily, September 10, 2010, www.myhealthnewsdaily.com/139-the-10-deadliest-cancers-and-why-theres-no-cure-.html, accessed May 16, 2013.

6. "Lung cancer—Small cell."

7. "Lung cancer—Small cell."

8. Georg Klemperer, *The Elements of Clinical Diagnosis* (London: Macmillan, 1904), chap. 1.

9. "Longitudinal study of multiple symptoms in advanced lung cancer," MD Anderson Cancer Center, www.clinicaltrials.gov/ct2/show/NCT00422500, accessed June 12, 2013.

10. National Center for Biotechnology Information, "Cancer," *PubMed Health*, September 3, 2012, www.ncbi.nlm.nih.gov/pubmedhealth/ PMH0002267, accessed May 25, 2013.

11. National Center for Biotechnology Information, "Cancer."

12. Mark Marinella, *Handbook of Cancer Emergencies* (Burlington, MA: Jones & Bartlett Learning, 2010), 8.

13. Marinella, *Handbook of Cancer Emergencies*, 8.

14. NATURAL AND NONPHARMACOLOGICAL LUNG CANCER APPROACHES

1. "Non-pharmacological," http://medical-dictionary.thefreedictionary. com/nonpharmacological, accessed April 13, 2013.

2. "Complementary and alternative medicine," National Cancer Institute, www.cancer.gov/cancertopics/cam, accessed April 14, 2013.

3. Edzard Ernst, "Patient information: Complementary and alternative medicine treatments (CAM) for cancer (beyond the basics)," www.uptodate. com/contents/complementary-and-alternative-medicine-treatments-cam-for-cancer-beyond-the-basics, accessed May 14 2013.

4. "CAM basics: What is complementary and alternative medicine?," National Center for Complementary and Alternative Medicine, http:// nccam.nih.gov/health/whatiscam, accessed May 12, 2013.

5. Barrie R. Cassileth, Gary E. Deng, Jorge E. Gomez, Peter A. S. Johnstone, Nagi Kumar, and Andrew J. Vickers, "Complementary therapies and integrative oncology in lung cancer: ACCP evidence-based clinical practice guidelines (2nd edition)," *Chest* 132, no. 3 (Suppl. 2007): 340S–354S.

6. "Complementary and alternative medicine," www.cancer.gov/ cancertopics/cam, accessed May 12, 2013; Cassileth et al., "Complementary therapies and integrative oncology in lung cancer."

7. Ernst, "Patient information."

8. "Complementary and alternative medicine"; R. B. Davis, D. M. Eisenberg, T. J. Kaptchuck, R. C. Kessler, M. Van Rompay, E. E. Walters, and S. A. Wilkey, "Long-term trends in the use of complementary and alternative medical therapies in the United States," *Annals of Internal Medicine* 135, no. 4 (2001): 262–68.

9. Cassileth et al., "Complementary therapies and integrative oncology in lung cancer."

10. J. A. Astin, "Why patients use alternative medicine: Results of a national study," *Journal of the American Medical Association* 279, no. 19 (1998): 1548–53.

11.   H. J. Burstein, S. Gelber, E. Guadagnoli, and J. C. Weeks, "Use of alternative medicine by women with early stage breast cancer," *New England Journal of Medicine* 340, no. 22 (1999): 1733–39; T. Risberg, S. Kaasa, E. Wist, and H. Melsom, "Why are cancer patients using non-proven complementary therapies? A cross-sectional multicentre study in Norway," *European Journal of Cancer* 33, no. 4 (1997): 575–80; K. J. Danielson, G. P. Lippert, and D. E. Stewart, "Unconventional cancer remedies," *Canadian Medical Association Journal* 138, no. 11 (1988): 1005–11; C. Crammer, T. Gansler, C. Kaw, and T. Smith, "A population-based study of prevalence of complementary methods use by cancer survivors: A report from the American Cancer Society's studies of cancer survivors," *Cancer* 113, no. 5 (2008): 1048–57.

12.   Cassileth et al., "Complementary therapies and integrative oncology in lung cancer."

13.   Cassileth et al., "Complementary therapies and integrative oncology in lung cancer."

14.   "Acupuncture: General information," National Cancer Institute, www.cancer.gov, accessed March 13, 2013.

15.   Cassileth et al., "Complementary therapies and integrative oncology in lung cancer."

16.   Cassileth et al., "Complementary therapies and integrative oncology in lung cancer."

17.   M. Broffman, J. M. Colford Jr., J. Gao, A. Hubbard, A. Kramer, A. Kushi, M. McCulloch, and M. van der Laan, "Lung cancer survival with herbal medicine and vitamins in a whole-systems approach: Ten-year follow-up data analyzed with marginal structural models and propensity score methods," *Integrated Cancer Therapy* 10, no. 3 (2011): 260–79.

18.   K. Boddy, E. Ernst, M. H. Pittler, and B. Wider, "The desktop guide to complementary and alternative medicine," www.uptodate.com/content/complementary-and-alternative-medicine-treatments-cam-for-cancer-beyond-the-basics, accessed April 17, 2013; "St. John's wort," Cancer Research UK, www.cancerresearchuk.org, accessed May 12, 2013.

19.   S. J. Arnott, M. M. Cody, S. M. Downer, T. A. Lister, P. McCluskey, M. L. Slevin, and P. D. Wilson, "Pursuit and practice of complementary therapies by cancer patients receiving conventional treatment," *British Medical Journal* 309, no. 6947 (1994): 86–89.

20.   Ernst, "Patient information."

21.   "Health risks," United States Environmental Protection Agency, www.epa.gov/radon/healthrisks.html, accessed April 25, 2013.

22.   "EPA map of radon zones," United States Environmental Protection Agency, www.epa.gov, accessed April 26, 2013.

23.   "EPA map of radon zones."

24. Natasja Sheriff, "Women's lung cancer deaths up in South and Midwest," Reuters, www.reuters.com, accessed April 25, 2013; "Lung cancer rates by state," Centers for Disease and Control Prevention, www.cdc.gov, accessed April 27, 2013.

25. "Rise in lung cancer deaths among southern, midwestern women in their 50s," Newsroom: The Partnership at Drugfree.org, www.drugfree.org, accessed April 25, 2013.

26. Sheriff, "Women's lung cancer deaths up in South and Midwest"; "Lung cancer rates by state."

27. Krisha McCoy, "How weather can affect your COPD," www.everydayhealth.com, accessed April 28, 2013.

28. "Cold weather effect breathing NSCLC?," Lung Cancer Survivors, www.inspire.com/groups/lung-cancer-survivors/discussion/cold-weather-effect-breathing-nsclc, accessed June 2, 2013.

29. Jane M. Martin, "COPD: Good days, bad days and weather," Health Central, www.healthcentral.com, accessed May 23, 2013; "Cold weather effect breathing NSCLC?"

30. McCoy, "How weather can affect your COPD."

31. "Cleanest cities," State of the Air 2013, www.stateoftheair.org/2013/city-rankings/cleanest-cities.html, accessed April 3, 2013.

32. "City rankings," State of the Air 2013, http://www.stateoftheair.org/2013/city-rankings, accessed April 3, 2013.

33. "Cleanest cities."

34. "City rankings."

35. "Particle pollution," State of the Air 2013, http://www.stateoftheair.org/2013/health-risks-particle.html, accessed March 25, 2013.

36. "Particulate matter," United States Environmental Protection Agency, www.epa.gov/pm/health.html, accessed April 23, 2013.

37. Douglas W. Dockery, "Health effects of particulate air pollution," *Annals of Epidemiology* 19, no. 4 (2009): 257–63.

38. "Particle pollution."

39. "Lung cancer and flying," NetDoctor, www.netdoctor.co.uk/ate/cancer/203359.html, accessed March 25, 2013.

40. "Air travel with a lung condition," British Lung Foundation, www.blf.org, accessed March 26, 2013.

41. "Travelling with cancer," Virtual Medical Centre, www.virtualmedicalcentre.com/healthandlifestyle/travelling-with-cancer/188, accessed March 27, 2013.

42. J. S. Aquinik, V. Cohen, G. Kasymjanova, D. Levi, D. Small, and V. Tagalakis, "High risk of deep vein thrombosis in patients with non-small cell

lung cancer: A cohort study of 493 patients," *Journal of Thoracic Oncology* 2, no. 8 (2007): 729–34.

43. "Deep vein thrombosis and travel," Federal Aviation Administration, www.faa.gov, accessed April 3, 2013.

44. "Air travel with a lung condition," Fit for Travel, www.fitfortravel.nhs. uk/advice/advice-for-travellers/air-travel-with-a-lung-condition.aspx, accessed April 3, 2013.

45. "Herbal medicine," Cancer Research UK, www.cancerresearchuk.org, accessed April 3, 2013.

46. Christine Gratus, Sheila M. Greenfield, Sarah Damery, Sally A. Warmington, Robert Grieve, Neil M. Steven, and Philip Routledge, "The use of herbal medicine by people with cancer: A qualitative study," *BMC Complementary and Alternative Medicine* 9 (2009): 14.

47. Ernst, "Patient information"; "Herbal Medicine"; "Herbs and supplements for lung cancer," University of Maryland Medical Center, www.umm.edu, accessed April 4, 2013; "Vitamins & supplements search," WebMD, www.webmd.com, accessed April 4, 2013.

48. "American ginseng," University of Maryland Medical Center, www.umm.edu, accessed April 5, 2013; "Ginseng (American)," Memorial Sloan-Kettering Cancer Center, www.mskcc.org/cancer-care/herb/ginseng-american, accessed April 5, 2013.

49. "Ginseng (American)."

50. "Find a vitamin or supplement," WebMD, www.webmd.com, accessed April 5, 2013.

51. "Green tea," University of Maryland Medical Center, www.umm.edu, accessed April 5, 2013.

52. "St. John's wort."

53. "St. John's wort."

54. "Quercetin," University of Maryland Medical Center, www.umm.edu, accessed April 5, 2013.

55. J. W. Choi, H. Liu, H. Song, J. H. Park, and J. W. Yun, "Plasma marker proteins associated with the progression of lung cancer in obese mice fed a high-fat diet," *Proteomics* 12, no. 12 (2012): 1999–2013.

56. Tina St. John, *With Every Breath: A Lung Cancer Guidebook* (Vancouver, WA: Lung Cancer Caring Ambassadors Program, 2005), 154–62.

57. "Cancer protective effect of fruits and vegetables may be modest at best," Science Daily, www.sciencedaily.com/releases/2010/04/100406162941.htm, accessed April 5 2013.

58. T. Norat and E. Riboli, "Epidemiologic evidence of the protective effect of fruit and vegetables on cancer risk," *American Journal of Clinical Nutrition* 78, no. 3 (Suppl. 2003): 559S–569S.

59. "Cancer protective effect of fruits and vegetables may be modest at best."

60. "Macrobiotic diet," American Cancer Society, www.cancer.org, accessed April 25, 2013.

61. Amott et al., "Pursuit and practice of complementary therapies by cancer patients receiving conventional treatment."

62. "Macrobiotic diet."

63. "Macrobiotic diet."

64. Peter Jaret, "Eating well during cancer treatment," WebMD, www.webmd.com/cancer/features/eating-treatment, accessed April 26, 2013.

65. L. C. Young, C. C. Brown, A. Schatzkin, C. M. Dresser, M. J. Slesinski, C. S. Cox, and P. R. Taylor, "Intake of vitamins E, C and A and the risk of lung cancer: The National Health and Nutrition Examination Survey I epidemiologic follow-up study," *American Journal of Epidemiology* 148 (1997): 231–43.

66. G. S. Omenn, G. E. Goodman, M. D. Thornquist, J. Balmes, M. R. Cullen, A. Glass, J. P. Keogh, E. L. Meyskens Jr., B. Valanis, J. H. Williams Jr., S. Barnhart, and S. Hammar, "Effects of a combination of beta carotene and vitamin A on lung cancer and cardiovascular disease," *New England Journal of Medicine* 334 (1996): 1150–55; Alpha Tocopherol, Beta Carotene Cancer Prevention Study Group, "The effect of vitamin E and beta carotene on the incidence of lung cancer and other cancers in male smokers," *New England Journal of Medicine* 330 (1994): 1029–35 ; C. H. Hennekens, J. E. Buring, J. E. Manson, M. Stampfer, B. Rosner, and N. R. Cook, "Lack of effect of long-term supplementation with beta carotene on the incidence of malignant neoplasms and cardiovascular disease," *New England Journal of Medicine* 18 (1996): 1145–49.

67. M. C. R. Alvanja, R. C. Brownson, and J. Benichou, "Estimating the effect of dietary fat on the risk of lung cancer in non-smoking women," *Lung Cancer* 14 (1996): S63–S74 .

68. Jeremy Barnes, "If a person's lung size cannot increase, how does exercise serve to improve lung function?," Scientific American, www.scientificamerican.com, accessed April 26, 2013.

69. I. Lee, H. Sesso, and R. S. Paffenbarger, "Physical activity and risk of lung cancer," *International Journal of Epidemiology* 28 (1999): 620–25.

70. M. A. Spruit, P. P. Janssen, S. C. Willemsen, M. M. Hochstenbag, and E. F. Wouters, "Exercise capacity before and after an 8-week multidisciplinary inpatient rehabilitation program in lung cancer patients: A pilot study," *Lung Cancer* 2, no. 52 (2006): 257–60.

71. Barnes, "If a person's lung size cannot increase, how does exercise serve to improve lung function?"

72. "Impaired glucose tolerance," www.patient.co.uk/health/impaired-glucose-tolerance, accessed April 26, 2013.

73. "Exercise for cancer patients: Fitness after treatment," WebMD, www.webmd.com, accessed April 26, 2013.

74. Iris Winston, "Researchers study benefits of exercise for lung cancer patients," www.canada.com, accessed April 26, 2013.

75. Cathleen Calkins, "Exercises for lung cancer patients," www.livestrong.com, accessed April 26, 2013.

76. Winston, "Researchers study benefits of exercise for lung cancer patients"; Calkins, "Exercises for lung cancer patients."

77. Lee W. Jones, Neil D. Eves, William E. Kraus, Anil Potti, Jeffrey Crawford, James A. Blumenthal, Bercedis L. Peterson, and Pamela S. Douglas, "The lung cancer exercise training study: A randomized trial of aerobic training, resistance training, or both in postsurgical lung cancer patients: rational and design," *BioMed Central Cancer* 10 (2010): 155.

78. Jones et al., "The lung cancer exercise training study."

79. A. H. Andersen, A. Vinthen, L. L. Poulsen, and A. Mellemgaard, "Do patients with lung cancer benefit from physical exercise?," *Acta Oncologica* 50, no. 2 (2011): 307–13.

80. Winston, "Researchers study benefits of exercise for lung cancer patients."

81. "Aerobic exercise," Cleveland Clinic, http://my.clevelandclinic.org/healthy_living/exercise/hic_aerobic_exercise.aspx, accessed April 26, 2013.

82. Calkins, "Exercises for lung cancer patients."

83. Barnes, "If a person's lung size cannot increase, how does exercise serve to improve lung function?"

84. "Resistance training," eMedicine Health, www.emedicinehealth.com/strength_training/article_em.htm, accessed April 26, 2013.

85. Lacey Meyer, "Lung cancer and exercise?," Cure, www.curetoday.com/index.cfm/fuseaction/article.show/id/2/article_id/1492, accessed April 26, 2013.

86. Laird Harrison, "High-intensity exercise best during lung cancer therapy," Medscape, www.medscape.com/viewarticle/752078, accessed April 26, 2013.

87. Harrison, "High-intensity exercise best during lung cancer therapy."

88. "Lung cancer patients: Post-surgery exercise beneficial," American Cancer Society, www.cancer.org, accessed April 26, 2013.

89. Meyer, "Lung cancer and exercise?"

90. A. Tardon, W. J. Lee, M. Delgado-Rodriguez, M. Dosemeci, D. Albanes, R. Hoover, and A. Blair, "Leisure-time physical activity and lung cancer: A meta-analysis," *Cancer Causes and Control* 16, no. 4 (2005): 389–97.

91. S. G. Wannamethee, A.G. Shaper, and M. Walker, "Physical activity and risk of cancer in middle-aged men," *British Journal of Cancer* 85, no. 9 (2001): 1311–16.

92. Penny Sinner, Aaron R. Folsom, Lisa Harnack, Lynn E. Eberly, and Kathryn H. Schmitz, "The association of physical activity with lung cancer incidence in a cohort of older women: The Iowa Women's Health Study," *Cancer Epidemiology, Biomarkers & Prevention* 15, no. 12 (2006): 2359–63; A. Kubik, P. Zatloukal, L. Tomasek, N. Pauk, L. Petruzelka, and I. Plesko, "Lung cancer risk among non-smoking women in relation to diet and physical activity," *Neoplasma* 51, no. 2 (2004): 136–43.

93. Centers for Disease Control and Prevention, "Racial/ethnic disparities and geographic differences in lung cancer incidence—38 states and the District of Columbia, 1998–2006," *Morbidity and Mortality Weekly Report* 59, no. 44 (2010): 1434–38.

94. C. Laroche, F. Wells, R. Coulden, S. Stewart, M. Goddard, E. Lowry, A. Price, and D. Gilligan, "Improving surgical resection rate in lung cancer," *Thorax* 53, no. 6 (1998): 445–49.

95. "Surgery for lung cancer," Lung Cancer Answers, www.lung-cancer.com/surgery.html, accessed April 26, 2013.

96. "Types of surgery for lung cancer," Cancer Research UK, www.cancerresearchuk.org, accessed April 26 2013; "Surgery for lung cancer."

97. "Types of surgery for lung cancer."

98. "Surgery for lung cancer"; "Types of surgery for lung cancer."

99. W. G. Langston, "Surgical resection of lung cancer," *Nursing Clinics of North America* 27, no. 3 (1992): 665–79.

100. "Cryotherapy for lung cancer," Cancer Research UK, www.cancerresearchuk.org/cancer-help/type/lung-cancer/treatment/cryotherapy-for-lung-cancer, accessed April 25, 2013.

101. "Cryotherapy," Cancer Treatment Centers of America, www.cancercenter.com, accessed April 26, 2013.

102. "Cryotherapy for lung cancer."

103. "Cryotherapy for lung cancer."

104. Lizhi Niu, Kecheng Xu, and Feng Mu, "Cryosurgery for lung cancer," *Journal of Thoracic Disease* 4, no. 4 (2012): 408–19.

105. Lizhi Niu et al., "Cryosurgery for lung cancer."

106. M. O. Maiwand and G. Asimakopoulos, "Cryosurgery for lung cancer," *Technology in Cancer Research and Treatment* 3, no. 2 (2004): 143–50.

107. "Non-small cell lung cancer treatment," National Cancer Institute, www.cancer.gov, accessed April 26, 2013.

108. "Lasers in cancer treatment," National Cancer Institute, www.cancer.gov/cancertopics/factsheet/Therapy/lasers, accessed April 26, 2013.
109. "Lasers in cancer treatment," National Cancer Institute.
110. "Lasers in cancer treatment," National Cancer Institute.
111. "Lasers in cancer treatment," American Cancer Society, www.cancer.org, accessed April 12, 2013.
112. "Lasers in cancer treatment," American Cancer Society.
113. "Lasers in cancer treatment," American Cancer Society.

15. PHARMACOLOGICAL LUNG CANCER APPROACHES

1. Frank V. Fossella, Ritsuko Komaki, and Joe B. Putnam Jr., eds., *Lung Cancer: M.D. Anderson Cancer Care Series* (New York: Springer-Verlag, 2003), 17–18.
2. Michael Braham, *Complementary, Natural and Alternative Small Cell Lung Cancer Treatments* (Chicago: Cancer Group Institute, 2011), 40–50.
3. Keith M. Bellizi and Margot Ann Gosney, eds., *Cancer and Aging Handbook: Research and Practice* (New York: Wiley, 2012), 478–80.
4. Bellizi and Gosney, *Cancer and Aging Handbook*.
5. Bellizi and Gosney, *Cancer and Aging Handbook*.
6. K. Tateishi, T. Ichiyama, K. Hirai, T. Agatsuma, S. Koyama, T. Hachiya, N. Morozumi, T. Shiina, and T. Koizumi, "Clinical outcomes in elderly patients administered gefitinib as first-line treatment in epidermal growth factor receptor-mutated non-small-cell lung cancer: Retrospective analysis in a Nagano Lung Cancer Research Group study," *Medical Oncology* 30, no. 1 (2013): 450.
7. G. Chen, J. Feng, C. Zhou, Y. L. Wu , X. Q. Liu, C. Wang, S. Zhang, J. Wang, S. Zhou, S. Ren, S. Lu, L. Zhang, C. P. Hu, C. Hu, L. Luo, L. Chen, M. Ye, J. Huang, X. Zhi, Y. Zhang, Q. Xiu, J. Ma, L. Zhang, and C. You, "Quality of life (QoL) analyses from OPTIMAL (CTONG-0802), a phase III, randomised, open-label study of first-line erlotinib versus chemotherapy in patients with advanced EGFR mutation-positive non-small-cell lung cancer (NSCLC)," *Annals of Oncology* 24, no. 6 (2013): 1615–22; Y. L. Wu, J. S. Lee, S. Thongprasert, C. J. Yu, L. Zhang, G. Ladrera, V. Srimuninnimit, V. Sriuranpong, J. Sandoval-Tan, Y. Zhu, M. Liao, C. Zhou, H. Pan, V. Lee, Y. M. Chen, Y. Sun, B. Margono, F. Fuerte, G. C. Chang, K. Seetalarom, J. Wang, A. Cheng, E. Syahruddin, X. Qian, J. Ho, J. Kurnianda, H. E. Liu, K. Jin, M. Truman, I. Bara, and T. Mok, "Intercalated combination of chemotherapy and erlotinib for patients with advanced stage non-small-cell lung cancer (FASTACT-2): A

randomised, double-blind trial," *Lancet Oncology* 13, no. S1470–2045 (2013): 70254–57.

8.   E. E. Vokes, R. Salgia, and T. G. Karrison, "Evidence-based role of bevacizumab in non-small cell lung cancer," *Annals of Oncology* 24, no. 1 (2013): 6–9.

9.   J. Zhou, W. Y. Zhao, X. Ma, R. J. Ju, X. Y. Li, N. Li, M. G. Sun, J. F. Shi, C. X. Zhang, and W. L. Lu, "The anticancer efficacy of paclitaxel liposomes modified with mitochondrial targeting conjugate in resistant lung cancer," *Biomaterials* 34, no. 14 (2013): 3626–38; Y. Tsubata, T. Okimoto, K. Miura, F. Karino, S. Iwamoto, M. Tada, T. Honda, S. Hamaguchi, M. Ohe, A. Sutani, T. Kuraki, A. Hamada, and T. Isobe, "Phase I clinical and pharmacokinetic study of bi-weekly carboplatin/paclitaxel chemotherapy in elderly patients with advanced non-small cell lung cancer," *Anticancer Research* 33, no. 2 (2013): 261–66.

10.   C. Gridelli, P. Maione, and A. Rossi, "The PARAMOUNT trial: A phase III randomized study of maintenance pemetrexed versus placebo immediately following induction first-line treatment with pemetrexed plus cisplatin for advanced nonsquamous non-small cell lung cancer," *Reviews on Recent Clinical Trials* 8, no. 1 (2013): 23–28; A. T. Shaw, A. M. Varghese, B. J. Solomon, D. B. Costa, S. Novello, M. Mino-Kenudson, M. M. Awad, J. A. Engelman, G. J. Riely, V. Monica, B. Y. Yeap, and G. V. Scagliotti, "Pemetrexed-based chemotherapy in patients with advanced, ALK-positive non-small cell lung cancer," *Annals of Oncology* 24, no. 1 (2013): 59–66.

11.   D. R. Camidge, N. Blais, D. L. Jonker, D. Soulières, R. C. Doebele, A. Ruiz-Garcia, A. Thall, K. Zhang, S. A. Laurie, R. C. Chao, and L. Q. Chow, "Sunitinib combined with pemetrexed and cisplatin: Results of a phase I dose-escalation and pharmacokinetic study in patients with advanced solid malignancies, with an expanded cohort in non-small cell lung cancer and mesothelioma," *Cancer Chemotherapy and Pharmacology* 71, no. 2 (2013): 307–19; M. P. Barr, S. G. Gray, A. C. Hoffmann, R. A. Hilger, J. Thomale, J. D. O'Flaherty, D. A. Fennell, D. Richard, J. J. O'Leary, and K. J. O'Byrne, "Generation and characterisation of cisplatin-resistant non-small cell lung cancer cell lines displaying a stem-like signature," *PLoS One* 8, no. 1 (2013): e54193; Q. Ashton Acton, ed., *Issues in Cancer Drugs and Therapies* (Atlanta: Scholarly Editions, 2012), 349–69.

12.   "Porfimer (injection)," U.S. National Library of Medicine, www.ncbi.nlm.nih.gov, accessed May 12, 2013.

13.   E. Kontopodis, D. Hatzidaki, I. Varthalitis, N. Kentepozidis, S. Giassas, N. Pantazopoulos, N. Vardakis, M. Rovithi, V. Georgoulias, and S. Agelaki, "A phase II study of metronomic oral vinorelbine administered in the second line and beyond in non-small cell lung cancer (NSCLC): A phase II study of the

Hellenic Oncology Research Group," *Journal of Chemotherapy* 25, no. 1 (2013): 49–55; Q. Lin, J. Wang, Y. Liu, H. Su, N. Wang, Y. Huang, C. X. Liu, P. Zhang, Y. Zhao, and K. Chen, "High-dose 3-dimensional conformal radiotherapy with concomitant vinorelbine plus carboplatin in patients with non-small cell lung cancer: A feasibility study," *Oncology Letters* 2, no. 4 (2011): 669–74.

14. I. Djerassi, C. J. Rominger, J. S. Kim, J. Turchi, U. Suvansri, and D. Hughes, "Phase I study of high doses of methotrexate with citrovorum factor in patients with lung cancer," *Cancer* 30, no. 1 (1972): 22–30; K. R. Hande, R. K. Oldham, M. F. Fer, R. L. Richardson, and F. A. Greco, "Randomized study of high-dose versus low-dose methotrexate in the treatment of extensive small cell lung cancer," *American Journal of Medicine* 73, no. 3 (1982): 413–39.

15. R. Wang, S. Qin, Y. Chen, Y. Li, C. Chen, Z. Wang, R. Zheng, and Q. Wu, "Enhanced anti-tumor and anti-angiogenic effects of metronomic cyclophosphamide combined with Endostar in a xenograft model of human lung cancer," *Oncology Reports* 28, no. 2 (2012): 439–45; Y. Watanabe, E. Ogo, H. Kaida, G. Suzuki, H. Eto, H. Suefuji, C. Hattori, C. Tsuji, and N. Hayabuchi, "Treatment with low-dose cyclophosphamide and radiation therapy for advanced non-small lung cancer in elderly patient [in Japanese]," *Gan To Kagaku Ryoho* 38, no. 9 (2011): 1503–5.

16. A. T. Shaw, D. W. Kim, K. Nakagawa, T. Seto, L. Crinó, M. J. Ahn, T. De Pas, B. Besse, B. J. Solomon, F. Blackhall, Y. L. Wu, M. Thomas, K. J. O'Byrne, D. Moro-Sibilot, D. R. Camidge, T. Mok, V. Hirsh, G. J. Riely, S. Iyer, V. Tassell, A. Polli, K. D. Wilner, and P. A. Jänne, "Crizotinib versus chemotherapy in advanced ALK-positive lung cancer," *New England Journal of Medicine* 368, no. 25 (2013): 2385–94; H. K. Ahn, K. Jeon, H. Yoo, B. Han, S. J. Lee, H. Park, M. J. Lee, S. Y. Ha, J. H. Han, J. M. Sun, J. S. Ahn, M. J. Ahn, and K. Park, "Successful treatment with crizotinib in mechanically ventilated patients with ALK positive non-small-cell lung cancer," *Journal of Thoracic Oncology* 8, no. 2 (2013): 250–53; A. Gröschel, A. Warth, and N. Reinmuth, "Crizotinib—Molecular therapy for lung cancer [in German]," *Pneumologie* 67, no. 4 (2013): 205–8.

17. Lorraine Johnston, *Lung Cancer: Making Sense of Diagnosis, Treatment, and Options* (Beijing: O'Reilly, 2001), 208–13.

18. M. I. Koukourakis, P. G. Tsoutsou, and I. Abatzoglou, "Computed tomography assessment of lung density in patients with lung cancer treated with accelerated hypofractionated radio-chemotherapy supported with amifostine," *American Journal of Clinical Oncology* 32, no. 3 (2009): 258–61; S. Wang, Y. Zhang, S. Zhang, and S. Ma, "Effect of amifostine on locally advanced non-small cell lung cancer patients treated with radiotherapy: A meta-

analysis of randomized controlled trials [in Chinese]," *Zhongguo Fei Ai Za Zhi* 15, no. 9 (2012): 539–44.

19. N. Peled, K. Yoshida, M. W. Wynes, and F. R. Hirsch, "Predictive and prognostic markers for epidermal growth factor receptor inhibitor therapy in non-small cell lung cancer," *Therapeutic Advances in Medical Oncology* 1, no. 3 (2009):137–44; J. W. Neal, R. S. Heist, P. Fidias, J. S. Temel, M. Huberman, J. P. Marcoux, A. Muzikansky, T. J. Lynch, and L. V. Sequist, "Cetuximab monotherapy in patients with advanced non-small cell lung cancer after prior epidermal growth factor receptor tyrosine kinase inhibitor therapy," *Journal of Thoracic Oncology* 5, no. 11 (2010): 1855–58.

20. Virginia Poole Arcangelo and Andrew M. Peterson, *Pharmacotherapeutics for Advanced Practice: A Practical Approach* (Philadelphia: Lippincott Williams and Wilkins, 2006), 816–28.

21. J. Garst J, "Topotecan: An evolving option in the treatment of relapsed small cell lung cancer," *Journal of Therapeutics and Clinical Risk Management* 3, no. 6 (2007): 1087–95; S. Agelaki, E. Kontopodis, A. Kotsakis, V. Chandrinos, I. Bompolaki, Z. Zafeiriou, E. Papadimitraki, D. Stoltidis, K. Kalbakis, and V. Georgoulias, "A phase I clinical trial of weekly oral topotecan for relapsed small cell lung cancer," *Cancer Chemotherapy and Pharmacology* 72, no. 1 (2013): 45–51.

22. I. Karam, S. Y. Jiang, M. Khaira, C. W. Lee, and D. Schellenberg, "Outcomes of small cell lung cancer patients treated with cisplatin-etoposide versus carboplatin-etoposide," *American Journal of Clinical Oncology* (April 3, 2013), published online ahead of print; R. Rezonja, L. Knez, T. Cufer, and A. Mrhar, "Oral treatment with etoposide in small cell lung cancer—Dilemmas and solutions," *Radiological Oncology* 47, no. 1 (2013): 1–13.

23. Mario Dicato, *Side Effects of Medical Cancer Therapy Prevention and Treatment* (London: Springer, 2013), 204–11.

24. C. Centeno Cortés, M. J. Borau Clavero, A. Sanz Rubiales, and F. López-Lara Martín, "Intestinal bleeding in disseminated non-small cell lung cancer," *Lung Cancer* 18, no. 1 (1997): 101–5.

25. Y. Qi, G. K. Dy, G. D. Nelson, S. E. Schild, S. J. Mandrekar, and A. A. Adjei, "Incidence of bleeding and thrombosis among elderly patients (pts) undergoing systemic chemotherapy in advanced non-small cell lung cancer (NSCLC): An analysis of North Central Cancer Treatment Group (NCCTG) trials," *Journal of Clinical Oncology* 28, no. 15 (2010): e18093.

26. L. Tamási, V. Müller, N. Eszes, T. Kardos, M. Budai, K. Vincze, G. Losonczy, and M. Szilasi, "Patterns of erythropoiesis-stimulating agent use for chemotherapy-induced anemia in lung cancer: results of a retrospective Hungarian real-life clinical data analysis," *Expert Opinions in Drug Safety* 10, no. 4 (2011): 503–7.

27. Mayo Clinic Staff, "Low blood cell counts: Side effect of cancer treatment," www.mayoclinic.com, accessed May 12, 2013.

28. Y. H. Lee, Y. F. Tsai, Y. H. Lai, and C. M. Tsai, "Fatigue experience and coping strategies in Taiwanese lung cancer patients receiving chemotherapy," *Journal of Clinical Nursing* 17, no. 7 (2008): 876–83.

29. Marylin J. Dodd, *Managing the Side Effects of Chemotherapy and Radiation Therapy* (San Francisco: UCSF Nursing Press, 2001), 247–54.

30. Dodd, *Managing the Side Effects of Chemotherapy and Radiation Therapy*.

31. R. Paus, I. S. Haslam, A. A. Sharov, and V. A. Botchkarev, "Pathobiology of chemotherapy-induced hair loss," *Lancet Oncology* 14, no. 2 (2013): e50–e59.

32. X. Zhang, P. Yue, B. D. Page, T. Li, W. Zhao, A. T. Namanja, D. Paladino, J. Zhao, Y. Chen, P. T. Gunning, and J. Turkson, "Orally bioavailable small-molecule inhibitor of transcription factor Stat3 regresses human breast and lung cancer xenografts," *Proceedings of the National Academy of Science U. S. A.* 109, no. 24 (2012): 9623–8; M. L. Stallings-Mann, J. Waldman, Y. Zhang, and E. Miller, "Matrix metalloproteinase induction of Rac1b, a key effector of lung cancer progression," *Science Translational Medicine* 4, no. 142 (2012): 142–95.

33. J. M. Tuscana, J. Kato, D. Pearson, C. Xiong, L. Newell, Y. Ma, D. R. Gandara, and R. T. O'Donnell, "CD22 antigen is broadly expressed on lung cancer cells and is a target for antibody-based therapy," *Cancer Research* 72, no. 21 (2012): 5556–65.

34. Vall d'Hebron Institute of Oncology, "Lung tumors eradicated in a preclinical mouse model," March 21, 2012, www.medicalnewstoday.com/releases/257371.php, accessed April 27, 2013.

35. Lung Foundation of Australia, *Better Living with Lung Cancer* (Sydney: Lung Foundation of Australia, 2012), 43.

16. ADDRESSING THE MENTAL ASPECTS OF LUNG CANCER

1. Madeline Mary E. Cooley, Julie Lynch, Kilah Fox, and Linda Sarna, *Psycho-Oncology*, 2nd ed. (New York: Oxford University Press, 2010), 152.

2. S. B. Artherholt and J. R. Fann, Psychosocial care in cancer," *Current Psychiatry Reports* 14, no. 1 (2012): 23–29.

3. L. A. Fashoyin-Aje, K. A. Martinez, and S. M. Dy, "New patient-centered care standards from the Commission on Cancer: Opportunities and challenges," *Journal of Supportive Oncology* 10, no. 3 (2012): 107–11.

4. S. Van Dooren, A. J. Rijnsburger, C. Seynaeve, H. J. Duivenvoorden, M. L. Essink-Bot, M. M. Tilanus-Linthorst, H. J. de Koning, and A. Tibben, "Psychological distress in women at increased risk for breast cancer: The role of risk perception," *European Journal of Cancer* 40, no. 14 (2004): 2056–63; J. L. Bayer-Cartera, D. Christensena, L. Dahmousha, M. L. McCormicka, K. DeGeesta, D. R. Spitza, A. Soodb, and S. K. Lutgendorfa, "Psychological risk factors are related to higher levels of antioxidant enzyme activity in ovarian cancer patients," *Brain, Behavior, and Immunity* 26, no. 1 (suppl. 2012): S34.

5. S. K. Lutgendorf, K. DeGeest, L. Dahmoush, D. Farley, F. Penedo, D. Bender, M. Goodheart, T. E. Buekers, L. Mendez, G. Krueger, L. Clevenger, D. M. Lubaroff, A. K. Sood , S. W. Cole, K. DeGeest, and L. Dahmoush, "Social isolation is associated with elevated tumor norepinephrine in ovarian carcinoma patients," *Brain, Behavior, and Immunity* 25, no. 2 (2011): 250–55.

6. "Psychological stress and cancer," National Cancer Institute, www.cancer.gov, accessed April 27, 2013.

7. "Psychological stress and cancer."

8. S. K. Lutgendorf, A. K. Sood, B. Anderson, S. McGinn, H. Maiseri, M. Dao, J. I. Sorosky, K. De Geest, J. Ritchie, and D. M. Lubaroff, "Social support, psychological distress, and natural killer cell activity in ovarian cancer," *Journal of Clinical Oncology* 23, no. 28 (2005): 7105–13.

9. S. K. Lutgendorf, A. K. Sood, and M. H. Antoni, "Host factors and cancer progression: Biobehavioral signaling pathways and interventions," *Journal of Clinical Oncology* 28, no. 26 (2010): 4094–99; P. G. McDonald, M. H. Antoni, S. K. Lutgendorf, S. W. Cole, F. S. Dhabhar, S. E. Sephton, M. Stefanek, and A. K. Sood, "A biobehavioral perspective of tumor biology," *Discovery Medicine* 5, no. 30 (2005): 520–26; A. Melhem-Bertrandt, M. Chavez-Macgregor, X. Lei, E. N. Brown, R. T. Lee, F. Meric-Bernstam, A. K. Sood, S. D. Conzen, G. N. Hortobagyi, and A. M. Gonzalez-Angulo, "Beta-blocker use is associated with improved relapse-free survival in patients with triple-negative breast cancer," *Journal of Clinical Oncology* 29, no. 19 (2011): 2645–52; M. Moreno-Smith, S. K. Lutgendorf, and A. K. Sood, "Impact of stress on cancer metastasis," *Future Oncology* 6, no. 12 (2010): 1863–81; S. C. Segerstrom and G. E. Miller, "Psychological stress and the human immune system: A meta-analytic study of 30 years of inquiry," *Psychological Bulletin* 130, no. 4 (2004): 601–30; E. K. Sloan, S. J. Priceman, B. F. Cox, S. Yu, M. A. Pimentel, V. Tangkanangnukul, J. M. Arevalo, K. Morizono, B. D. Karanikolas, L. Wu, A. K. Sood, and S. W. Cole, "The sympathetic nervous system induces a metastatic switch in primary breast cancer," *Cancer Research* 70, no. 18 (2010): 7042–52.

10. M. Y. Smith, W. H. Redd, C. Peyser, and D. Vogl, "Post-traumatic stress disorder in cancer: A review," *Psychooncology* 8, no. 6 (1999): 521–37;

K. Hodgkinson, P. Butow, A. Fuchs, G. E. Hunt, A. Stenlake, K. M. Hobbs, A. Brand, and G. Wain, "Long-term survival from gynecologic cancer: Psychosocial outcomes, supportive care needs and positive outcomes," *Gynecologic Oncology* 104, no. 2 (2007): 381–89.

11. Li, Sarah Hales, and Gary Rodin, *Psycho-Oncology*, 2nd ed. (Oxford University Press, 2010), 303.

12. Li et al., *Psycho-Oncology*, 304.

13. Li et al., *Psycho-Oncology*, 305.

14. Li et al., *Psycho-Oncology*, 307.

15. Wasan Ali, *Best Practice Intervention for the Management of Adjustment Disorders (AD): Annotated Information Package* (Christchurch: Department of Public Health, 2007), 2.

16. Naoki Nakaya, Kumi Saito-Nakaya, Tatsuo Akechi, Shinichi Kuriyama, Masatoshi Inagaki, Nobutaka Kikuchi, Kanji Nagai, Shoichiro Tsugane, Yutaka Nishiwaki, Ichiro Tsuji and Yosuke Uchitomi, "Negative psychological aspects and survival in lung cancer patients," *Psychooncology* 17, no. 5 (2008): 466–73; Jeffrey E. Young, Jaynel Rygh, Arthur D. Weingberger, and Aaron T. Beck, *Clinical Handbook of Psychological Disorders* (New York: Guilford Press, 2008), 250.

17. David Semple, Roger Smyth, Jonathan Burns, Rajan Darjee, and Andrew McIntosh, *The Oxford Handbook of Psychiatry* (New York: Oxford University Press, 2005), 242.

18. Penelope Hopwood and Richard J. Stephens, "Depression in patients with lung cancer: Prevalence and risk factors derived from quality-of-life data," *Journal of Clinical Oncology* 18, no. 4 (2000): 893–903.

19. Hopwood and Stephens, "Depression in patients with lung cancer."

20. Elly Trepman, Lorren Sandt, and Cindy Langhorne, eds., *Lung Cancer Choices* (Vancouver, WA: Caring Ambassadors Program, 2012), 84.

21. H. Faller, H. Bülzebruck, P. Drings, and H. Lang, "Coping, distress, and survival among patients with lung cancer," *Archives of General Psychiatry* 56, no. 8 (1999): 756–62, G. Buccheri, "Depressive reactions to lung cancer are common and often followed by a poor outcome," *European Respiratory Journal* 11, no. 1 (1998): 173–78.

22. Naoki Nakaya, Kumi Saito-Nakaya, Tatsuo Akechi, Shinichi Kuriyama, Masatoshi Inagaki, Nobutaka Kikuchi, Kanji Nagai, Shoichiro Tsugane, Yutaka Nishiwaki, Ichiro Tsuji, and Yosuke Uchitomi, "Negative psychological aspects and survival in lung cancer patients," *Psychooncology* 17, no. 5 (2008): 466–73.

23. Trepman et al., *Lung Cancer Choices*, 84; Haley Pessin, Lia Amakawa, and William S. Breitbart, *Psycho-Oncology*, 2nd ed. (New York: Oxford University Press, 2010), 319.

24. Jameson K. Hirsch, Andrea R. Floyd, and Paul R. Duberstein, "Perceived health in lung cancer patients: the role of positive and negative effect," *Quality of Life Research* 21, no. 2 (2102): 187–94.

25. Pessin et al., *Psycho-Oncology*, 319.

26. Pessin et al., *Psycho-Oncology*, 320; I. Spoletini, W. Gianni, C. Caltagirone, R. Madaio, L. Repetto, and G. Spalletta, "Suicide and cancer: Where do we go from here?," *Critical Reviews in Oncology/Hematology* 78, no. 3 (2011): 206–19.

27. Pessin et al., *Psycho-Oncology*, 319.

28. Pessin et al., *Psycho-Oncology*, 319.

29. A. Davis, "Jack Kevorkian: A medical hero? His actions are the antithesis of heroism," *British Medical Journal* 313, no. 7051 (1996): 228.

30. D. Stark, M. Kiely, A. Smith, G. Velikova, A. House, and P. Selby, "Anxiety disorders in cancer patients: Their nature, associations, and relation to quality of life," *Journal of Clinical Oncology* 20, no. 14 (2002): 3137–48.

31. Tomer T. Levin and Yesne Alici, *Psycho-Oncology*, 2nd ed. (New York: Oxford University Press, 2010), 324.

32. Levin and Alici, *Psycho-Oncology*, 325.

33. M. M. Byrne, J. Weissfeld, and M. S. Roberts, "Anxiety, fear of cancer, and perceived risk of cancer following lung cancer screening," *Medical Decision Making* 28, no. 6 (2008): 917–25; D. Buchanan, R. Milroy, L. Baker, A. M. Thompson, and P. A. Levack, "Perceptions of anxiety in lung cancer patients and their support network," *Supportive Care in Cancer* 1, no. 18 (2010): 29–36; S. Li, Y. Wang, S. Xin, and J. Cao, "Changes in quality of life and anxiety of lung cancer patients underwent chemotherapy [in Chinese]," *Zhongguo Fei Ai Za Zhi* 15, no. 8 (2012): 465–70.

34. C. A. Schag and R. L. Heinrich, "Anxiety in medical situations: Adult cancer patients," *Journal of Clinical Oncology* 45, no.1 (1989): 20.

35. S. K. Inouye, "Delirium in older persons," *New England Journal of Medicine* 354, no. 11 (2006): 1157–65.

36. William S. Breitbart and Yesne Alici, *Psycho-Oncology*, 2nd ed. (New York: Oxford University Press, 2010), 332–38.

37. N. K. LoConte, N. M. Else-Quest, J. Eickhoff, J. Hyde, and J. H. Schiller, *Assessment of Guilt and Shame in Patients with Non-Small-Cell Lung Cancer Compared with Patients with Breast and Prostate Cancer* (Madison: University of Wisconsin Paul Carbone Comprehensive Cancer Center, 2008), 1.

38. P. Christo and D. Mazloomdoost, *Interventional Pain Treatments for Cancer Pain* (New York: Annals of the New York Academy of Sciences, 2008), 299–328.

39. Howard S. Smith and Steven D. Passik, *Pain and Chemical Dependency* (New York: Oxford University Press, 2008), 19.

40. E. Bruera, J. Moyano, L. Seifert, R. L. Fainsinger, J. Hanson, and M. Suarez-Almazor, "The frequency of alcoholism among patients with pain due to terminal cancer," *Journal of Pain Symptom Management* 10, no. 8 (1995): 599–603.

41. J. Nagano, Y. Ichinose, H. Asoh, J. Ikeda, A. Ohshima, N. Sudo, and C. Kubo, "A prospective Japanese study of the association between personality and the progression of lung cancer," *Internal Medicine* 45, no. 2 (2006): 57–63; Y. Kim, P. R. Duberstein, S. Sörensen, and M. R. Larson, "Levels of depressive symptoms in spouses of people with lung cancer: Effects of personality, social support, and caregiving burden," *Psychosomatics* 46, no. 2 (2005): 123–30; N. Nakaya, Y. Tsubono, Y. Nishino, T. Hosokawa, S. Fukudo, D. Shibuya, N. Akizuki, E. Yoshikawa, M. Kobayakawa, M. Fujimori, K. Saito-Nakaya, Y. Uchitomi, and I. Tsuji, "Personality and cancer survival: The Miyagi cohort study," *British Journal of Cancer* 92, no. 11 (2005): 2089–94.

42. S. Mellon, L. L. Northouse, and L. K. Weiss, "A population-based study of the quality of life of cancer survivors and their family caregivers," *Cancer Nursing* 29, no. 2 (2006): 120–31.

43. "Better Living with Lung Cancer," The Lung Foundation, www.lungfoundation.com.au, accessed April 27, 2013.

44. S. Fischer Verlag, *Healing through Exercise* (Cambridge: Lifelong Books, 2009), 15.

45. S. Fischer Verlag, *Healing through Exercise*, 15.

46. S. Fischer Verlag, *Healing through Exercise*, 90.

47. S. Fischer Verlag, *Healing through Exercise*, 90.

17. LUNG CANCER AT HOME

1. Kemp H. Kernstine and Karen L. Reckamp, *Lung Cancer: A Multidisciplinary Approach to Diagnosis and Management* (New York: Demos Medical Publishing, 2010), 27.

2. John P. Caughlin, Sylvia L. Mikucki-Enyart, Ashley V. Middleton, Anne M. Stone, and Laura E. Brown, "Being Open without Talking about It: A Rhetorical/Normative Approach to Understanding Topic Avoidance in Families after a Lung Cancer Diagnosis," *Communication Monographs* 78, no. 4 (2011): 409–36.

3. B. J. Kramer, M. Kavanaugh, A. Trentham-Dietz, M. Walsh, and J. A. Yonker, "Predictors of family conflict at the end of life: The experience of

spouses and adult children of persons with lung cancer," *Gerontologist* 50, no. 2 (2010): 215–25.

4. "Living with a diagnosis of lung cancer, 3rd edition," National Lung Cancer Partnership, last updated November 13, 2012, www.nationallungcancerpartnership.org, accessed May 8, 2013.

5. . "Advanced cancer care planning," American Society of Clinical Oncology, www.cancer.net/coping/advanced-cancer-care-planning, accessed May 8, 2013.

6. K. S. Van Campen and C. A. Marshall, "How families cope with cancer," *McClelland Institute Publications Research Link* 2, no. 4 (2010): 1–4.

7. Van Campen and Marshall, "How families cope with cancer."

8. . Connie Yarbro, Debra Wujcik, and Barbara Holmes Gobel, *Cancer Nursing: Principles and Practice*, 7th ed. (Boston: Jones & Bartlett Learning, 2010), 1785–93.

9. Tina St. John, *With Every Breath: A Lung Cancer Guidebook* (Vancouver, WA: Lung Cancer Caring Ambassadors Program, 2005), 154–62.

10. "Family life," American Society of Clinical Oncology, www.cancer.net/coping/relationships-and-cancer/family-life, accessed May 8, 2013.

11. I. Henoch, B. Bergman, M. Gustafsson, F. Gaston-Johansson, and E. Danielson, "The impact of symptoms, coping capacity, and social support on quality of life experience over time in patients with lung cancer," *Journal of Pain and Symptom Management* 34, no. 4 (2007): 370–79.

12. Y. Chida, M. Harner, J. Wardle, and A. Steptoe, "Do stress-related psychosocial factors contribute to cancer incidence and survival?," *Nature Clinical Practice Oncology* 5, no. 8 (2008): 1–3.

13. F. Hansen and Jo-Ann Sawatzky, "Stress in patients with lung cancer: A human response to illness," *Oncology Nursing Forum* 35, no. 2 (2008): 217–23.

14. Hansen and Sawatzky, "Stress in patients with lung cancer."

15. "Mind-body medicine for lung cancer," Cancer Treatment Centers of America, www.cancercenter.com, accessed May 8, 2013.

16. G. R. Hunter, C. S. Bickel, G. Fisher, W. Neumeier, and J. McCarthy, "Combined aerobic/strength training and energy expenditure in older women," *Medicine in Science in Sports and Exercise* 45, no. 7 (2013): 1386–93.

17. Marilyn Haas, *Contemporary Issues in Lung Cancer*, 2nd ed. (Boston: Jones & Bartlett Learning, 2010), 125–27.

18. M. Vera-Llonch, D. Weycker, A. Glass, S. Gao, R. Borker, B. Barber, and G. Oster, "Healthcare costs in patients with metastatic lung cancer receiving chemotherapy," *BioMed Central Health Services Research* 11 (2011): 305.

18. FINDING MOTIVATION AS A LUNG CANCER PATIENT

1. J. E. Nelson, E. B. Gay, A. R. Berman , C. A. Powell, J. Salazar-Schicchi, and J. P. Wisnivesky, "Patients rate physician communication about lung cancer," *Cancer* 117, no. 22 (2011): 5212–20.

2. D. Berendes, F. J. Keefe, T. J. Somers, S. M. Kothadia, L. S. Porter, and J. S. Cheavens, "Hope in the context of lung cancer: Relationships of hope to symptoms and psychological distress," *Journal of Pain and Symptom Management* 40, no. 2 (2010): 174–82.

3. K. S. Clay, C. Talley, and K. B. Young, "Exploring spiritual well-being among survivors of colorectal and lung cancer," *Journal of Religion and Spirituality in Social Work* 29, no. 1 (2010): 14–32.

4. E. A. Cho and H. E. Oh, "Effects of laughter therapy on depression, quality of life, resilience and immune responses in breast cancer survivors [in Korean]," *Journal of the Korean Academy of Nursing* 41, no. 3 (2011): 285–93; S. Noji and K. Takayanagi, "A case of laughter therapy that helped improve advanced gastric cancer," *Journal of the Japan Hospital Association* 29 (2010): 59–64.

5. L. S. Porter, F. J. Keefe, J. Garst, D. H. Baucom, C. M. McBride, D. C. McKee, L. Sutton, K. Carson, V. Knowles, M. Rumble, and C. Scipio, "Caregiver-assisted coping skills training for lung cancer: Results of a randomized clinical trial," *Journal of Pain and Symptom Management* 41, no. 1 (2011): 1–13.

6. N. Prasertsri, J. Holden, F. J. Keefe, and D. J. Wilkie, "Repressive coping style: Relationships with depression, pain, and pain coping strategies in lung cancer out patients," *Lung Cancer* 71, no. 2 (2011): 235–40.

7. B. L. Andersen, "Psychological interventions for cancer patients to enhance the quality of life," *Journal of Consulting and Clinical Psychology* 60, no. 4 (1992): 552–68.

8. A. Floyd, E. Dedert, S. Ghate, P. Salmon, I. Weissbecker, J. L. Studts, B. Stetson, and S. E. Sephton, "Depression may mediate the relationship between sense of coherence and quality of life in lung cancer patients," *Journal of Health Psychology* 16, no. 2 (2011): 249–57.

9. B. J. Kramer, M. Kavanaugh, A. Trentham-Dietz, M. Walsh, and J. A. Yonker, "Complicated grief symptoms in caregivers of persons with lung cancer: The role of family conflict, intrapsychic strains, and hospice utilization," *Omega* 62, no. 3 (2010): 201–20.

10. M. S. Vos, H. Putter, H. C. van Houwelingen, and H. C. de Haes, "Denial in lung cancer patients: A longitudinal study," *Psychooncology* 17, no. 12 (2008): 1163–71.

11.   Pedro T. Sánchez, Gema Peiró, Miguel de Lamo, Nieves del Pozo, Francisco Palmero, Ana Blasco, and Carlos Camps, "From emotion to psychopathology in lung cancer: The role of the anger experience [in Spanish]," *Revista Electronica de Motivación y Emoción* 11, no. 29–30 (n.d.).

12.   M. M. Byrne, J. Weissfeld, and M. S. Roberts, "Anxiety, fear of cancer, and perceived risk of cancer following lung cancer screening," *Medical Decision Making* 28, no. 6 (2008): 917–25.

13.   K. Milbury, H. Badr, and C. L. Carmack, "The role of blame in the psychosocial adjustment of couples coping with lung cancer," *Annals of Behavioral Medicine* 44, no. 3 (2012): 331–40.

14.   A. Rokach, L. Findler, J. Chin, S. Lev, and Y. Kollender, "Cancer patients, their caregivers and coping with loneliness," *Psychology, Health and Medicine* 18, no. 2 (2013): 135–44.

19. PREVENTION AND COLLECTIVE EFFORTS

1.   D. M. Parkin, P. Pisani, A. D. Lopez, and E. Masuyer, "At least one in seven cases of cancer is caused by smoking: Global estimates for 1985," *International Journal of Cancer* 59 (1994): 494–504.

2.   World Health Organization, *The World Health Report 2002, Reducing Risks, Promoting Healthy Life* (Geneva: World Health Organization, 2002).

3.   A. R. Collins, "Carotenoids and genomic stability," *Mutation Research* 18 (2001): 21–28.

4.   S. Mannisto, S. A. Smith-Warner, and D. Spiegelman, "Dietary carotenoids and risk of lung cancer in a pooled analysis of seven cohort studies," *Cancer Epidemiology, Biomarkers and Prevention* 13 (2004): 40–48.

5.   A. Tardon, W. J. Lee, M. Delgado-Rodriguez, M. Dosemeci, D. Albanes, R. Hoover, and A. Blair, "Leisure-time physical activity and lung cancer: A meta-analysis," *Cancer Cause and Control* 16 (2005): 389–97.

6.   I. Thune and E. Lund, "The influence of physical activity on lung cancer risk: A prospective study of 81516 men and women," *International Journal of Cancer* 70 (1997): 57–62.

7.   P. Vineis, T. Thomas, R. B. Hayes, W. J. Blot, T. J. Mason, L. W. Pickle, P. Correa, E. T. Fontham, and J. Schoenberg, "Proportion of lung cancers in males due to occupation in different areas of the US," *International Journal of Cancer* 42 (1998): 851–56; P. Vineis and L. Simonato, "Proportion of lung and bladder cancers in males resulting from occupation: A systematic approach," *Archives of Environmental Health* 46 (1991): 6–15.

8. Robert Longly, "Smoking Deaths Cost U.S. $92 Billion a Year," http://usgovinfo.about.com/od/medicalnews/a/smokingcosts.htm, accessed May 22, 2013.

9. National Center for Chronic Disease Prevention and Health Promotion (US) Office on Smoking and Health, *Preventing Tobacco Use among Youth and Young Adults: A Report of the Surgeon General* (Atlanta: Centers for Disease Control and Prevention, 2012).

10. National Center for Chronic Disease Prevention and Health Promotion (US) Office on Smoking and Health, *Preventing Tobacco Use Among Youth and Young Adults*; American Lung Association Research and Program Services Epidemiology and Statistics Unit, *Trends in Tobacco Use* (Los Angeles: American Lung Association, 2011).

11. P. M. Cinciripini, S. S. Necht, J. E. Henningfield, M. W. Manley, and B. S. Kramer, "Tobacco addiction: Implications for treatment and cancer prevention," *Journal of the National Cancer Institute* 89, no. 24 (1990): 1852–67; U.S. Department of Health and Human Services, Public Health Services, Centers for Chronic Disease Prevention and Health Promotion, Office on Smoking and Health, Department of Health and Human Services, *The Health Benefits of Smoking Cessation: A Report of the Surgeon General* (Rockville, MD: Centers for Disease Control, 1990), 90–8416; M. C. Fiore, W. C. Bailey, and S. J. Cohen, *Smoking Cessation: Clinical Practice Guidelines No. 18* (Rockville, MD: U.S. Department of Health and Human Services, Public Health Service, Agency for Health Care Policy and Research, 1996).

12. R. T. Greenlee, T. Murray, and S. Bolden, "Cancer Statistics, 2000," *CA: A Cancer Journal for Clinicians* 50, no. 1 (2000): 7–33.

13. Fiore et al., *Smoking Cessation* .

14. A. Sanders-Jackson, M. Gonzalez, B. Zerbe, A. V. Song, and S. A. Glantz, "The pattern of indoor smoking restriction law transitions, 1970–2009: Laws are sticky," *American Journal of Public Health* 103, no. 8 (2013): e44–e51; J. Gruber, "Government policy towards smoking: A view from economics," *Yale Journal of Health, Policy, Law, and Ethics* 3, no. 1 (2002): 119–26; P. A. Wingo, L. A. Ries, G. A. Giovino, D. S. Miller, H. M. Rosenberg, D. R. Shopland, M. J. Thun, and B. K. Edwards, "Annual report on the nation on the status of cancer, 1973–1996, with a special section on lung cancer and tobacco smoking," *Journal of the National Cancer Institute* 91, no. 8 (1999): 675–90; H. K. Koh, "The end of 'tobacco and cancer' century," *Journal of the National Cancer Institute* 91, no. 8 (1999): 660–61.

15. J. E. Callinan, A. Clarke, K. Doherty, and C. Kelleher, "Legislative smoking bans for reducing secondhand smoke exposure, smoking prevalence and tobacco consumption," *Cochrane Database of Systematic Reviews* 4 (2010): CD005992; C. S. Carpenter, "The effects of local workplace smoking

laws on smoking restrictions and exposure to smoke at work," *Journal of Human Resources* 44, no. 4 (2009): 1023–46; C. Carpenter, *How Do Workplace Smoking Laws Work? Quasi-Experimental Evidence from Local Laws in Ontario*, working paper no. 13133 (Cambridge, MA: National Bureau of Economic Research, 2007); C. L. Miller and J. A. Hickling, "Phased-in smoke-free workplace laws: Reported impact on bar patronage and smoking, particularly among young adults in South Australia," *Australian and New Zealand Journal of Public Health* 30, no. 4 (2006): 325–27.

16. S. Glantz and A. Charlesworth, "Tourism and hotel revenues before and after passage of smoke-free restaurant ordinances," *Journal of the American Medical Association* 281 (1999): 1911–18.

17. Centers for Disease Control and Prevention, "Disparities in second-hand smoke exposure—United States, 1988–1994 and 1999–2004," *Morbidity and Mortality Weekly Report* 57, no. 27 (2008): 744–47.

18. Y. Anzai, T. Ohkubo, Y. Nishino, I. Tsuji, and S. Hisamichi, "Relationship between health practices and education level in the rural Japanese population," *Journal of Epidemiology* 10, no. 13 (2000): 149–56.

19. M. Saatchi, "How can an act of parliament cure cancer?," *Journal of the Royal Society of Medicine* 106, no. 5 (2013): 169–72.

20. C. J. Bradley, B. Dahman, and H. D. Bear, "Insurance and inpatient care: Differences in length of stay and costs between surgically treated cancer patients," *Cancer* 118, no. 20 (2012): 5084–91.

20. CONCLUSION

1. Jackie Ellis, "The impact of lung cancer on patients and caregivers," *Chronic Respiratory Disease* 9, no. 1 (2012): 39–47.

2. A. Jemal, F. Bray, M. M. Center, J. Ferlay, E. Ward, and D. Forman, "Global cancer statistics," *CA: A Cancer Journal for Clinicians* 61, no. 2 (2011): 69–90.

3. David Berendes, Francis J. Keefe, Tamara J. Somers, Sejal M. Kothadia, Laura S. Porter, and Jennifer S. Cheavens, "Hope in the context of lung cancer: Relationships of hope to symptoms and psychological distress," *Journal of Pain and Symptom Management* 40, no. 2 (2010): 174–82.

4. Sally Moore, Mary Wells, Hilary Plant, Frances Fuller, Majella Wright, and Jessica Corner, "Nurse specialist led follow-up in lung cancer: The experience of developing and delivering a new model of care," *European Journal of Oncology Nursing* 10, no. 5 (2006): 364–77; Sally Moore, Amanda Sherwin, Jibby Medina, Emma Ream, Hilary Plant, and Alison Richardson, "Caring for caregivers: A prospective audit of nurse specialist contact with families and

caregivers of patients with lung cancer," *European Journal of Oncology Nursing* 10, no. 3 (2006): 207–11.

5. "Cancer topics," National Cancer Institute, posted September 17, 2012, www.cancer.gov/cancertopics, accessed May 23, 2013.

6. R. L. Street Jr. and P. Haidet, "How well do doctors know their patients? Factors affecting physician understanding of patients' health beliefs," *Journal of General Internal Medicine* 26, no. 1 (2011): 21–27.

7. "Drugs information online," last modified March 18, 2013, www.drugs.com/enc/lung-cancer.html, accessed May 23, 2013.

BIBLIOGRAPHY

PREFACE

Hammerman, P. S. "My take on . . . comprehensive Genomic Survey of Squamous Cell Lung Cancer." *Oncology Times* 34, no. 20 (2012): 12.

McCann, S., MacAuley, D., Barnett, Y., Bunting, B., Bradley, A., Jeffers, L., and Morrison, P. J. "Cancer genetics: Consultants' perceptions of their roles, confidence and satisfaction with knowledge." *Journal of Evaluation in Clinical Practice* 13, no. 2 (2007): 276–86.

Partridge, M., Ramos, M., Sardaro, A., and Brada, M. "Dose escalation for non-small cell lung cancer: analysis and modelling of published literature." *Radiotherapy and Oncology* 99, no. 1 (2011): 6–11.

Steginga, S. K., Dunn, J., Dewar, A. M., McCarthy, A., Yates, P., and Beadle, G. "Impact of an intensive nursing education course on nurses' knowledge, confidence, attitudes, and perceived skills in the care of patients with cancer." *Oncology Nursing Forum* 32, no. 2 (2005): 375–81.

Wassenaar, C. A., Dong, Q., Wei, Q., Amos, C. I., Spitz, M. R., and Tyndale, R. F. "Relationship between CYP2A6 and CHRNA5-CHRNA3-CHRNB4 variation and smoking behaviors and lung cancer risk." *Journal of the National Cancer Institute* 103 no. 17 (2011): 1342–46.

CHAPTER I

Alberts, B., Johnson, A., Lewis, J., Raff, M., Roberts, K., and Walter, P. "Desmosomes connect intermediate filaments from cell to cell." In *Molecular Biology of the Cell*, 4th ed. New York: Garland Science, 2002.

Alberts, B., Johnson, A., Lewis, J., Raff, M., Roberts, K., and Walter, P. "The lipid bilayer." In *Molecular Biology of the Cell*, 4th ed. New York: Garland Science, 2002.

Alberts, B., Johnson, A., Lewis, J., Raff, M., Roberts, K., and Walter, P. "Most cancers derive from a single abnormal cell." In *Molecular Biology of the Cell*, 4th ed. New York: Garland Science, 2002.

Alberts, B., Johnson, A., Lewis, J., Raff, M., Roberts K., and Walter, P. "The universal features of cells on earth." In *Molecular Biology of the Cell*, 4th ed. New York: Garland Science, 2002.

Atsuta, J., Sterbinsky, S. A., Plitt, J., Schwiebert, L. M., Bochner, B. S., and Schleimer, R. P. "Phenotyping and cytokine regulation of the BEAS-2B human bronchial epithelial cell: Demonstration of Esme H, Cemek M, Sezer M, Saglam H, Demir A, Melek H, Unlu M. High levels of oxidative stress in patients with advanced lung cancer." *Respirology* 13, no. 1 (2008): 112–16.

Berg, J. M., Tymoczko, J. L., and Stryer, L. "Mutations involve changes in the base sequence of DNA." In *Biochemistry*, 5th ed. New York: W. H. Freeman, 2002, sec. 27.6.

Bloom, M., Evans, E., and Mouritsen, O. G. "Physical properties of the fluid lipid-bilayer component of cell membranes: A perspective." *Quarterly Reviews of Biophysics* 24, no. 3 (1991): 293–397.

Gutschner, T., Hämmerle, M., Eissmann, M., Hsu, J., Kim, Y., Hung, G., Revenko, A., Arun, G., Stentrup, M., Gross, M., Zörnig, M., MacLeod, A. R., Spector, D. L., and Diederichs, S. "The noncoding RNA MALAT1 is a critical regulator of the metastasis phenotype of lung cancer cells." *Cancer Research* 73, no. 3 (2013): 1180–89.

Nasser, M. W., Datta, J., Nuovo, G., Kutay, H., Motiwala, T., Majumder, S., Wang, B., Suster, S., Jacob, S. T., and Ghoshal, K. "Down-regulation of micro-RNA-1 (miR-1) in lung cancer: Suppression of tumorigenic property of lung cancer cells and their sensitization to doxorubicin-induced apoptosis by miR-1." *Journal of Biological Chemistry* 283, no. 48 (2008): 33394–405.

Pryor, J. W. "Difference in the ossification of the male and female skeleton." *Journal of Anatomy* 62, no. 4 (1928): 499–506.

CHAPTER 2

American Society of Clinical Oncology. "Progress against cancer." Last modified June 8, 2012. www.cancer.net. Accessed March 25, 2013.

Blow, J. J. "Cell multiplication: Editorial overview." *Current Opinions in Cell Biology* 12, no. 6 (2000): 655–57.

Hartwell, L., Hood, L., Goldberg, M. L., Reynolds, A. E., Silver, L. M., and Veres, R. *Genetics: From Genes to Genomes*. New York: McGraw-Hill, 2000.

Hartwell, L., and Weinert, T. A. "Checkpoints: Controls that ensure the order of cell cycle events." *Science* 246 (1989): 629–34.

Lüdtke, T. H., Farin, H. F., Rudat, C., Schuster-Gossler, K., Petry, M., Barnett, P., Christoffels, V. M., and Kispert, A. "Tbx2 controls lung growth by direct repression of the cell cycle inhibitor genes Cdkn1a and Cdkn1b." *PLOS Genetics* 9, no. 1 (2013): e1003189.

Zhao, J., Bacolla, A., Wang, G., and Vasquez, K. M. "Non-B DNA structure-induced genetic instability and evolution." *Cellular and Molecular Life Sciences* 67, no. 1 (2010): 43–62.

Zoidl, G., Olk, S., Tuchinowitz, A., and Dermietzel, R. "Cell-to-cell communication in astroglia and the cytoskeletal impact." *Neuromethods* 79 (2013): 283–97.

CHAPTER 3

Aiba, M., Asaka, S., Ide, H., Isohata, N., Katsube, T., Konno, S., Murayama, M., Naritaka, Y., Ogawa, K., Shimakawa, T., Brambilla, C., Brambilla, E., Brichon, P. Y., Gazzeri, S., Jacrot, M., Morel, F., Moro, D., and Nagy-Mignotte, H. "Cytotoxic chemotherapy induces cell differentiation in small-cell lung carcinoma." *Journal of Clinical Oncology* 9, no. 1 (1991): 50–61.

Cooper, G. M. "Chromosomes and chromatin." In *The Cell: A Molecular Approach*, 2nd ed. Sunderland, MA: Sinauer Associates, 2000.

Demetriou, T., Papavramidis, T., and Papavramidou, N.. "Ancient Greek and Greco-Roman methods in modern surgical treatment of cancer." *Annals of Surgical Oncology* 17, no. 3 (2010): 665–67.

Lew, D. J., and Rout, M. P. "Cell structure and dynamics: Editorial overview." *Current Opinion in Cell Biology* 21 (2009): 1–3.

Martins, I., Galluzzi, L., and Kroemer, G. "Hormesis, cell death and aging." *Aging* 3, no. 9 (2011): 821–28.

Shiozawa, S., and Yoshimatsu, K. "Occult lung cancer incidentally found during surgery for esophageal and gastric cancer." *Anticancer Research* 28 (2008): 1841–48.

William, J., Variakojis, D., Yeldandi, A., and Raparia, K. "Lymphoproliferative neoplasms of the lung: A review." *Archives of Pathology and Laboratory Medicine* 137, no. 3 (2013): 382–91.

CHAPTER 4

Audesirk, T., and Audesirk, G. *Biology: Life on Earth*. 5th ed. Upper Saddle River, NJ: Prentice Hall, 1999.

Cotran, R., Kumar, V., and Robbins, S. *Robbins Pathologic Basis of Disease*. 4th ed. Philadelphia: Saunders; 1989.

Devita, V. T., Jr., and Rosenberg, S. A. "Two hundred years of cancer research." *New England Journal of Medicine* 366 (2012): 2207–14.

Diamandopoulus, G. T. "Cancer: An historical perspective." *Anticancer Research* 16, no. 4 (1996): 1595–602.

Feinberg, A. P., and Tycko, B. "The history of cancer epigenetics." *Nature Reviews Cancer* 4, no. 2 (2004): 143–53.

Gallucci, B. B. "Selected concepts of cancer as a disease: From the Greeks to 1900." *Oncology Nursing Forum* 12 (1985): 67–71.

Goeckenjan, G. "Lung cancer—Historical development, current status, future prospects [in German]." *Pneumologie* 64, no. 9 (2010): 555–59.

Harvey, A. M. "Early contributions to the surgery of cancer: William S. Halsted, Hugh H. Young and John G. Clark." *Johns Hopkins Medical Journal* 135, no. 6 (1974): 399–417.

Houston, T. P. "Lung cancer and tobacco: Historical issues, epidemiology, and intervention." In *Malignant Tumors of the Lung*. New York: Springer, 2004.

Reck, M., and Gatzemeier, U. "Advanced non-small cell lung cancer therapy: Historical and future perspectives." *Targeted Oncology* 3, no. 3 (2008): 135–47.

Skuladottir, H., Olsen, J. H., and Hirsch, F. R. "Incidence of lung cancer in Denmark: Historical and actual status." *Lung Cancer* 27, no. 2 (2000): 107–18.

CHAPTER 5

Adonis, M., Chahuan, M., Zambrano, A., Avaria, P., Díaz, J., Miranda, R., Campos, M., Benítez, H., and Gil, L. "Relationship between toxicogenomic, environment and lung cancer." In *Oncogenesis, Inflammatory and Parasitic Tropical Diseases of the Lung*. New York: InTech, 2013.

Hart, C. L., Hole, D. J., Gillis, C. R., Smith, G. D., Watt, G. C., and Hawthorne, V. M. "Social class differences in lung cancer mortality: Risk factor explanations using two Scottish cohort studies." *International Journal of Epidemiology* 30, no. 2 (2001): 268–74.

Haugen, A., Ryberg, D., Mollerup, S., Zienolddiny, S., Skaug, V., and Svendsrud, D. H. "Gene-environment interactions in human lung cancer." *Toxicology Letters* 112–113 (2000): 233–37.

Takata, Y., Xiang, Y. B., Yang, G., Li, H., Gao, J., Cai, H., Gao, Y. T., Zheng, W., and Shu, X. O. "Intakes of fruits, vegetables, and related vitamins and lung cancer risk: Results from the Shanghai Men's Health Study (2002–2009)." *Nutrition and Cancer* 65, no. 1 (2013): 51–61.

Thun, M. J. "The evolving relationship of social class to tobacco smoking and lung cancer." *Journal of the National Cancer Institute* 101, no. 5 (2009): 285–87.

CHAPTER 6

Gabrielson, E. "Worldwide trends in lung cancer pathology." *Respirology* 11, no. 5 (2006): 533–38.

Little, A. G., Gay, E. G., Gaspar, L. E., and Stewart, A. K. "National survey of non-small cell lung cancer in the United States: Epidemiology, pathology and patterns of care." *Lung Cancer* 57, no. 3 (2007): 253–60.

Suh, J. H. "Current readings: Pathology, prognosis, and lung cancer." *Seminars in Thoracic and Cardiovascular Surgery* 25, no. 1 (2013): 14–21.

Travis, W. D. "Pathology of lung cancer." *Clinics in Chest Medicine* 23, no. 1 (2002): 65–81.

CHAPTER 7

Bach, P. B. "Lung cancer screening." *Journal of the National Comprehensive Cancer Network* 6, no. 3 (2008): 271–75.

Brunnström, H., Johansson, L., Jirström, K., Jönsson, M., Jönsson, P., and Planck, M. "Immunohistochemistry in the differential diagnostics of primary lung cancer: An investigation within the southern Swedish lung cancer study." *American Journal of Clinical Pathology* 140, no. 1 (2013): 37–46.

Göke, F., and Perner, S. "Translational research and diagnostics in lung cancer [in German]." *Pathologe* 33, no. 2 (Suppl. 2012): 269–72.

Harewood, G. C., Wiersema, M. J., Edell, E. S., and Liebow, M. "Cost-minimization analysis of alternative diagnostic approaches in a modeled patient with non-small cell lung cancer and subcarinal lymphadenopathy." *Mayo Clinic Proceedings* 77, no. 2 (2002): 155–64.

Querings, S., Altmüller, J., Ansén, S., Zander, T., Seidel, D., Gabler, F., Peifer, M., Markert, E., Stemshorn, K., Timmermann, B., Saal, B., Klose, S., Ernestus, K., Scheffler, M., Engel-Riedel, W., Stoelben, E., Brambilla, E., Wolf, J., Nürnberg, P., and Thomas, R. K. "Benchmarking of mutation diagnostics in clinical lung cancer specimens." *PLoS One* 6, no. 5 (2011): e19601.

Sugiyama, T., Frazier, D. P., Taneja, P., Morgan, R. L., Willingham, M. C., and Inoue, K. "Role of DMP1 and its future in lung cancer diagnostics." *Expert Reviews in Molecular Diagnostics* 8, no. 4 (2008): 435–47.

CHAPTER 8

Jacobsen, J., Jackson, V., Dahlin, C., Greer, J., Perez-Cruz, P., Billings, J. A., Pirl, W., and Temel, J. "Components of early outpatient palliative care consultation in patients with metastatic nonsmall cell lung cancer." *Journal of Palliative Medicine* 14, no. 4 (2011): 459–64.

Jones, D. R., Vaughters, A. B., Smith, P. W., Daniel, T. M., Shen, K. R., and Heinzmann, J. L. "Economic assessment of the general thoracic surgery outpatient service." *Annals of Thoracic Surgery* 82, no. 3 (2006): 1068–71.

Roulston, A., Bickerstaff, D., Haynes, T., Rutherford, L., and Jones, L. "A pilot study to evaluate an outpatient service for people with advanced lung cancer." *International Journal of Palliative Nursing* 18, no. 5 (2012): 225–33.

CHAPTER 9

Bettio, D., Cariboni, U., Venci, A., Valente, M., Spaggiari, P., and Alloisio, M. "Cytogenetic findings in lung cancer that illuminate its biological history from adenomatous hyperplasia to bronchioalveolar carcinoma to adenocarcinoma: A case report." *Experimental and Therapeutic Medicine* 4, no. 6 (2012): 1032–34.

Carneiroa, C., and Guptab, N. "Broncheoalveolar carcinoma associated with pulmonary lymphangioleiomyomatosis and tuberous sclerosis complex: Case report." *Clinical Imaging* 35, no. 3 (2011): 225–27.

Farasat, S., Yu, S. S., Neel, V. A., Nehal, K. S., Lardaro, T., Mihm, M. C., Byrd, D. R., Balch, C. M., Califano, J. A., Chuang, A. Y., Sharfman, W. H., Shah, J. P., Nghiem, P., Otley, C. C., Tufaro, A. P., Johnson, T. M., Sober, A. J., and Liégeois, N. J. "A new American Joint Committee on Cancer staging system for cutaneous squamous cell carcinoma: Creation and rationale for inclusion of tumor (T) characteristics." *Journal of the American Academy of Dermatology* 64, no. 6 (2011): 1051–59.

Liao, R. G., Jung, J., Tchaicha, J. H., Wilkerson, M. D., Sivachenko, A., Beauchamp, E. M., Liu, Q., Pugh, T. J., Pedamallu, C. S., Hayes, D. N., Gray, N. S., Getz, G., Wong, K. K., Haddad, R. I., Meyerson, M., and Hammerman, P. S. "Inhibitor-sensitive FGFR2 and FGFR3 mutations in lung squamous cell carcinoma." *Cancer Research* (2013 June 20): [Published online ahead of print].

Roggli, V. L., Vollmer, R. T., Greenberg, S. D., McGavran, M. H., Spjut, H. J., and Yesner, R. "Lung cancer heterogeneity: A blinded and randomized study of 100 consecutive cases." *Human Pathology* 16, no. 6 (1985): 569–79.

Zuyderduyn, S. D., Lonergan, K., Vatcher, G. P., II, Jones, S. J., Lam, S., Lam, W., Macaulay, C., Marra, M. A., Ng, R., and Ling, V. "A machine learning approach to finding gene expression signatures of the early developmental stages of squamous cell lung carcinoma." *97th Annual AACR Conference Proceedings* 2006: 431–34.

CHAPTER 10

Baldi, A., Groger, A. M., Esposito, V., Di Marino, M. P., Ferrara, N., and Baldi, F. "Neuroendocrine differentiation in non-small cell lung carcinomas." *In Vivo* 14, no. 1 (2000): 109–14.

Churg, A. "The fine structure of large cell undifferentiated carcinoma of the lung: Evidence for its relation to squamous cell carcinomas and adenocarcinomas." *Human Pathology* 9, no. 2 (1978): 143–56.

Jung, J. H., Jung, C. K., Choi, H. J., Jun, K. H., Yoo, J., Kang, S. J., and Lee, K. Y. "Diagnostic utility of expression of claudins in non-small cell lung cancer: different expression profiles in squamous cell carcinomas and adenocarcinomas." *Pathology—Research and Practice* 295, no. 6 (2009): 409–16.

Mayer, J. E., Jr., Ewing, S. L., Ophoven, J. J., Sumner, H. W., and Humphrey, E. W. "Influence of histologic type on survival after curative resection for undifferentiated lung cancer." *Journal of Thoracic and Cardiovascular Surgery* 84, no. 5 (1982): 641–48.

Shim, H. S., Lee, H., Park, E. J., and Kim, S. H. "Histopathologic characteristics of lung adenocarcinomas with epidermal growth factor receptor mutations in the International Association for the Study of Lung Cancer/American Thoracic Society/European Respiratory Society lung adenocarcinoma classification." *Archives of Pathology and Laboratory Medicine* 135, no. 10 (2011): 1329–34.

Skarda, J., Uberall, I., Tichý, T., and Matej, R. "News in the classification of pulmonary adenocarcinomas and potential prognostic and predictive factors in non-small lung cancer [in Czech]." *Ceskoslovenska Patologie* 47, no. 4 (2011): 168–72.

Sundaresan, V., Reeve, J. G., Stenning, S., Stewart, S., and Bleehen, N. M. "Neuroendocrine differentiation and clinical behaviour in non-small cell lung tumours." *British Journal of Cancer* 64, no. 2 (1991): 333–38.

CHAPTER 11

Boffetta, P., and Trichopoulos, D. "Cancer of the lung, larynx, and pleura." In *Textbook of Cancer Epidemiology*, 2nd ed. New York: Oxford University Press, 2008.

Braun, C., and Anderson, C. *Pathophysiology: Functional Alterations in Human Health.* Philadelphia: Lippincott Williams & Wilkins, 2007.

Cagle, P. T., Farver, C. F., Fraire, A. E., and Tomashefski, J. E., Jr. *Dail and Hammar's Pulmonary Pathology.* Cleveland, OH: Springer Science, 2008.

Ung, Y. C., Maziak, D. E., Vanderveen, J. A., Smith, C. A., Gulenchyn, K., Lacchetti, C., and Evans, W. K. "18-fluorodeoxyglucose positron emission tomography in the diagnosis and staging of lung cancer: A systematic review." *Journal of the National Cancer Institute* 99, no. 23 (2007): 1753–67.

Yousem, S., and Beasley, M. B. "Bronchioloalveolar carcinoma." *Archives of Pathology and Laboratory Medicine* 131 (2007): 1027.

CHAPTER 12

Althoen, M. C., Siegel, A., Tsapakos, M. J., and Seltzer, M. A. "Lung cancer metastasis to an adrenal myelolipoma detected by PET/CT." *Clinical Nuclear Medicine* 36, no. 10 (2011): 922–94.

Brown, J. E., Cook, R. J., Major, P., Lipton, A., Saad, F., Smith, M., Lee, K. A., Zheng, M., Hei, Y. J., and Coleman, R. E. "Bone turnover markers as predictors of skeletal complications in prostate cancer, lung cancer, and other solid tumors." *Journal of the National Cancer Institute* 91, no. 1 (2005): 59–69.

Fukushima, K., Kido, M., Fukumoto, T., Hori, Y., Kusunoki, N., Tsuchida, S., Takahashi, M., Tanaka, M., Kuramitsu, K., Tsugawa, D., Gon, H., Chuma, M., Urade, T., Matsumoto, I., Ajiki, T., Ku, Y., Kanzawa, M., and Ito, T. "A case report of intrahepatic cholangiocarcinoma diagnosed as lung cancer with liver metastasis treated with radiofrequency ablation [in Japanese]." *Gan To Kagaku Ryoho* 38, no. 12 (2011): 2030–32.

Hsu, J. W., Chiang, C. D., Hsu, W. H., Hsu, J. Y., and Chiang, C. S. "Superior vena cava syndrome in lung cancer: An analysis of 54 cases." *Gaoxiong Yi Xue Ke Xue Za Zhi* 11, no. 10 (1995): 568–73.

Iwanami, T., Uramoto, H., Baba, T., Takenaka, M., Yokoyama, E., Oka, S., So, T., Ono, K., So, T., Takenoyama, M., Hanagiri, T., Iwata, T., Inoue, M., and Yasumoto, K. "Treatment recommendations for adrenal metastasis of non-small cell lung cancer [in Japanese]." *Kyobu Geka* 63, no. 13 (2010): 1101–6.

Iwase, A., Onuma, E., Nagashima, O., Yae, T., Kunogi, M., and Hirai, S. "Long-term survival of adrenal metastasis from non-small cell lung cancer." *International Cancer Conference Journal* 2, no. 1 (2013): 1–3.

Jian, G., Songwen, Z., Ling, Z., Qinfang, D., Jie, Z., Liang, T., and Caicun, Z. "Prediction of epidermal growth factor receptor mutations in the plasma/pleural effusion to efficacy of gefitinib treatment in advanced non-small cell lung cancer." *Journal of Cancer Research and Clinical Oncology* 136, no. 9 (2010): 1341–47.

Landry, C. S., Perrier, N. D., Karp, D. D., Xing, Y., Lee, J. E., and Grubbs, E. G. "Outcome of patients with adrenal metastasis from lung cancer: Selection criteria for surgery." *Journal of Clinical Oncology* 28, no. 15 (Suppl. 2010): e18071.

Miyaaki, H., Ichikawa, T., Taura, N., Yamashima, M., Arai, H., Obata, Y., Furusu, A., Hayashi, H., Kohno, S., and Nakao, K. "Diffuse liver metastasis of small cell lung cancer causing marked hepatomegaly and fulminant hepatic failure." *Internal Medicine* 49, no. 14 (2010): 1383–86.

Morris, P. G., Reiner, A. S., Szenberg, O. R., Clarke, J. L., Panageas, K. S., Perez, H. R., Kris, M. G., Chan, T. A., DeAngelis, L. M., and Omuro, A. M. "Leptomeningeal metastasis from non-small cell lung cancer: Survival and the impact of whole brain radiotherapy." *Journal of Thoracic Oncology* 7, no. 2 (2012): 382–85.

Pancoast, H. K. "Superior pulmonary sulcus tumor characterized by pain, Horner's syndrome, destruction of bone atrophy and hand muscles: Chairman's address." *Journal of the American Medical Association* 99, no. 17 (1932): 1391–96.

Rodríguez-Piñeiro, A. M., Blanco-Prieto, S., Sánchez-Otero, N., Rodríguez-Berrocal, F. J., and de la Cadena, M. P. "On the identification of biomarkers for non-small cell lung cancer in serum and pleural effusion." *Journal of Proteomics* 73, no. 8 (2010): 1511–22.

Seike, T., Fujita, K., Yamakawa, Y., Kido, M. A., Takiguchi, S., Teramoto, N., Iguchi, H., and Noda, M. "Interaction between lung cancer cells and astrocytes via specific inflammatory cytokines in the microenvironment of brain metastasis." *Clinical and Experimental Metastasis* 28, no. 1 (2011): 13–25.

Terasaki, K., Ohkubo, K., and Kanekura, T. "Facial edema as a clue to superior vena cava syndrome associated with lung cancer." *European Journal of Dermatology* 22, no. 4 (2012): 546–47.

Wu, Y. K., Chen, K. T., Kuo, Y. B., Huang, Y. S., and Chan, E. C. "Quantitative detection of surviving in malignant pleural effusion for the diagnosis and prognosis of lung cancer." *Cancer Letters* 273, no. 2 (2009): 331–35.

CHAPTER 13

Gorham, J., Ameye, L., Berghmans, T., Sculier, J. P., and Meert, A. P. "The lung cancer patient at the emergency department: A three-year retrospective study." *Lung Cancer* 80, no. 2 (2013): 203–8.

Hagenbeek, A. "A passion to cure cancer." *Nature Medicine* 17, no. 3 (2011): 277.

Joshi, P., Berry, M., and Bowen, F. "When do patients with known lung cancer present to emergency services?" *Thorax* 67 (2012): A132–33.

Wilcock, A., Crosby, V., Freer, S., Freemantle, A., Caswell, G., and Seymour, J. "Lung cancer diagnosed following emergency admission: A mixed methods study protocol to improve understanding of patients' characteristics, needs experiences and outcomes." *BioMed Central Palliative Care* 12, no. 1 (2013): 24.

CHAPTER 14

Agarwal, M., Brahmanday, G., Chmielewski, G. W., Welsh, R. J., and Ravikrishnan, K. P. "Age, tumor size, type of surgery, and gender predict survival in early stage (stage I and II) non-small cell lung cancer after surgical resection." *Lung Cancer* 68, no. 3 (2010): 398–402.

Blot, W. J., and Fraumeni, J. F., Jr. "Geographic patterns of lung cancer: industrial correlations." *American Journal of Epidemiology* 103, no. 6 (1976): 539–50.

Byers, T. E., Graham, S., Haughey, B. P., Marshall, J. R., and Swanson, M. K. "Diet and lung cancer risk: Findings from the Western New York Diet Study." *American Journal of Epidemiology* 125, no. 3 (1987): 351–63.

Colditz, G. A., Stampfer, M. J., and Willett, W. C. "Diet and lung cancer: A review of the epidemiologic evidence in humans. *Archives of Internal Medicine* 147, no. 1 (1987): 157–60.

Crabtree, T. D., Denlinger, C. E., Meyers, B. F., El Naqa, I., Zoole, J., Krupnick, A. S., Kreisel, D., Patterson, G. A., and Bradley, J. D. "Stereotactic body radiation therapy versus surgical resection for stage I non-small cell lung cancer." *Journal of Thoracic Cardiovascular Surgery* 140, no. 2 (2010): 377–86.

De Matteis, S., Consonni, D., and Bertazzi, P. A. "Exposure to occupational carcinogens and lung cancer risk: Evolution of epidemiological estimates of attributable fraction." *Acta Bio Medica* 79, no. 1 (Suppl. 2008): 34–42.

Granger, C. L., McDonald, C. F., Berney, S., Chao, C., and Denehy, L. "Exercise intervention to improve exercise capacity and health related quality of life for patients with non-small cell lung cancer: A systematic review." *Lung Cancer* 72, no. 2 (2011): 139–53.

Jack, R. H., Gulliford, M. C., Ferguson, J., and Møller, H. "Geographical inequalities in lung cancer management and survival in South East England: Evidence of variation in access to oncology services?" *British Journal of Cancer* 88, no. 7 (2003): 1025–31.

Jain, R., Kosta, S., and Tiwari, A. "Ayurveda and cancer." *Pharmacognosy Research* 2, no. 6 (2010): 393–94.

Kasymjanova, G., Grossman, M., Tran, T., Jagoe, R. T., Cohen, V., Pepe, C., Small, D., and Agulnik, J. "The potential role for acupuncture in treating symptoms in patients with lung cancer: An observational longitudinal study." *Current Oncology* 20, no. 3 (2013): 152–57.

Pass, H. I. *Adjunctive and Alternative Treatment of Bronchogenic Lung Cancer.* Philadelphia: Saunders, 1991.

Ruan, W. J., Lai, M. D., and Zhou, J. G. "Anticancer effects of Chinese herbal medicine, science or myth?" *Journal of Zhejiang University Science B* 7, no. 12 (2006): 1006–14.

Svoboda, R. E. "Life, health and longevity through the science of Ayurveda: A case study of cancer." *International Journal of Yoga Therapy* 5, no. 1 (1994): 38–41.

Vanderpool, R. C. "Severe weather, band practice, coal trucks, and other real-world experiences in conducting focus group research in central Appalachia." *Preventing Chronic Disease* 6, no. 2 (2009): A70.

Wan, C., You, S., Quan, P., Song, Y., Liu, T., Lu, J., and Zheng, P. "Development and validation of the quality-of-life assessment system for lung cancer based on traditional Chinese medicine." *Evidence Based Complementary Alternative Medicine* 2012: 1–10.

CHAPTER 15

Lindley, C., McCune, J. S., Thomason, T. E., Lauder, D., Sauls, A., Adkins, S., and Sawyer, W. T. "Perception of chemotherapy side effects cancer versus noncancer patients." *Cancer Practice* 7, no. 2 (1999): 59–65.

MacDonald, V. "Chemotherapy: Managing side effects and safe handling." *Canadian Veterinary Journal* 50, no. 6 (2009): 665–68.

Partridge, A. H., Burstein, H. J., and Winer, E. P. "Side effects of chemotherapy and combined chemohormonal therapy in women with early-stage breast cancer." *Journal of the National Cancer Institute Monographs* 30 (2001): 135–42.

Ramsey, S. D., Martins, R. G., Blough, D. K., Tock, L. S., Lubeck, D., and Reyes, C. M. "Second-line and third-line chemotherapy for lung cancer: Use and cost." *American Journal of Managed Care* 14, no. 5 (2008): 297–306.

Ramsey, S. D., Martins, R. G., Blough, D. K., Tock, L. S., Lubeck, D., Reyes, C. M., Frank, S. J., Forster, K. M., Stevens, C. W., Cox, J. D., Komaki, R., Liao, Z., Tucker, S., Wang, X., Steadham, R. E., Brooks, C., and Starkschall, G. "Treatment planning for lung cancer: Traditional homogeneous point-dose prescription compared with heterogeneity-corrected dose-volume prescription." *International Journal of Radiation Oncology Biology Physics* 56, no. 5 (2003): 1308–18.

CHAPTER 16

Al-Wadei, H. A., Plummer, H. K., III, Ullah, M. F., Unger, B., Brody, J. R., and Schuller, H. M. "Social stress promotes and γ-aminobutyric acid inhibits tumor growth in mouse models of non–small cell lung cancer." *Cancer Prevention Research* 5, no. 2 (2012): 189–96.

Carlsen, K., Jensen, A. B., Jacobsen, E., Krasnik, M., and Johansen, C. "Psychosocial aspects of lung cancer." *Lung Cancer* 47, no. 3 (2005): 293–300.

Cohen, B. E., Marmar, C. R., Neylan, T. C., Schiller, N. B., Ali, S., and Whooley, M. A. "Posttraumatic stress disorder and health-related quality of life in patients with coronary heart disease: Findings from the Heart and Soul Study." *Archives of General Psychiatry* no. 66, no. 11 (2009): 1214–20.

Nakaya, N., Saito-Nakaya, K., Akechi, T., Kuriyama, S., Inagaki, M., Kikuchi, N., Nagai, K., Tsugane, S., Nishiwaki, Y., Tsuji, I., and Uchitomi, Y. "Negative psychological aspects and survival in lung cancer patients." *Psycho-Oncology* 17, no. 5 (2008): 466–73.

Ryan, L. S. "Psychosocial issues and lung cancer: A behavioral approach." *Seminars in Oncology Nursing* 12, no. 4 (1996): 318–23.

Siminoff, L. A., Wilson-Genderson, M., and Baker, S., Jr. "Depressive symptoms in lung cancer patients and their family caregivers and the influence of family environment." *Psycho-Oncology* 19, no. 12 (2010): 1285–93.

Weiss, T., Weinberger, M., Schwerd, A. M., and Holland, J. "A 30-year perspective on psychosocial issues in lung cancer: How lung cancer 'came out of the closet.'" *Thoracic Surgery Clinics* 22, no. 4 (2012): 449–56.

CHAPTER 17

Chen, Y.-J., Narsavage, G. L., Sterns, A. A., Petitte, T. M., and Coole, C., Jr. "Outcomes of home telemonitoring for patients with lung cancer using intention-to-treat approach." https://stti.confex.com/stti/bc42/webprogram/Paper58935.html. Accessed May 20, 2013.

Fujita, A., Igami, Y., Takabatake, H., Tagaki, S., Yamamoto, R., and Sekine, K. "Period of time patients with advanced non-small cell lung cancer could remain at home during CIC therapy (cisplatin + ifosfamide + CPT-11) [in Japanese]." *Gan To Kagaku Ryoho* 26, no. 6, (1999): 805–11.

Gabrijel, S., Grize, L., Helfenstein, E., Brutsche, M., Grossman, P., Tamm, M., and Kiss, A. "Receiving the diagnosis of lung cancer: Patient recall of information and satisfaction with physician communication." *Journal of Clinical Oncology* 26, no. 2 (2008): 297–302.

Leppert, W., Turska, A., Majkowicz, M., Dziegielewska, S., Pankiewicz, P., and Mess, E. "Quality of life in patients with advanced lung cancer treated at home and at a palliative care unit." *American Journal of Palliative Care* 29, no. 5 (2012): 379–87.

McCorkle, R., Benoliel, J. Q., Donaldson, G., Georgiadou, F., Moinpour, C., and Goodell, B. "A randomized clinical trial of home nursing care for lung cancer patients." *Cancer* 64, no. 6 (1989): 1375–82.

White, E. J. "Home care of the patient with advanced lung cancer." *Seminars in Oncology Nursing* 3, no. 3 (1987): 216–21.

CHAPTER 18

Butler, K. M., Rayens, M. K., Zhang, M., and Hahn, E. J. "Motivation to quit smoking among relatives of lung cancer patients." *Public Health Nursing* 28, no. 1 (2011): 43–50.

Carmack Taylor, C. L., Badr, H., Lee, J. H., Fossella, F., Pisters, K., Gritz, E. R., and Schover, L. "Lung cancer patients and their spouses: Psychological and relationship functioning within 1 month of treatment initiation." *Annals of Behavioral Medicine* 36, no. 2 (2008): 129–40.

Faller, H., Lang, H., and Schilling, S. "Emotional distress and hope in lung cancer patients, as perceived by patients, relatives, physicians, nurses and interviewers." *Psycho-Oncology* 4, no. 1 (1995): 221–31.

McBride, C. M., Pollak, K. I., Garst, J., Keefe, F., Lyna, P., Fish, L., and Hood, L. "Distress and motivation for smoking cessation among lung cancer patients' relatives who smoke." *Journal of Cancer Education* 18, no. 3 (2003): 150–56.

CHAPTER 19

Aitio, A., Attfield, M., Cantor, K. P., Demers, P. A., Fowler, B. A., Fubini, B., Gerín, M., Goldberg, M., Grandjean, P., Hartwig, A., Heinrich, U., Henderson, R., Ikeda, M., Infante, P., Kane, A., Kauppinen, T., Landrigan, P., Lunn, R., Merletti, F., Muhle, H., Rossman, T., Samet, J., Siemiatycki, J., Stayner, L., Waalkes, M. P., Ward, E. M., and Ward, J. M. *IARC Monographs—100C, a review of human carcinogens. Part C: Arsenic, metals, fibres, and dusts.* Lyon: International Agency for Research on Cancer, 2009.

American Cancer Society. *Cancer Facts and Figures 2013.* Atlanta: American Cancer Society, 2013.

Bellizzi, K. M., and Gosney, M. *Cancer and Aging Handbook: Research and Practice.* Hoboken, NJ: Wiley, 2012.

Schottenfeld, D., and Fraumeni, J. F., Jr. *Cancer Epidemiology and Prevention.* 2nd ed. New York: Oxford University Press, 1996.

Stewart, D. J. *Lung Cancer: Prevention, Management and Emerging Therapies,* New York: Humana Press, 2010.

CHAPTER 20

Arora, N. K., and Gustafson, D. H. "Perceived helpfulness of physicians' communication behavior and breast cancer patients' level of trust over time." *Journal of General Internal Medicine* 24, no. 2 (2009): 252–55.

Berendes, D., Keefe, F. J., Somers, T. J., Kothadia, S. M., Porter, L. S., and Cheavens, J. S. "Hope in the context of lung cancer: Relationships of hope to symptoms and psychological distress." *Journal of Pain Symptom Management* 40, no. 2 (2010): 174–82.

Kersey-Cantril, C. A. "Nursing care of the elderly patient with cancer: The critical blend of science and art—Back to basics." *Frontiers of Radiation Therapy and Oncology* 20 (1986): 173–77.

Sato, T. "Confidence intervals for effect parameters common in cancer epidemiology." *Environmental Health Perspectives* 87 (1990): 95–101.

Wall, L. M. "Changes in hope and power in lung cancer patients who exercise." *Nursing Science Quarterly* 13, no. 3 (2000): 234–42.

Wenger, N. S., and Vespa, P. M. "Ethical issues in patient-physician communication about therapy for cancer: Professional responsibilities of the oncologist." *Oncologist* 15, no. 1 (Suppl. 2010): 43–48.

INDEX

Achong, Bert, 40
acinar adenocarcinoma, 103, 277
actinic keratosis, 98
adenocarcinomas, 299n5–299n7
adenomatous hyperplasia, 101
adenosine triphosphate (ATP), 297n7
adenosquamous carcinomas, 314n10
adenylatecyclase, 302n70
adjustment disorder, 335n11
adrenal cortex, 295n48
affect: in adrenal glands, 33, 139; in
    brachial plexus, 301n47; in breathing,
    300n35; in liver, 301n54; in
    personality, 300n28, 300n37; in social
    isolation, 306n4. *See also* thoracic
    outlet syndrome
air pollution: arising from cooking, 51,
    315n20; causes of lung adeno
    carcinomas and, 111; environmental
    factors of, 106; forms of, 153; health
    effects of, 324n37
airways, 30
alveoli, 9; in adult human lungs, 294n41;
    in mammals, 294n40; type I cells in,
    295n42–295n43; type II cells in, 10
American Cancer Society, 40, 83
amifostine, 177
aminopterin, 303n8
amirubicin, 123
anamnesis, 71
anger, 227

antiemetics, 195
antihistamines, 195
anxiety, 194
apoptosis (cell death), 16; beginning of,
    15–16; mutation and, 52; process of,
    28, 278; results of, 282
asbestos, 49
aseptic, 39
asymptomatic, 309n14

Barr, Yvonne, 40
basal cell carcinomas, 96
basaloid carcinoma, 106, 278
Beatson, Thomas, 39
benign tumors: growth of, 20;
    Hippocrates and, 37; lung adeno-
    carcinomas and, 28, 112; lung cancer
    and, 62
benzodiazepines, 195
beta-carotene supplements, 53
beta-integrin, 114
bevacizumab : agents and, 123; avastin
    and, 278; indications for, 173; role of,
    330n8
biopsy, 311n49
bone cancer, 135–136
Boveri, Theodor, 39
breath analysis, 74, 279
British Medical Bulletin, 292n1
brain: in cerebrum, 137; lung cancer and,
    29, 137; parts of, 136–137

epithelial cells, 2; basis of, 293n8; carcinomas and, 299n4
Epstein, Anthony, 40
Epstein-Barr virus, 303n9
erlotinib, 172
erythropoietin, 301n58
esophagus, 30; abnormalities of, 130; gastrointestinal region and, 182, 282; reflux and, 62
estrogen, 295n52; breast cancer and, 296n57; effects of, 295n54. *See also* somatic cells
etoposide, 118, 178, 282
euthanasia, 193
ezrin-radixin-moesin, 114, 282

Fabray, Wilhelm, 38
Family: beliefs of, 210; mental aspects of, 199; personalized care plan and, 208; restabilization within, 199; role of, 210, 211, 214, 215; stuck points in, 199
fear, 227
field cancerization, 121
fight-or-flight response system, 188
filamins A and B, 114
fine-needle aspiration biopsy, 109
fistula : development of, 165; lumps and, 282
fluorescence differential gel electrophoresis, 114

Galen, 303n5
Galileo, 38
galactorrhea, 300n44
gas chromatography, 310n25
gastrooesophageal reflux, 62
gefitinib, 123, 172, 283
gemcitabine, 178
germ cell tumors, 27
glutamate : amounts of, 18; neurotransmitters, 282, 283
golgi apparatus, 5
government: for children and adolescents, 238; in economic losses, 234; interventions of, 234–235; smoking guidelines of, 236; strategies against smoking of, 237, 341n14
Graz, Medical University of, 110
grief, 226

guilt, 196, 228, 292n17; tips for, 228
gynecological oncologists, 313n6
gynecomastia, 300n43

Halsted, William Stewart, 39
Harrison, George, 44
Hawaii, University of, 184
Health, National Institutes of, 322n5
heart, 31
hematemesis, 307n10
hemoptysis, 300n33, 307n9
Hippocrates, 303n3
Hodgkin's disease, 52. *See also* lymphomas
hope, 222, 243; after the diagnosis, 245; living with, 245; survivors of, 244; tips for, 222
Horner's syndrome, 131–132, 283, 319n9
humor, 223; tips for, 223
humoral theory, 41
Hunter, John, 38, 303n12
hyaline cartilages : composition of, 7; c-shaped, 8, 283
hypercalcemia, 34, 148
hyperplasia, 19, 64
hypoxemia, 302n79

immunohistochemistry, 109, 113
inappropriate antidiuretic hormone syndrome (SIADH), 306n3
infectious disease theory, 42
inner strength, 222
insomnia, 67; avoid, 201; condition, 67; or loss, 191; pain and, 67; placed on, 201; problems, 193; symptoms of, 196
internists, 86
invasion, process of, 133; in staging and grading, 134. *See also* metastasis; tumor-node metastasis
iron nanoparticles, 73

Jennings, Peter, 43

Kansas State University, 309n20
kidneys, 33

Lambert-Eaton myasthenic syndrome, 34
Lane-Claypon, Janet, 40

ABOUT THE AUTHOR

Naheed Ali, MD, PhD, is the author of *Diabetes and You* (Rowman & Littlefield, 2011), *The Obesity Reality* (Rowman & Littlefield, 2012), *Understanding Alzheimer's* (Rowman & Littlefield, 2012), *Arthritis and You* (Rowman & Littlefield, 2013), and *Understanding Parkinson's Disease* (Rowman & Littlefield, 2013). For years, Dr. Ali taught at colleges in the United States, where he lectured on various biomedical topics. Visit him online at NaheedAli.com.